From readers and patients, praise for Dr. Vliet's books

"As mothers we are very in-tune with our kids. Our intuitions tell us when there is something wrong. Even at a young age your daughters can be experiencing the side-effects of hormonal imbalance. Thank goodness for Dr. Vliet, the knowledge she possesses, and her application of the hormonal sciences. She has changed our lives. This book could change your life too."

—S.A. (mother of daughter with PCOS)

"I saw Dr. Vliet on TV and was very intrigued with the hormone connections she attributes to many symptoms. For years I've questioned doctors as to my severe PMS symptoms, reoccurring yeast and bladder infections, and depression after the birth of my children. All of them seem to think it is just a matter of time for my hormones to readjust but deny any real connection. No one has ever done a hormone analysis on me. I immediately went to the book store to purchase Dr. Vliet's book to help me know which questions to ask when I do see the doctor again."

—S.R.

"For the last few months my daughter has felt tired, swollen, constipated, had gained 8 lbs even though she works out and eats healthy, shaky, anemic, her hands and feet feel like they are tingling or feel numb, headaches, eyes go blurry and her mind is foggy. Her doctors have dismissed any suggestion of hormonal problems. She is so tired and discouraged. This from a woman that has always been active and alive…thank you for your book…we now have hope."

—L.A.

"Every woman in America should read Dr. Vliet's books. After bouncing from doctor to doctor for well over a year with symptoms of anxiety, insomnia and heart palpitations, Dr. Vliet correctly diagnosed my hormonal problems. She gave me my life back!"

It's My
OVARIES,
Stupid!

Elizabeth Lee Vliet, M.D.

One of
The Savvy Woman's Health Guide™
Series

℗
HER Place Press
www.herplace.com

It's My Ovaries, Stupid! Revised Edition
One of The Savvy Woman's Health Guide™ series
by Elizabeth Lee Vliet, M.D.

Copyright © 2007 Elizabeth Lee Vliet, M.D.

Published by:
ΨP HER Place Press
PO Box 64507
Tucson AZ 85728-4507
www.herplace.com

Notice of Rights:

Disclaimer

Cover Design:	New West Agency and Kitty Werner
Book Design:	Kitty Werner, RSBPress
Production and Prepress:	Kitty Werner, RSBPress

Printed by Central Plains Book Manufacturing, Winfield KS
Printed on New Life Opaque 100% recycled paper

ISBN 1-933213-03-5
ISBN 978-1-933213-03-3
Printed and bound in the United States of America
0 9 8 7 6 5 4 3 2 1

Introduction To Revised Edition

Health risks to your ovaries and your hormones continue to escalate every year. The headlines have become even more ominous in the years since I wrote the first edition of *It's My Ovaries, Stupid!*

One recent example is *Mercury Rising,* a TIME report about the alarming increase in mercury in our environment. Mercury is highly toxic and is now found *everywhere,* not just in seafood. Levels have been *increasing in recent years,* and it is far more dangerous than we had thought, causing everything from fatigue to tremors, circulatory and reproductive disorders, and adverse effects on the brain, kidney and liver.

Mercury is just *one* of hundreds of toxic chemicals that damage women's hormones, fertility and health. Even cosmetics and personal care products are now a concern due to an exponential increase in use of *nanoparticle* technology. Nanoparticle ingredients are potentially more damaging because smaller particles can penetrate cells to a greater degree than larger particles in older products. Secondhand cigarette smoke has been linked to more and more health problems. The latest? Its role in rising rates of autism in children.

Everywhere we turn, there is more information from environmental science and wildlife research to show how our hormone pathways can be disrupted by chemicals we are exposed to daily. But medical education and health services are still not equipped to deal with these new threats, especially as they relate to the rising incidence of ovarian hormone disorders in women. That's one reason I felt I had to do a new edition of *It's My Ovaries, Stupid!*

This edition also starts a new approach in my efforts to make cutting edge health information more accessible to more women: *The Savvy Women's Health Guide*™ paperback books, using the more user-friendly format that I began with my earlier books in *The Savvy Woman's Guide*™ series. There are color highlights and pullouts throughout the book to help you busy women find important information and health tips more quickly.

I included some of the cutting edge research from international conferences I attend every year. There has been an explosion of incredible recent research to show the powerful and crucial effects of our ovarian hormones on all body systems, in particular brain pathways that regulate memory, mood, sleep, pain and other critical functions. Studies continue to show the importance of optimal hormone levels for women.

Yet contrast this positive worldwide research with the maelstrom of negative, frightening headlines about "hormones" and "hormone replacement therapy" (HRT) that has prevailed in the United States since 2002.

Negative media reports from the Women's Health Initiative (WHI) and Heart and Estrogen/ progestin Replacement Study (HERS) hit like a nuclear explosion in July 2002. Each of these clinical trials used only Premarin—estrogens derived from the urine of pregnant horses, and a synthetic progestin—Provera—hormones not identical to anything our bodies ever made naturally, a point rarely mentioned in the coverage.

But the damage was done. Ever since the first WHI media reports, women have been led to believe that all hormone therapy caused breast cancer, heart attacks, strokes and blood clots. Women are now afraid to even take birth control pills, and millions have stopped menopausal hormone therapy.

The benefits were lost in the media furor that exaggerated hormone risks. Women were led to think *all* hormones and all ways to deliver them have the same risks. That is simply not the case.

It wasn't *human* "estrogen" that led to the problems reported from the WHI —it was a combination of horse estrogens and the synthetic progestin Provera (Prempro), or horse estrogens (Premarin) used alone that led to the increased risks reported initially. There are many well-studied, alternative, bioidentical (or "natural") forms of hormones available, with fewer negative effects documented in studies from many different countries including the United States. And none of the media stories have accurately presented the higher risk with oral hormones compared to lower risks for transdermal options using patches, for example.

Headlines continue to scream that "estrogen" increases risk of breast cancer, even though the WHI showed that women taking estrogen alone had *lower* risk of breast cancer than those taking *no hormones*. The National Toxicology Program decided to add "estrogen" to the list of human carcinogens. Never mind world experts who felt that data did not warrant such an extreme classification.

Why did damage found with Premarin and Prempro, the non-human forms of hormones, get applied to all hormone preparations, even though they are chemically as different as night and day? We haven't

seen this broad-brush warning for all medicines in a class after *one* study of *one* product happening in any other field of medicine, or with any other class of medications. Why has it continued to be the case with women's hormones?

The WHI was presented in the press as a study of "healthy" menopausal women.

Healthy? I don't think so! Look at these statistics:

- 35% of these women were already under treatment for high blood pressure
- 35% were overweight
- another 34% were *obese* by the medical definition of obesity
- 12.5% had high enough cholesterol to require medication
- 4% had diabetes
- 16% had a family history of breast cancer
- 40% were former smokers, 10% continued to smoke during the study

"Typical" American maybe, but *not* "healthy."

The average age of women in the WHI was about 64 years, and almost 30% were over 70. This is 10–15 years *later* than most menopausal hormone therapies are started. These women, like the older women in the HERS study, already had evidence of heart disease, high cholesterol and high blood pressure.

Professor A. R. Genazzani, a world-renown physician researcher and the President of the International Society of Gynecological Endocrinology said, ***"We would never choose that kind of combination for our elderly patients with those clinical characteristics."***[1] Older women with such health risks need much lower doses of hormones and preferably a non-oral form to help minimize risks seen with the oral ones.

The International Menopause Society position paper, published in September, 2002, concluded: ***"The WHI results, and particularly the data on cardiovascular disease risk, should only be related to the continuous combined treatment of 0.625 mg CEE (conjugated equine estrogens) together with 2.5 mg MPA (medroxy-progesterone acetate), prescribed to elderly, obese women with characteristics similar to those depicted in the WHI study".***[2]

These comments and the WHI findings, validate concerns I have raised about Premarin and Prempro in my previous books and medical articles *for more than a decade.* I will explain these issues further in upcoming chapters.

Why are the negative results trumpeted and crucial positive findings down-played or ignored? The press shouted there was a 26% increase in risk of breast cancer. What they *didn't* say was that the statistical increase was *minute*: of 10,000 women taking Prempro, only 8 more would develop breast cancer than women not taking Prempro, or only 7 more heart attacks.

The WHI authors indicated that the average risk in an individual woman is 0.1% per year for breast cancer or heart attacks.[3] Most media stories don't report that number.

The alarmist headlines made it appear that more women died taking hormones. This was not so. **Articles neglected to say that the death rate in the Prempro group from breast cancer or heart disease was no higher than women taking placebo.**

The focus on fear of breast cancer appears to sell newspapers and magazines. That same fear is also used to sell everything from herbs and soy supplements to new and expensive "designer estrogen" prescription products. Instead of balanced information, we are bombarded with poorly researched and hastily presented stories with a biased focus on breast cancer to the exclusion of other serious disorders—osteoporosis, diabetes, and cardiovascular disease are prime examples—that kill many times more women every year.

We are made to feel terrified about hormones our bodies make naturally our entire reproductive life. Estrogen seems to have become an "axis of evil"—something we are to fear, something that "causes cancer." All you hear about is the slight increase in risk of breast cancer that may occur with some—not all—types of estrogen-progestin therapy after menopause. There are far more ominous links to breast cancer.

For instance, in 1990, researchers in Finland found that women with breast cancer had higher concentrations of pesticide chemical residues (*lindane*) in their breasts. Women with the highest lindane residues were 10 times more likely to have breast cancer than women with lower levels. The blood from all the women with breast cancer was analyzed and had 50% more of this pesticide residue than the blood from women without breast cancer.

A 1992 analysis of Connecticut women showed similar trends: levels of PCB, DDE and DDT in the breast tissue of women with breast cancer were 50–60 % higher than in women without cancer.

You need sound facts about these other factors in the hormone-breast cancer link before you "throw the baby out with the bath water" on prescription hormones.

My "mission" is to give you straight talk and sound information. I also discuss more of the story behind the headlines, such as:

- ❧ **Environmental endocrine disruptors interfere with function and production of human hormones and increase cancer risk.** We need to recognize and research, expose and identify, these hormone saboteurs and toxins that are often ignored.

- ❧ **The "cookie-cutter" approach cannot continue.** Estrogen derived from pregnant horse's urine has been used for about 85% of all HRT prescriptions in the United States for over 50 years. You wouldn't see 85% of men with heart disease given the same drug, and same dose. Women deserve better!

- ❧ **FDA-approved bioidentical copies of human hormones became available in the United States as far back as 1976. Even more have come on the market since the first edition of this book.** These need to be used instead of horse-derived or synthetic progestins that have very different—and often negative—effects in the human body. FDA approved products containing bioidentical 17-beta estradiol include Estrace (and generic) tablets, Vivelle DOT and Climara patches, Estrogel, Estasorb, Femring, Estring, and bioidentical progesterone products Prochieve and Prometrium.

- ❧ **Doctors are *still* using Premarin and Prempro more often than available human forms of estrogen and progesterone,** even after the risks identified in the WHI and HERS! You need to speak up and insist on other options.

- ❧ **"One-size-fits-all" is not acceptable any longer.** Women are individuals, with individual body chemistries. Women vary in response to hormones just as they do with all other classes of medicines we use. Women must have hormone options individually tailored to their needs for optimal response.

- ❧ **We must measure hormone response with objective tests.** The "gold standard" serum (blood) tests for hormone levels are reliable for management of *infertility* in younger women. We need these same reliable objective tests for management of midlife and menopausal hormone issues. Saliva tests and hair analysis are not adequate for the complexity of women's hormones.

I revised and updated *It's My Ovaries, Stupid!* to bring you a science-based focus from the international research studies that form the basis of my clinical work. My goal is to strip away the myths surrounding hormones and hormone therapy, including such misconceptions as hormones cause cancer, all estrogens are the same, all progestins are the same, and how you take them doesn't matter.

This book answers questions raised by the barrage of alarming stories, sheds light on the complex puzzle of our female hormones, uncovers new information about risks to your ovaries, and gives you a guide to get properly tested and identify ways to feel better and reduce future disease risk.

I do not have any financial interest in any of the products I recommend in my books. I have no financial ties to any pharmaceutical company or compounding pharmacy. I do not recommend something that I would not use myself, or would not feel comfortable recommending to a family member if the need arose.

My goal is to give you the most up-to-date, reliable, and medically sound information I am able to find so you have the tools to effectively demand optimal care for *your* health and the health of the world you live in.

I am also writing this book in hopes it will be helpful to those in the community of health professionals who are genuinely interested in improving health care for women, and who want to understand the crucial ways that our ovary hormones affect body systems and functions.

For even more information on the "estrogen" story and the problems with the WHI, I encourage you to read *The Savvy Woman's Guide*™ *to Estrogen*, and *The Savvy Woman's Guide*™ *to Hormone Headlines*.

Elizabeth Lee Vliet, M.D.
January, 2007

Overview of the Problem
How I Came to Write This Book

My Medical Journey as a "Hormone Detective"

Hormones and their connections in how we think and feel and function has been my life's work in medicine. During more than 25 years of medical practice, I have evaluated countless women of all ages—from 9 to 90—who were convinced their hormones were wreaking havoc with their health and sanity, but other physicians had simply dismissed them as "neurotic" or "psychosomatic."

I had so many patients, of many different ages, describe the same physical and emotional experience at similar times of their menstrual cycles, that I began to look at these ovarian hormone patterns more closely. Since I knew that thyroid hormones caused mood and anxiety problems as well as the usual physical symptoms, I wondered what "brain" symptoms might be triggered by the changing levels of estradiol, progesterone, testosterone and DHEA during the menstrual cycle.

When I started this work in 1983, few physicians took "PMS" seriously. Yet I was convinced that it was real, and it was caused by hormone ups and downs, not just life stress, wrong diet or bad marriage.

My background in Internal Medicine and interest in endocrinology—especially the effects of hormones on the brain—gave me a framework in which to think about and track symptoms. Before my medical career, I taught Chemistry and Biology, and later, psychopharmacology for health professionals.

Fortunately, I also had formal specialty training in Psychiatry at Johns Hopkins, one of the top programs in the country that focused on the biological underpinnings of behavioral and mood syndromes. This experience provided an extraordinary depth of clinical experience that laid the foundation for my later work in these neuroendocrine effects on women's total health.

With this combined "mind-body" medicine background, I had an excellent education in how to differentiate a purely psychiatric disorder from one with similar symptoms but with an underlying endocrine cause. I could begin the detective work to uncover the mood, behavioral and physical symptoms that appeared at predictable times of the menstrual cycle, then disappeared the rest of the month.

It seemed logical to me that if a woman's symptoms were clearly happening at the same time of her menstrual cycle each month, they were *more likely* to have endocrine, or hormonal triggers. This pattern was *different* from similar problems in women who experienced their mood or physical symptoms most all the time: i.e., mood and anxiety problems present every day, on a sustained basis that don't change with the menstrual cycle, are more typical of true primary psychiatric syndromes.

Menstrual cycle effects on women's physical and emotional health have been described in medical literature since the time of the ancient Greeks. Twenty-five hundred years ago Hippocrates recognized that when women had scant or absent bleeding cycles, they had more joint and muscle pain and other problems.

After treating thousands of women and checking their cycle-specific ovarian hormone levels, I now see the staggering and costly problems for women when the health care system casually ignores these hormone effects.

I have also come to see the enormous health risks to women's ovaries and fertility that result from exposure to environmental endocrine disrupting chemicals, food additives in everything from soft drinks to "health food," rising mercury and other heavy metals in our environment, and destructive modern lifestyles—smoking, chronic dieting, alcohol and drug use, lack of sleep, and toxic stress.

There is another dimension to my background that is just as important as the "professional" me. As a woman, I have dealt with these same confusing, capricious, and frustrating hormone changes. None of us are immune to these problems. I connect, at a very personal level, with what you are experiencing. I will share some of my own story as we walk this hormonal road together in the pages ahead.

Since the medical establishment can be slow to change, I decided I wanted to write for *women who want to become empowered to make positive changes in their health and lives.* I want to reach women who want answers, who want to know about the good science that explains how our hormones work, who want to know constructive and medically sound approaches to feeling healthy and energetic.

Because I am still actively seeing "real-life" women in my Tucson and Dallas medical offices, I have kept up with new developments from international research to find solutions to help solve these problems for my patients. If my approaches to treatment aren't working in the real world of women's lives, then I must refine my recommendations to find more effective ways to help women feel better.

You aren't just reading theory here—you are reading about approaches I have found that *work*. I do my own literature research and read original articles and sources carefully; I also attend the major international conferences each year to bring you the latest information.

Getting well and *staying well* is a process, a journey. It isn't a quick fix using one magic bullet or hormone recipe for everybody. For some, it is easy and quick; for others, it is more difficult, slow and even arduous. I hope this book will be your guide to answers, tests, and treatments that will help you on your journey.

Now, What About YOU?

Have you ever thought to yourself "What's wrong with me? My body feels like an alien creature. I don't seem to be handling things as well as I used to. I don't feel good. I feel soooo tired. I don't accomplish as much as I once did. I'm not the *me* I once knew. What's going on?"

Something is different. It may have started out with little things: bone-tired fatigue, waking up in the middle of the night, body aches, forgetfulness, going to the bathroom more frequently, more noticeable PMS, headaches coming more often and lasting longer, no interest in sex, feeling blue and anxious for no apparent reason.

You wonder: "Is this all in my head? My doctor hasn't found anything physically wrong with me. He tells me I'm just stressed and need to take an antidepressant and do relaxation exercises. Is this just how it is? I am *too young* to feel *this old!* What is causing this? What can I do?"

Maybe your symptoms are more severe. Maybe you are undergoing medical treatment, seeing various physicians and specialists, taking lots of medication, or herbs and teas you can't even pronounce, yet you're still not getting better or finding answers that make sense. You may still be thinking "My doctor says I don't have anything wrong…I must be imagining all this after all."

NO. The problem is not in your head. These problems can be very real, and commonly may be caused by changes in the balance of your body's ovarian hormones.

This book is to help those of you who have not reached the "typical" age of perimenopause or menopause—but who may be having various health

Dr. Vliet's Guide to the Most Common Reasons for Consults

What do I see most commonly in the women coming to us for consults? Here's a typical list:

- *fatigue, to the point of exhaustion*
- *weight gain that's out of control*
- *loss of sex drive*
- *difficulty getting pregnant*
- *heart palpitations, racing or pounding heartbeat*
- *memory problems, difficulty concentrating, feeling scattered*
- *headaches*
- *restless, fragmented sleep*
- *pelvic, vaginal and/or external genital (vulvar) pain*
- *painful intercourse, difficulty having an orgasm*
- *cyclic, severe acne*
- *mood swings*
- *increasingly severe PMS*
- *painful periods, severe cramping with bleeding*
- *heavy bleeding*
- *irregular menstrual cycles*
- *"irritable" bowel or chronic constipation*
- *sensitivity to strong smells and chemicals*
- *worsening allergies*
- *chronic yeast infections*
- *thinning scalp hair*
- *excess facial and body hair growth*
- *dry skin*
- *dry eyes*
- *low-body temperature*
- *aching joints*
- *muscle pain*
- *marked pain with urination*

These are not "fun-time" symptoms, and this is just a partial list. All of these problems may have many causes, but how do we find out a possible *hormonal* cause if we don't have a reliable measure of your ovarian hormones?

problems—understand your ovaries and their hormones and what they do throughout your brain and body to keep you well and vibrant. I'll explain what happens when your hormones go awry, and the many ways they can be disrupted, putting women's ovaries on overload and causing them to "shut down" at earlier and earlier ages.

Your Hormone Web: Effects Throughout Your Body

It's a difficult to keep a symptom list *short* when looking at everything that can be affected by changes in ovarian hormones.

Estradiol alone is involved in over 400 functions in a woman's body. That doesn't even take into account the profound effects of testosterone, progesterone and DHEA throughout the brain and body.

Is it any wonder, then, that women have a whole panoply of problems when their ovarian hormones go awry?

How Does This Relate to ME? I Am Too Young for Menopause.

We have all been taught to think of menopause, or the end of menstruation, as the only time in a woman's life when the ovaries are no longer producing hormones. In our usual life progression, *menopause* affects women who are usually much older than most of you reading this book.

Doctors generally don't consider hormone loss as a possibility in women younger than 40. *"It can't be hormonal, you're too young,"* is a standard phrase you may have heard time and again when seeking medical care for these problems.

These "mysterious" symptoms are often severe and plague women even in their teens, twenties, and thirties. Young women may experience symptoms one would "expect" in older perimenopausal or menopausal women. What about hormone problems that can occur in young women after a serious viral illness, a tubal ligation, or exposure to environmental chemicals?

Doctors—and most women—don't tend to think about the possibility of hormone imbalances in girls *before* puberty. What about the alarming increase in premature puberty in girls as young as 6, 7 and 8 years old? Today this serious problem is happening more and more in younger women for reasons I'll talk about in chapters 4–7.

These young women desperately need good evaluation and treatment now, to prevent later serious health problems like infertility, obesity, insulin resistance, and even early onset diabetes.

There are several different, but overlapping, syndromes that affect your ovaries: *premature ovarian decline* (POD), *premature ovarian failure* (POF), *polycystic ovary syndrome* (PCOS), *endometriosis, premenstrual syndrome* (PMS) and the "new" more severe form now called *premenstrual dysphoric disorder* (PMDD), *post-partum depression* (PPD) and several types of autoimmune, viral and inflammatory illnesses that affect the ovaries (*oophoritis*).

These different conditions share a common feature: *the ovaries are not producing an optimal balance of estradiol and testosterone, even though they may still be producing healthy levels of progesterone.*

Even though there are important medical distinctions among these conditions, *all* are **overlooked** and **under-treated**. Underlying hormone causes of common health problems for women are not taken into account in health care today.

As a result, they cost women—and our society—countless billions of dollars in misspent health care costs, substance abuse, lost productivity in the workplace, and premature disability claims.

At a more personal level, they cost individual women in staggering and profound ways:

- lost quality of life from the adverse side effects from medications
- frequent doctor's visits
- decreased function and/or missed time from work
- family discord
- breakdown of personal relationships

Women should have access to a medical system that sees our hormone fluctuations are important and relevant, not something to be overlooked or trivialized.

Physicians are even *less* aware of the way that synthetic chemicals in our environment may be contributing to serious health problems in younger and younger women.

Women are facing a *silent* health crisis similar in magnitude to the environmental damage that Rachel Carson first documented in 1962 with her landmark book, *Silent Spring.* Her efforts focused world attention on the damage from DDT.

Today we face even more threats from newly developed chemicals, permutations of the old DDT. While these new compounds may satisfy legal limits, they are still present in quantities that can seriously damage our bodies.

Women's ovaries and thyroid glands are especially vulnerable to these "chemical disruptors," whether we are exposed in our mother's womb, or during infancy, childhood, or as adults. This is a ticking time bomb, waiting to explode in health problems for today's young women and girls as they grow older. The health of your ovaries is so much more at risk today than ever before in history as a result of environmental "hormone disrupters."

As a biology student at the College of William and Mary, I was interested in the developing field of animal behavior and studied what happened to young animals whose mothers were given various drugs and chemicals during pregnancy. In the 1950s and 1960s, research had shown that chemicals given to a pregnant female could disrupt sexual behavior, fertility, and reproductive tract development in the developing offspring. My master's thesis explored different aspects of these issues, based on work done in rats, mice and hamsters.

For example, female offspring displayed male mating behavior or were infertile. Male offspring engaged in female sexual behaviors and had abnormally small testicles. I was fascinated by these ominous findings, but little did I know how significant this would become to my later work in women's health.

Over the years, as I have worked with patients to solve their puzzling health changes, I have returned to this basic science as well as wildlife studies and new research on human health problems creatively connect the dots. The picture that has unfolded is an alarming one, and one we desperately need to understand better and take seriously.

A Flaw in the Medical Model for Women

Most physicians, regardless of specialty, do not check women's ovarian hormone levels. The one exception is fertility specialists who are helping women get pregnant. Why aren't these same hormones checked when women have other problems? Seems like a shocking oversight, doesn't it?

For one thing, in the United States, women's healthcare has been mainly focused on reproductive issues, traditionally handled by the *surgical* specialty of Obstetrics and Gynecology (Ob-Gyn), which includes ovarian (i.e., reproductive) hormones. But most of the focus in training is on surgical skills. My friends in gynecology are quick to tell me that their training didn't focus much on the nuances of hormone medication management, or on hormone effects on the body above the waist!

Internal medicine, on the other hand, is a specialty that teaches doctors to do detailed medical histories of the patterns of symptoms, and use various lab tests to check for what is out of balance when the symptoms appear.

Diabetes is an example. Internists look at the pattern of symptoms—abnormal weight gain, increased thirst, increased trips to the bathroom to urinate, and increased appetite for sweets, to name a few. They measure glucose and insulin levels at set times relative to meals, and several other lab tests. They use this information to make decisions about medications. Internists are also taught to *recheck* blood tests after starting new medications to monitor a person's response and to determine a proper dose. Doses are individualized for each person.

I was accustomed to this approach in evaluating problems described by my patients.

- ֍ Was diabetes causing depressed, lethargic mood? Check the blood glucose level and see if it is too high.
- ֍ Was hypothyroidism causing depressed mood, slowed thinking, memory loss? Check the level of *thyroid stimulating hormone* (TSH) and see if it is too high or too low.

Even before I started working with the ovarian hormones in the early 1980s, I correlated appropriate blood tests with patients' history and physical findings to determine the medical problems that explained symptoms my patients described.

I was struck by the recurring patterns of symptoms that often came at the same time in the menstrual cycle, but then menses would start and symptoms got better. I began to wonder whether these problems were being caused by the predictable changes in ovarian hormones.

As I researched the medical literature to learn more about hormone effects beyond our reproductive system. I was excited to find a wealth of research about how ovarian hormones affects the brain, altering mood, sleep and a host of other targets in the body. I began to measure ovarian hormone at different times of the cycle.

That's when the "Aha" light bulb went on! Women were too often being told by other doctors, most without any formal training in psychiatry, that they were just *depressed, anxious or stressed*. I did not feel that most of these women actually had a psychiatric disorder, but they weren't "imagining" their symptoms either. The lab test results helped me show my patients that their ovarian hormones were in fact significantly out of balance when their symptoms were happening.

Physicians often forget that psychological symptoms from effects on brain pathways can be caused by physical changes, such as low or fluctuating hormones. These endocrine causes of mood and behavioral symptoms are not the same thing as a purely psychiatric disorder. But if no one is checking a woman's hormones, how can we find an endocrine cause?

Doctors have not been adequately trained in the role of ovarian hormones beyond their obvious reproductive function. Far-reaching mind-body effects of ovarian hormones are basically ignored.

It is staggering that systematic measurements of the unique female endocrine system are completely absent in most medical work-ups and testing procedures for women.

Expensive, and often less effective medications, some with risky side effects, are typically the only approach offered to these women. Ads on TV focus on a new drug or herb supplement for every symptom. Vast numbers of women with hormone-related health problems suffer needlessly, in spite of the safe and effective prescription hormone options that could help relieve a variety of symptoms.

"Gender-based" medicine is a current buzzword used in place of "women's health" but it also *fails to advocate testing of the very hormones that make us biologically female or male.* How can it then be *gender-based?* This must change —it is the next needed frontier in medical care for women.

Taking Care of the Ovaries: Whose Job is It, Really?

Our current specialty-based health care system is incredibly fragmented:

- Neurologists check your headaches
- Rheumatologists check your muscle pain
- Orthopedists check your bones and joints
- Dermatologists check skin problems like acne
- Urologists check bladder problems
- Physiatrists treat muscle pain syndromes
- Otolaryngologists check your ears and sinuses.
- Endocrinologists are trained to diagnose and treat "hormonal disorders." But in the U.S. they tend to focus on diabetes, thyroid disorders, and pituitary problems. They typically do not view the ovaries as "their" area. Endocrinologists often tell women that they need to see their gynecologist for "hormone" problems suspected to be due to ovarian hormone disorders.
- Obstetrician-gynecologists are surgeons who deliver babies, address surgical problems of the female reproductive organs, and provide annual pelvic and Pap exams. It is a surgical, not a medical-endocrine specialty. A typical Ob-Gyn may tell a woman that her non-reproductive symptoms, such as mood swings, insomnia or low energy, are not "gynecological," and she should see a psychiatrist or therapist.
- Psychiatrists treat depression and anxiety but don't check ovarian hormone levels in their evaluation of causes for mood or anxiety symptoms.

So when it comes to the non-reproductive effects of ovarian hormones… *whose job is it? So far this crucial question remains unanswered.*

There really is no identified specialty that focuses on the ovaries, the hormones they produce, and their multiple connections and effects on the multiple non-reproductive functions of a woman's body and brain. The only time women's ovarian hormones are checked is during treatment for infertility. Even many "women's health" specialists don't check ovarian hormone levels!

It seems clear to me if a man lost his testosterone, he wouldn't feel normal. Yet very few doctors tell a man that "it's just stress" if he lost the function of his testicles due to injury, disease, or surgery. Testosterone is the powerful hormone that "sets" a man's biology. **The ovarian hormones "set" the patterns of a woman's biology and are major metabolic regulators that affect every cell and tissue in our brain and bodies.**

Ovaries just can't be removed, have wedges cut out, tied off, suppressed or otherwise impaired with impunity. There are far-reaching consequences throughout the body if a woman's ovaries aren't up to par in their hormone production. These are very real health problems that, left unrecognized and untreated, can have devastating effects.

From your teens onward, you need to become informed about your body; about what your ovaries are and what they do besides help you have a baby. You also need to know the early clues that indicate a decline in these important ovarian hormones.

You need to understand the symptoms, the serious health problems, and the conditions that affect ovarian hormone production, as well as what treatments are available, and the consequences of your decisions.

I believe that if you have this knowledge, then you will be able to make *appropriate, intelligent choices* to feel better and enjoy this time of your life.

As one 30 year-old aspiring actress said recently during her first visit: "I am tired of feeling so bad and so *old*. I am tired of being told by doctors that I am just stressed and need to slow down. I am tired of not having a life! **I want my life back!** That's why I am here!"

It IS Possible—and Desirable—to Test Ovarian Hormones

Doctors often refuse to check hormones and say "it isn't necessary," or "it's too expensive." *I disagree.*

Doctors also say "there is "no way to check your hormones," or "hormone tests aren't reliable." *I disagree.*

We have a multi-billion dollar infertility industry in this country that is based on reliably measuring women's ovarian hormones with blood tests that have been available since the 1960's. If fertility specialists did not monitor women's ovarian hormones, they would not succeed in helping infertile women get pregnant.

If we can reliably check blood tests for women's hormones when they are trying to get *pregnant*, why can't physicians use the same tests to help answer other *health* problems? In my view, *other health needs of women* are just as important as trying to become pregnant.

I often get answers to health questions that other doctors don't because I include a thorough measurement of women's hormone levels in every new patient evaluation.

My patients tell me that other doctors have said "Ovarian hormones levels vary so much, the information isn't useful." But in medicine, *everything* in our body changes from moment-to-moment, so it seems totally illogical to me that you can't test women's hormone levels because they change!

No test in medicine is perfect, and every test we use has variability. Glucose, insulin, cholesterol, and all of our other blood chemicals are varying minute to minute throughout our days. Yet, doctors do not treat diabetes without measuring glucose and insulin levels. Doctors don't treat high cholesterol problems without measuring the complete blood fat (lipid) profile.

Bottom line: *Doctors deal with this variation in all other tests and they can learn to deal with the variation in women's ovarian hormones too.*

I explain my patients' hormone results, along with history and physical findings. I point out that *all* of our medical tests have a built-in day-to-day, hour-to hour, minute-to-minute variation. Nothing in the body is static. I help patients see how symptoms *change* as the hormone levels go up and down. Then we work together on a systematic, individualized treatment plan to integrate all this. To me, this approach is key to a truly *woman-centered* healthcare model.

Hormones Alone Are Not the Answer...

Is this book just about taking hormones? Do hormones fix everything?

Of course not.

Hormones are not the only, or necessarily the best, course of treatment for every woman. There are lots of books on other solutions to relieve symptoms. There are very few books, however, that focus primarily on these hormone pieces of the puzzle.

That is why I have focused on hormones in this book. I will discuss the pros and cons of various hormone balancing options, talk about ways to help you find the right type of hormones to minimize unwanted side effects, and help you understand the flaws and misinterpretations of the scientific studies that have created an unwarranted fear of hormones, especially estrogens, in the minds of women young and old.

Dietary, lifestyle, and environmental influences can have an adverse effect on healthy ovarian function. Some unsuspected culprits are the overuse of soy supplements, too much exercise, chronic dieting, and exposure to environmental chemicals. Television and the Internet bombard us with "cures" that make the quackery of 19th Century health hustlers look tame. And some actually damage women's fertility and hormones.

I will talk about the "excitotoxins" in food and beverages that are potent neurological disrupters of the pituitary-ovarian pathways and can lead to hormonal imbalance, particularly in women. Diets high in processed foods with these chemical additives are another factor that leads to increasing ovarian hormone problems seen in younger and younger women today.

I have done my best to write *It's My Ovaries, Stupid!* in simple terms to make the medical explanations and "chemical soup" easier to understand. It may sound complicated at times, but women are smart, savvy and persistent when it comes to their health. Many women tell me they like to understand the science that explains their experiences. They feel their observations are validated when the science explains what they have been going through. I also find that women who are experiencing puzzling health problems are hungry for as much information as possible, and feel frustrated when books are too sketchy or superficial in their descriptions.

Is this book for you? Take the Self Test that follows. Then let's get started on understanding your "marvelous and maddening" hormones, and what they do.

Elizabeth Lee Vliet, M.D.
January 2007

Your Road Map to this Book

Section I: Body Basics describes how the ovaries work, what they do, what their "life cycle" is, how they interact with other hormone systems, and how to recognize symptoms of faltering hormone production. Your ovarian hormones are a tapestry of pathways interwoven throughout your body, affecting every aspect of your health. You need to know how they work throughout your life.

Section II: Ovaries At Risk describes the dietary, environmental, and lifestyle "toxins" that damage your ovaries, as well as the wide variety of medical conditions, illnesses and surgeries that can cause hormone imbalances.

Section III: Your Ovaries and Your Body shows how hormone imbalances can result in a bewildering array of health problems affecting just about every system in the body—from hair loss, brittle nails, to anxiety, insomnia, memory loss, low energy, and loss of sex drive!

Section IV: Getting Well—Your Hormone Power Life Plan® gives you a list of tests you may request from your doctors, the hormone levels that should be tested, and when in the menstrual cycle it is most meaningful to have them done. I explain what the "numbers" mean, and the differences between "optimal" and "normal" levels and ranges. I show you what hormonal and other medication options you might consider along with mind–body strategies that help you regain your energy and zest. I teach you ways to clean up your home and work environment to eliminate toxic chemicals that affect you and your family and describe ways to improve your lifestyle choices so that you don't unwittingly sabotage your fertility or overall health.

Appendix I lists common medical abbreviations, and **Appendix II** lists medical references. Included are many older studies to show just how long many of these connections have been known. Some of these well-done studies go back several decades, which is why it is even more incomprehensible to me that doctors still don't address these issues in women's heath care thirty or forty years later. Finding these older references took me a lot of effort, which you will not have time to do. Don't think that because they are "old" they no longer hold true. These "basics" still hold, even if overlooked. Included are up-to-the-minute references to illustrate how our knowledge is increasing.

I used patient stories, first-hand experiences and feedback from the women I have seen as patients. Each one is a real person, with real struggles. Even though I have changed the names to protect their privacy, I have accurately portrayed their descriptions, lab results, and treatment approaches used. I hope their stories help you not feel quite so alone and frightened. You deserve answers and sound approaches to help solve problems. Hormones are not to be feared, they are Mother Nature's gift to keep our bodies and minds vibrant and healthy!

Dr. Vliet's Self-test: "Is This Me?"

Take the Self-Test that follows to see what health problems you may be experiencing that may be linked to your ovarian hormones. As you read further, I will provide explanations and helpful options so you can begin to feel better! But first, write down your answers below.

Answer the following questions honestly with a YES or NO. Then total the number of yes and no answers and write the totals below.

_____ I feel tired and I barely have energy to get through a normal day

_____ I have trouble sleeping through at night and feeling rested when I awake in the morning

_____ I feel more irritable and edgy than is usual for me

_____ I have angry outbursts that seem out of proportion to events

_____ I feel nervous and tense, especially a week or so before my period

_____ I feel depressed, especially a week or so before my period

_____ I have crying spells for no obvious reason

_____ I have more mood swings than I used to

_____ I am gaining weight even though I haven't changed my eating habits

_____ I have lost more than 10 pounds without trying to diet or change my eating habits

_____ I crave sweets or chocolate or carbohydrates more than I used to

_____ I crave salty or fatty foods

_____ I drink more than 1 alcoholic beverage a day

_____ I find myself craving alcohol and have a hard time resisting it

_____ I drink more than 1 soft drink (colas, etc.) a day

_____ I eat processed and prepared foods daily or quite often

_____ I have trouble with chronic constipation or diarrhea

_____ My muscles and/or joints ache, or frequently feel stiff

_____ I am sensitive to perfumes and chemical smells (i.e. get headaches, feel dizzy, can't think clearly, or have other symptoms when around strong smells)

_____ I have more allergies than I used to

Dr. Vliet's Self-test: "Is This Me?"

_____My menstrual cycles are more irregular

_____My menstrual flow is much lighter, or much heavier, than usual for me

_____I have been skipping a lot of menstrual periods lately

_____I have gone more than 2 months without a period

_____I have tried to get pregnant and haven't been successful

_____I don't have my usual sex drive

_____I have trouble having an orgasm

_____I am losing hair, or my hair is getting quite thin and brittle

_____I feel lethargic, sluggish and slowed down a lot of the time

_____I frequently have problems with my memory and concentration

_____I have trouble making decisions, or feel like my thinking is scattered, or have trouble focusing

_____I have swelling of my hands or feet

_____I have more headaches than I used to

_____I have been having palpitations or racing heartbeat, especially around the time of my menstrual bleeding

_____I have dizzy spells

_____My skin is itchy, or dry, or feels like ants crawling inside

_____My family or I use pesticides at home, either inside or outside

_____I/We use chemical cleaners for bathrooms, kitchens, carpets, etc.

_____My mother took, or may have taken, DES or other hormones during pregnancy.

Total number YES_____ NO_____

If you have answered YES to more than 4 or 5 of these questions, you may be experiencing damaging effects of endocrine disruptors around you, or having premature ovarian decline causing lower than desirable levels of your estradiol, testosterone and other key hormones.

Kristi's Poem

"Dear Dr. Vliet,

I just wanted to take a moment and thank you for your help and dedication. While I have felt challenged seemingly beyond capacity since my twins were born, I have also felt very blessed. I am married to the most wonderful man and we share the privilege of parenting six amazing kids.

Throughout the years, as I have struggled with my health and emotions, it has felt like a roller coaster that never stops. My life brings me such joy, yet it overwhelmed me just the same. I felt guilt and shame. And when I was unwell, sadness for my family as they had essentially lost their mom to her unnamed problem. No one could possibly understand. No doctor could alleviate it. No therapist could probe it. No remedy could emolliate it.

When I first came to see you I was at a point where I realized I had to accept the possibility that I had a supreme moral flaw in my character or mental illness, both of which I feared and denied for years. So it was that my initial few months on hormone therapy were healing to more than just my body. As we have sought to remedy the various aspects of my ailments, it has been difficult and even frustrating, but despite the ups and downs, I have felt so hopeful. I thank you for giving me that renewal. I also want to share with you something I wrote after I started treatment with you:

For years I felt plagued
By a monster
Silently lurking inside,
Slowly ravaging my body
Torturing my mind
Tormenting my loved ones.

No one could see it.
Was it real?
Was it the figment of
A depraved mind?
Perhaps... so
I hid the monster.

I told no one
But my dearest,
My only earthly confidant.
We fought it
Unwittingly fed it
And still it grew.

It occasionally left open
Wounds in its wake
To be treated superficially

by experts
Who still couldn't see
The monster.

A life so young,
So full and blessed
It seemed I had much
For which to live
And yet
I could not

And now
A ray of hope.
Someone who sees
The monster!
Balm both to heal the body
And quiet the mind.

I am renewed
The monster's bane
So long unseen
Now no longer felt.
The monster is vanquished.'
  And I live—"

Contents

Chapter 1

When Ovaries Go Awry: Women's Lives, Women's Stories

Younger and younger women are being hit by the hormone syndromes I listed in the Introduction—Premature Ovarian Decline (POD), Premenopausal Syndrome (PMS), and Polycystic Ovary Syndrome (PCOS).

Why is this?

Women today are under much more stress than our mothers and grandmothers and lead very complex, demanding lives... burning the candle at both ends and in the middle. Women today are also immersed in more chemicals than ever before, with insidious consequences for our hormone pathways.

Yes... such stress *does* affect your ovaries and decrease your hormones!

At the same time, however, women are living lives that require a higher level of functioning, both physical and mental, than ever before. Disruptive symptoms or health problems that once might have gone unnoticed when women rarely worked outside the home can now seriously get in your way when you are holding down a full-time job in addition to your homemaking.

POD and menopause: symptoms can be similar for both—restless sleep, crawly skin, and hot flashes. But POD isn't technically menopause because younger women still have follicles that can become eggs. Menstrual periods are still occurring, even if lighter and more irregular.

Women who reach *natural menopause* have exhausted their lifetime supply of follicles in the ovary, and can't produce normal levels of ovarian hormones. If your follicles are depleted, you don't ovulate, you can't produce estrogen and progesterone, so the lining of the uterus doesn't build up, and you no longer have monthly periods. That's *menopause.*

Many women don't mind the end of menstruation. But what they do mind are symptoms: insomnia, low energy, loss of sex drive, foggy thinking, or constant hot flashes.

It's Not All In Your Head—It Can Be Hormones!

Women's Lives, Women's Stories

A common thread runs through each story: *confusion, self-doubt, and feelings of being betrayed by one's own body and by the medical system.* What's going on? Do these women just need to get a grip, simplify their lives, take a break, relax? Is this mental or physical? What are options to treat the underlying cause?

The following stories illustrate an intriguing variety of the effects hormone imbalance and hormone decline can have on a woman's body. Some are devastating; most caused the patient to seek medical help. All are disruptive and unacceptable, particularly when they hit at a young age.

The last seven months have been strange for *Rebecca.* Although she's only 31, her body aches as if she's much older. Her joints hurt, she feels stiff and sore. It's hard for her to get out of bed in the morning. She just doesn't have the same level of energy she used to. In the past she could stay up late and really push herself to get all of her work done. Now it takes her a week to recover from even one late night.

She had one ectopic pregnancy, plus an early miscarriage, and she has not been able to conceive again. She has totally lost interest in sex and this is affecting her marriage. She's started to get excruciating headaches and is battling a low-grade depression. She's heard about perimenopause but she feels she is too young for that. She is able to go through the motions of her life, but feels as if she's missing out on a lot and aging much too quickly. What's going on? Her doctor said she is depressed and recommended an antidepressant, but Rebecca isn't convinced. She thinks there is more to it.

What her doctor doesn't know is that Rebecca's mother had been treated with DES, a potent synthetic estrogen used to help prevent miscarriage. DES affects a baby's development in the womb, leading to ovarian hormone problems in adulthood. This plays a role in Rebecca's problems.

Don't we know! Symptoms of low hormones can drastically affect the *quality* of your life.

Wisdom: The patterns of hormone decline effects are individual for each woman.

For 17-year-old *Cathie*, "that time of the month" has been a nightmare. Since her periods began at age 11, she has experienced migraines, vomiting and excruciating cramps every month with the onset of her menstrual bleeding.

Various physicians prescribed a range of medications, including Prozac and beta-blockers, but nothing seemed to help. Cathie and her mother figured that since these episodes always came when her periods started, her hormones must trigger the headaches and cramps.

They asked the doctors to check her menstrual cycle hormones, but their requests were dismissed. It seems obvious to them there is a connection and they felt "put down" by her doctor's dismissal of their opinions about a hormone link.

Now Cathie is getting desperate. She's missing too much school because of the headaches and she's on so much medication that it is hard to stay alert when she does attend.

When I checked her ovarian hormones, I found clues to what set off her menstrual migraines. Her estradiol on the first day of bleeding dropped to an abnormally low 10 pg/ml. She didn't need so many medications every day. She needed a way to keep her estradiol from dropping sharply and setting off the headaches.

Peggy sought medical help when she realized that at age 28 she had the same symptoms as her 80-year-old grandmothers! For the last two years she felt "foggy" and would forget such simple things as her social security number and friend's phone number.

At first she blamed her failing memory and emotional difficulties on stress and sleep deprivation. But when her hair started falling out, her skin felt crawly, her menstrual periods became irregular, the flow became very light, and her constipation got worse, she realized something else must be happening.

Her food allergies were also getting worse, so she gave up foods with wheat, dairy products, sugar, or stimulants, but this didn't seem to help. She decided it was time to see her doctor.

He said her symptoms were caused by stress and for her to get more rest and scale back her workload. How could she? She had two young children, a full-time job and an ailing grandmother to care for. She had handled stress before and didn't have these problems. She was certain something else was going on.

Warning: Anti-depressants are prescribed too often for women—without even checking their hormones!

Hunh? Hormone links are often obvious to women… but often *dismissed* by doctors. This has got to change!

Peggy realized that she never had these problems until after her tubal ligation following the birth of her second child. She noticed her periods were lighter and her cycles shorter. Though her friends say they feel tired, they seem to be handling their life demands much better than Peggy feels she is.

"What's wrong with me?" she wonders. "Is this all in my head? I tried seeing a new doctor and she didn't find anything physically wrong with me. She tells me I'm just stressed and to do relaxation exercises. I think there is something else. I think getting my tubes tied must have affected my hormones, but my doctor says that can't happen…I wonder how I find out?"

Peggy was correct: tubal ligations can decrease blood flow to the ovary, resulting in lower hormone levels. When I evaluated her, her blood levels of estradiol and testosterone were extremely low. Her doctors missed it because they didn't check her hormone levels.

Leah, a 26-year-old, was experiencing similar symptoms to the others I described, but hers had a different culprit. For two years Leah had been on a synthetic progestin, Depo-Provera, for contraception.

She felt like her life was "going down the tubes" with loss of energy, depressed mood, loss of sex drive, and irritable, angry feelings much of the time. She said, *"I saw the title of your book and it was me! My main concern right now is just feeling better. I had a happy life until all this hit me. This is hard on my marriage. It's hanging on by a thread."*

Depo-Provera is a *progestin-only* synthetic contraceptive that *contains no estrogen*. This progestin typically suppresses the ovarian cycles, and decreases all ovarian hormone levels.

But this wasn't quite the situation with Leah. Her ovaries were still producing a healthy rise in progesterone, typical of that seen with ovulation. But her estradiol levels were significantly below optimal levels, an effect of the Depo-Provera. The cyclic rise in progesterone from her own ovaries was added to the negative side effects of the Depo-Provera.

Her total progesterone/progestin load was much too high relative to her very low estradiol for the second half of her ovarian cycle. The E:P ratio was all wrong. The progesterone/progestin dominance was the primary trigger for her severe PMS, headaches and terrible mood swings. Needless to say, she changed to a different contraceptive and is doing much better! She said, "*I feel like myself—I have my life back!*"

All of these younger women had low hormone levels or abnormal ratios of estradiol and progesterone that caused very disruptive symptoms. The good news is, there is help!

The Hidden Epidemic: What is Happening to Young Women Today?

Premature ovarian decline (POD) is the early phase of decrease in ovarian hormone production, primarily affecting estradiol, our most active form of estrogen. In some women this early phase also shows a decline in testosterone as well, even though progesterone and Follicle Stimulating Hormone (FSH) may still be quite normal.

There isn't a formal "medical" definition of this first phase of hormone decline, and there is no well-accepted diagnosis or insurance code for it. Doctors today don't check hormone levels so they don't recognize it exists.

What is Premature Ovarian Decline POD?

Over the past twenty years I have systematically checked ovarian hormone levels in thousands of women of all ages, in different phases of the menstrual cycle. I can clearly document that this early phase of ovarian decline exists. Earlier researchers have also described this pattern but it does not get much attention in today's health care.

Doctors are taught that estrogen doesn't decline until after women lose their ovulatory cycles. This turns out to be incorrect.

Our "standard" teaching was not based on any systematic tests of ovarian hormone levels correlated with women's symptoms; it was based on the observation that some women developed irregular cycles. The problem is that *very few physicians ever looked back to see what came before the irregular cycles to trigger the changes.*

POD, in the women I have tested, is characterized by estradiol levels *typically less than half the normal, optimal healthy level* for a young woman still in her reproductive years. Progesterone is usually maintained in the healthy ovulatory ranges until much later in the course of ovarian decline.

Caution: Depo-Provera can cause irritable, depressed moods, weight gain, headaches and low sex drive.

Alert: We cannot just focus on age and then assume someone is too young to have hormone problems.

You know better! POD does exist. This is real. You are not imagining these changes.

POD

I call the first phase of this decline in your ovaries' hormone production POD, or *Premature Ovarian Decline*.

POD/POF

POD differs slightly from premature ovarian *failure...* but the symptoms are similar.

Attention:

It isn't "adrenal exhaustion": it's your ovaries!

There may also be lower than normal testosterone levels, higher levels of markers of bone breakdown, high or low DHEA levels, and the adrenal cortisol levels are higher than would be expected.

What helped me uncover the early stages of this process? I explored the detailed health history of women prior to their cycles becoming irregular. What happened in their lives before they developed these menstrual changes and bothersome symptoms? Had they been sick with a virus? Had they been through serious situational stresses? Did they have any other illnesses, surgery, new medications, new supplements, occupational, or environmental chemical exposures? Did they start smoking cigarettes or using alcohol or marijuana or cocaine? Did their mothers take DES or other hormones during pregnancy? Had they been exposed to pesticides? Did they drink excessive amounts of soft drinks? What was their diet like?

Most of the women I see are able to identify many pieces of their health puzzle. No one else took them seriously or thought their observations were important. I value my patients' insights and I use their observations to guide me as I think through their problems, and the tests we need to reach a diagnosis. *And most importantly, I check hormone levels.*

One reason that many doctors don't take women's hormone questions more seriously is the popular idea that pregnancy cravings and PMS mood swings are comical. The topics of sitcoms and mainstream jokes, we don't think they are real.

For many women, "that time of month" lasts only for a few days with little significant disruption. For many other women, however, symptoms are more severe. We should not tell these women to "just accept it" when there are a number of straightforward approaches to help them feel better.

Why shouldn't women's menstrual cycle symptoms be given as much attention as other health issues?

Health care can no longer afford to ignore women's ovarian hormones and the role they play in the health of our entire body.

I check hormone levels at specific phases of the menstrual cycle and correlate these levels with symptoms, and with what we know to be optimal levels for a fertile cycle.

In all these years of testing, I don't think I have seen anyone with symptoms clearly occurring with the menstrual cycle who had a truly normal, optimal level of estradiol.

I also do detailed thyroid testing, including thyroid antibodies. Medical wisdom says that menstrual disruption is frequently caused by thyroid problems, but I find that the usual thyroid tests often do not detect subtle abnormalities that affect the ovaries. I go a step further and look for clues to autoimmune thyroid disorders by also checking the thyroid antibodies. (See Chapters 9, 17).

Some women have both a thyroid disorder and ovarian decline; some have only one. Many women think they have a thyroid disorder, but actually have an ovarian problem with significantly diminished estradiol production.

Over time, low estradiol leads to increased risk of serious quality-of-life problems such as infertility, fibromyalgia, chronic fatigue, vulvodynia, depression, panic attacks, migraines, loss of sexual function, high cholesterol, high blood pressure, arthritis, diabetes, heart attacks, stroke, bone loss, and others. It's important to know which type of hormone problem you have, since health risks and treatments are different.

To me, it is incomprehensible to insist that it isn't necessary to check ovarian hormone levels, especially today when we know how intertwined these hormones are with the function of every other organ system including our brain.

I don't mean to say that all of these women need hormone treatment. Those with symptoms disrupting their quality of life who have abnormally low hormone levels deserve effective help rather than one "band-aid" medicine after another or being loaded up with anti-depressants and mood stabilizers!

POD is a phase we must learn to recognize and address early to avoid these preventable health problems among young women. I will describe these further in Section II. It is important for you to take charge of this problem now, while you are young enough to prevent permanent damage to your ovaries, your fertility, and your overall health.

What is Premature Ovarian Failure POF?

Premature ovarian failure (POF) or premature menopause refers to the *actual end of menstrual periods before the age of forty-two.*

Again!
Contrary to what doctors have been taught, it is *not* progesterone that declines first… it is *estradiol.*

Caution:
Elevated thyroid antibodies can cause enough thyroid gland dysfunction to affect your ovaries, even if the TSH is still normal.

POF
POF is characterized by an FSH greater than 20 and low ovarian hormone levels characteristic of menopause

POF is a devastating condition that has profound consequences on every dimension of a young woman's life, emotionally and physically. POF causes infertility, a dramatic increase in bone loss, lower sexual responsiveness, chronic insomnia, headaches, allergies and immune changes, abnormal weight gain, marked fatigue, and often, depressed mood and memory problems.

Causes:
POF has many causes, such as early loss of follicles, autoimmune illnesses, viruses or chemicals that damage the ovaries.

Later in the process, if not properly diagnosed and treated, POF leads to more severe health consequences, including diabetes, early heart attacks, strokes, osteoporosis and early death.

In both POD and POF the ovaries do not produce the proper amounts or balance of estradiol, progesterone and testosterone needed for your body to function and for you to feel your best, or to be fertile. If you are a young woman experiencing the loss of your ovarian hormones, it is ultimately less relevant what name you give it. The symptoms rob you of your quality of life and your ability to function at peak performance.

Almost:
POD and POF are different problems... linked by similar symptoms due to low hormone levels.

What are the basic differences between POD, POF, perimenopause and menopause?

Menopause is a natural progression of the aging process. We are born with all the follicles, or potential eggs, we will ever have. We lose follicles with every menstrual cycle. When we get older, and all the follicles have been used, we no longer make our ovarian hormones, and menstruation ends. *We call this menopause.*

Perimenopause is the stage prior to the end of menstruation, when we still have some follicles, but not enough to keep our cycles regular or to ovulate each month, or enough follicles to make optimal levels of ovarian hormones.

It's You:
The key point isn't the name... it's whether you have hormone levels you need to feel *well*.

POD and POF refer to conditions in which women still have their follicles, but the ovaries are not working properly. They don't make optimal levels of the ovarian hormones, even though follicles are still available to do so.

Again, it may not be critical what you call it. The fundamental issue is what hormones are you making, how much are you making, and whether those amounts are what your body needs.

The Hidden Epidemic: What's Different Now?

Precocious puberty. Girls developing breasts at age 6 or 7. Childhood obesity. Adolescent obesity. Infertility. PMS. PCOS. Post Partum Depression. Post Partum Psychosis. Diabetes epidemic.

Eating Disorders. Drug Use. Attention-deficit disorders. Hyper-activity disorders. Learning Disorders. Autism.

These topics all make been headline news on TV and maga-zines for the past few years. Why are they all so common now? What's happening to cause this? Is there something different for women of the 21st century from what our grandmothers and great-grandmothers experienced?

Yes. There are hidden saboteurs of your health that are new for women today.

You, and millions of other young women today, are growing up in a sea of chemicals in foods you eat, beverages you drink, and the environment you live in, both indoors and out. Most of were developed during and since the industrial boom after World War II.

Your grandmothers and great-grandmothers never faced the threat of these massive numbers of chemicals. Your mother may have been exposed to many of them, but because of her age, it is likely that much of her exposure would have occurred *after puberty*, which is a less critical time for these adverse health effects.

Younger women, however, have been exposed to these ubiquitous chemicals as early as the womb. They are called *endocrine disruptors*: hidden dangers to your ovaries, your thyroid, your fertility, and ultimately, the health of all your body systems affected by these crucial hormones.

If your brain, ovaries, and other endocrine organs are exposed to these endocrine disruptors during critical periods of your devel-opment in infancy and childhood, you are far more vulnerable to their insidious damage.

From animal studies, we find that miniscule amounts of hor-mone-like substances and other chemicals have a profound impact on a developing fetus.

For example, studies from around the world show that these chemicals disrupt brain function, cause abnormal sexual and mating behavior, damage the developing structures of the reproductive system, alter function of the immune system and thyroid gland and damage the ovaries in women and testicles in men, just to name a few of the disturbing findings.

Fact:
Endocrine disrupting chemicals have affected you since the womb can insidiously rob you of your health and fertility!

Too Late
Damage is greater when you are exposed to such chemicals in the womb.

Many endocrine disruptors are known carcinogens and can cause increased risk of various types of cancers.

Bitter tea
You have been steeped in these chemicals since conception. Like a teabag that has been steeped too long, these chemicals can leave bitter after-effects

Endocrine disruptors have some positives—such as the reduction of cholesterol caused by various plant-based estrogenic compounds found in many grains and soy. Others, such as pesticides that act at hormone receptors, are seriously toxic to the body and your fertility.

Still other types of endocrine disruptors, such as genistein found in soy, have mixed effects: it is beneficial at some concentrations, and has significant adverse effects at other concentrations, such as stimulating growth of breast cancers.

So how do you get exposed to these chemicals? The chemicals are dispersed throughout your environment. How do they get there?

Some endocrine disruptors occur as by-products of industrial manufacturing and use of fossil fuels like gasoline, jet fuel, and heating oil. They are spewed into the atmosphere and pollute our air. Then they come back to earth in rainwater to foul the water we drink and the soil that provides our food.

Where are they?
Endocrine disrupters are found in the foods you eat, the air you breathe, the water you drink, soft drinks you consume, and in household products.

These endocrine disruptors are insidious. You may not even know you have been exposed until you discover that you can't get pregnant, or you have problems with your menstrual cycle, or find yourself feeling so fatigued and sluggish you can't get through your day, or you begin to lose hair, or you develop serious allergies and chemical sensitivities.

At this point, you may be thinking, well if these chemicals are in everything as you say, how can I change that? How do I escape the negative effects? What can I, as one individual, do about it? There are many positive answers to those questions, which will be addressed throughout this book.

But before you can take these positive steps, you have to know more about how healthy ovarian cycles should work, and what happens to your body as you age. You need to know more about where these chemicals are, how they work, and what health problems they may aggravate. You will then see ways to avoid them and reduce their negative impact on your body. I explain these aspects in Section II: *Ovaries at Risk*.

Summary

In the cases I presented at the beginning of the chapter, all of these women got their lives back on track and are doing well. In most cases, it was a matter of addressing hormonal imbalances, primarily low estradiol levels, and in some cases, thyroid imbalances.

It all starts with proper testing, good detective work tracking symptom patterns together with laboratory information, common sense, diligence, persistence, and an innate curiosity to solve the mystery. In Section IV, I will talk more about ways to do this, and show you how to develop your own health action plan. You, and those who love you, deserve it.

Chapter 2

Your Ovaries:
An Owner's Manual

One of the delights of the study of medicine is learning about all of the wonderful and miraculous things that occur to create us and keep everything going, balancing, responding, and accommodating as we live each day.

We are all so similar, but at the same time, so different, with the most minute subtleties making us distinct from other creatures, and different from each other.

Well Designed
One has to marvel at *what* we are as well as *who* we are.

As a woman I continue to marvel at the intricacies of our bodies, and our rhythms. We are constantly in flux yet in balance and, while our ovaries define us as female from the very beginning, they are so much more than an 'egg factory.'

Our ovarian hormones play many roles in our overall health and well-being: maintaining bone and muscle strength, keeping our brain sharp, maintaining sleep, overseeing immune function, regulating blood pressure and heart function, and of course, our sexuality—not only its reproductive function, but our sexual thoughts, feelings and actions.

Our ovaries are inextricably involved with our entire endocrine system, with the hypothalamus, pituitary gland, parathyroid, thyroid, adrenal gland, and pancreas.

Each of these glands secretes its unique hormones, which interact with ovarian hormones in many ways, as you will see in upcoming chapters.

Our ovaries also have receptors, or docking sites, for chemical messengers that are made in the immune and nervous systems linking our female hormones to *all* of our other body systems.

The ovaries are dullish gray, pitted, lumpy, irregular in shape, and a little larger than an unshelled almond. They are partially attached to the uterus by arteries, veins, and connective tissue, yet they are also semi-floating in space in the pelvis. Their real connection to the uterus, *the fallopian tubes*, hover nearby, barely touching the ovaries.

Ugly, but...
The ovaries are not our most attractive internal organs.

Our ovaries hang in there month after month, year after year, part of a beautifully coordinated hormonal symphony. The process is perfectly orchestrated and intertwined.

Most of us think of *"eggs"* when we think of our ovaries, so let's begin there. Our supply of eggs begins forming virtually at conception. By about week 20, we will have built our maximum number of eggs, approximately six to seven million. During the next 15 to 20 weeks before birth, we lose about five million.

Naturally
The more menstrual periods a woman has, the sooner she depletes her supply of "eggs."

At birth we have approximately 20% of our eggs left, and by puberty we have approximately 20% of that last 20%, still somewhere between 200,000 and 400,000 follicles. At each ovulation we can lose 20 to 1,000 eggs, usually towards the smaller number.

For most of human evolution, women became pregnant in their teens. They also had many years of breastfeedings that suppressed ovulations, and they died at much younger ages, often before they even reached menopause.

We probably learn about our menstrual cycle first from our older girlfriends, then our mothers, and later in health classes at school. We often don't pay much more attention to what's happening with our monthly fluctuations. We become more aware of having periods, and whatever premenstrual problems we might experience, but we usually don't focus on the specifics of which hormone is doing what at any given point during our cycle.

Modern
The average woman today who has fewer pregnancies will have approximately 400–450 menstrual periods in her lifetime.

During early childhood, before age three or four, an area of the brain called the hypothalamus occasionally releases small bursts, or pulses, of reproductive hormones to support early female development.

Then the hypothalamus seems to take a sabbatical from its female cycle management role until about age 9 or 10, on average, when it then resumes its command central role.

Around this time—age 8–10—the adrenal gland gears up production of the adrenal androgens. It is the adrenal androgens, not the ovary, that trigger the start of pubic hair growth. By age eleven or so, the hypothalamus is fully up and running.

We don't yet know with certainty all of the triggers for the onset of puberty and periods. Menses generally begin about mid-way through the physiological process of puberty, when a girl reaches approximately 100 lbs in body weight and about 25% body fat.

These "magic numbers" seems to signal the brain that the body has sufficient fat as reserve energy, about 87,000 calories, to support a pregnancy, which requires approximately 80,000 calories.

We see further evidence for this "set point" of weight and percent fat as heavier girls begin menstruating earlier than thin or athletic girls with less body fat.

It may be that the brain is responding to a hormone called leptin that comes from the fat stores, or it may be that there are other chemical messengers that govern this process.

The *hypothalamus* begins sending out *gonadotrophin-releasing hormone* (GnRH) and when that level gets high enough, it stimulates the pituitary to release a hormone called *follicle-stimulating hormone* (FSH) and *luteinizing* (literally, "yellowing") *hormone* (LH).

The long awaited signal goes out to the ovaries, they rev up and send out the sex hormones that stimulate breast development, put fat on hips, and widen the pelvic bones.

FSH and LH wake up the follicles that are to become eggs (*ova*). Your early menstrual cycles may be a bit erratic while all the systems are getting organized, but usually within six to twelve months, the rhythms are humming along in a flow that will carry on for another forty-some years.

The menstrual cycle itself is a dynamic process, part of the complex and carefully timed procedure of fertility. We mark the "beginning" of the cycle with the sloughing of the uterine lining (bleeding) from the previous month's cycle.

The brain senses the fall in estradiol and progesterone levels to their low point; it signals the pituitary gland to start the cycle all over. The pituitary first sends out FSH to stimulate new follicles ("egg cells") to grow and start making estrogen, mainly estradiol, again.

Historically

Earlier generations may have had as few as 50 menstrual cycles, because they had multiple pregnancies.

Mystery

We don't know what governs which follicles stay and which go; some just quietly burst their membranes, die, and are reabsorbed into the bloodstream.

FSH & LH
These two will continue their work together for the rest of your menstrual life.

Beginning
Progesterone is at a very low level throughout the first half of the cycle, and doesn't start rising significantly until after ovulation.

Ready, set, go...
On about day 12 to 14, the LH signal arrives from the pituitary and tells the egg it's time to pop out.

This primes the follicles to develop for ovulation and stimulates the growth of the lining of the uterus. Each month about 20 or so follicles in each ovary start to expand and ripen. On day 5 or 6 or so, one of these is somehow chosen, and it becomes the *dominant* follicle. Occasionally, more follicles will develop, which can lead to twins, triplets, or other multiples.

When the FSH gets to its highest point of the cycle, this rise signals release of the egg, in the process we call *ovulation*. If multiple eggs are released it appears to be due to a higher FSH level than usual.

The dominant follicle, destined to become the egg, prepares for ovulation by growing a bubble-like sac to protect itself, and forces its way to the surface of the ovary. The other follicles recruited at the beginning seem to know which one has been picked, start to shrivel, then die and are reabsorbed into the bloodstream, a process called *atresia*.

The chosen follicle matures and grows, producing significant amounts of estradiol that triggers many changes, including the rapid growth and thickening of the uterine lining (*endometrium*). Thickening of the endometrium helps prepare the uterus for the arrival of a fertilized egg.

When the levels of estradiol reach about six times the usual level, the hypothalamus again nudges the pituitary and this time it cuts back on the release of FSH, which keeps any more eggs from developing.

Meanwhile the fallopian tubes wave their fimbria, delicate hair-like fronds, similar to the beautiful soft corals I have seen scuba diving. Anticipating the egg's arrival, the fimbria begin to brush the surface of the ovary looking for the large follicle that delivers the egg. At ovulation when the egg is released, many women feel a brief, sharp prick of pain we call *mittelschmertz*.

The cervical fluid changes quickly, often in a few hours or so, after the rapid rise in estradiol just prior to release of the egg. Sperm need a friendly, alkaline, nutrient-rich environment in which to survive during the long journey from the vagina, up through the uterus, and into the Fallopian tube. Women only need these estrogen-triggered changes in cervical fluid at ovulation in order to protect sperm from an otherwise acidic vagina. To further the preparation for fertilization, the cervix also changes its position, hugging the uterus closer, and becoming softer and more open to receive sperm.

Meanwhile, the egg literally bursts from the ovary, into the vast openness of the pelvic cavity. The arms of the fallopian tubes are waiting and waving, with their hair like projections, to quickly move the egg into the funnel of the fallopian tube. Fertilization, if it occurs, normally takes place in the fallopian tube, not in the uterus.

The follicle has still more work to do after the egg is released. Just after the egg pops free, the cells lining the cavity in the follicle begin filling with cholesterol, turning all soft and yellow, and become the *corpus luteum* (or "yellow body").

The corpus luteum makes more estradiol and starts pumping out progesterone to stimulate an even lusher thickening of the lining of the uterus. Everything is ready to receive the fertilized egg that should soon be coming down the fallopian tube.

For the first 42 days or so, the mother's ovarian hormones are essential to the survival of the fetus, until it gets its own hormone support system built, the *placenta*, which takes over synthesizing estrogen and progesterone to support pregnancy.

Even after the placenta takes over, however, the corpus luteum continues producing progesterone to prevent further development of eggs in the ovary, and continues sending hormones out to the mother's body. If the egg isn't fertilized by a sperm the corpus luteum stops all hormone production, begins to shrivel, and dies. Both estradiol and progesterone fall abruptly. The whole process begins again. Another menstrual cycle is underway.

The brief cramps at mid-cycle are likely the result of irritation of the abdominal lining cause by leaking blood or follicular fluid from the rupturing egg follicle, and/or the contractions of the fallopian tube.

In the luteal phase, many of the typical PMS symptoms you experience are caused by the rise in progesterone that triggers metabolic changes to prepare for pregnancy.

As we get older and our follicles become depleted, egg production stops. We no longer have our ovarian "hormone factory" to produce enough estrogen and progesterone to support menstruation. The end of menstruation is called *menopause*.

Signals
The rise in estradiol also changes the cervical fluid, which functions much like seminal fluid does in men.

Period
It is the drop in progesterone that triggers shedding of the uterine lining to begin your menstrual bleeding.

Midcycle
"Twinges" or a dull achiness is probably caused by the swelling of the follicles in each ovary in the race to be the chosen one.

Ovaries

As a "female" organ, they have multiple responsibilities.

But the menstrual cycle is only part of the job description of the ovaries. Ovaries are the primary producers of sex steroids: progesterone, testosterone, and estrogens, especially the primary premenopausal active form, 17-beta estradiol.

Estrone is another estrogen also made by the ovary and body fat. It is less active than estradiol. It serves as our reservoir, or storage, form of estrogen, and is the only form of estrogen present in measurable amounts after menopause.

That's why overweight women are said to have "too much estrogen." They may actually be *low in estradiol* but have *excess estrone*. This can make a huge difference in your health risks.

Very small amounts of testosterone, other androgens, and progesterone are also made in the adrenal glands, and our body fat also makes androgens and significant amounts of estrone.

Steroids

An umbrella group of hormones that includes *sex hormones* made by our ovaries.

Your Ovary As Hormone Factory

Hormones are a major heading included under a bigger umbrella called steroids. The basic chemical structure is four rings of carbon atoms. There are literally thousands of varieties of steroids and steroid-like hormones throughout nature, and they all have the cholesterol molecule as their basic building block.

Cholesterol serves as a building block for many hormones, including all the estrogens, progesterone and testosterone, as well as vitamin D.

Needed Fat

If you eat too little fat, you can't make cholesterol, or your ovarian hormones.

The body can make its own cholesterol from the fat in our diet, provided you eat the right amount of fat. If you eat too much fat, this will shift the hormone balance toward more estrone, the remaining form of estrogen after menopause, as well as male hormones that interfere with the normal production of your biologically active premenopausal estrogen, estradiol.

The function of a hormone is to circulate in body fluids (primarily in the bloodstream) and arouse or urge targeted body tissues to do, or not do, that which they are supposed to. Hormones are messengers, *chemical communicators* carrying messages to and from all organs of the body. They serve to connect one organ's function with others. We would die if we did not have this signaling system to keep our organs functioning in a balanced, integrated, and coordinated manner.

also see p. 386 to interpret labs

Dr. Vliet's Guide to the Menstrual Cycle Hormone Rhythm

Brain Hormone Levels

LH

FSH

Ovary Hormone Levels

350-500 pg/ml

PROGESTERONE
5-25 ng/ml

ESTROGEN
(ESTRADIOL)

ESTRADIOL
200-250 pg/ml

80-90 pg/ml

PROGESTERONE
0.3-0.9 ng/ml

Ovary

Follicular Phase

Ovary

Luteal Phase

Follicle ⟶ Egg

Corpus Luteum

Uterus

Endometrium thickening

OVULATION

Bleeding

Endometrium growing

Menstrual Phase | Proliferatory Phase | Secretory Phase

© Elizabeth Lee Vliet, MD and Gordon C. Vliet 1995, revised 2001–2007

Day 1   Day 4   Day 14   Day 21?   Day 28

History

The word hormone was coined in 1905, from a Greek word meaning to excite or to arouse.

Castrati

In 17th and 18th Century Italy, castrated men were known as castrati. Their high-pitched, feminine voices and ability to hit the high soprano notes were greatly desired in opera houses before women singers were allowed.

Fact

Hormone receptors, in untold numbers, are found throughout the body.

In a woman the secretion and interaction of hormones throughout the body is an exceptionally complex process. Because of the intertwining of the glands of the endocrine system, if the ovaries aren't functioning properly *any and all* of the body's systems may be affected by losing these powerful messengers.

The power of hormones in the body was evident long before we understood so many of their specific actions. The ancients knew that castration removed something of maleness, even if they didn't know exactly what it was that was gone.

Eunuchs were men castrated to guard harems of kings and sultans in ancient times. The eunuchs no longer had their male sexual urges, so they were "safe" to guard the women.

The converse is also true: if other endocrine systems are malfunctioning, this causes suppression, or failure of the ovary's ability to produce hormones and develop eggs normally. This is another reason the "endocrine disrupting" chemicals are such a threat to our entire hormonal balance and function.

The chart following shows some of the many body changes with every menstrual cycle. Body functions change with the ebb and flow of our ovarian hormones every day of our cycle. These are *profound* relationships!

How Do Hormones Trigger Actions?

Hormones have "docking sites" we call *receptors* made of proteins and located either on the surface or inside the cells themselves, usually in the nucleus. Cells throughout the body are like little manufacturing plants, making chemicals the body needs to function. Hormones may act like "purchasing agents" in some instances, and or as "team facilitators" in others.

Hormone actions can be faster than the blink of an eye as when acting at receptors located on cell membranes, or they can promote action more slowly as when they act on cell nuclei to direct production of specific enzymes and proteins.

In any given cell, there may be thousands of receptors, in some many more. Perhaps that is why it doesn't take much to get a major response. There are two types of estrogen receptors, *alpha* and *beta*. Some tissues of the body have alpha, some have beta, and some have both types of receptors.

There can be a such a wide variety of symptoms when estradiol levels decline because so many different organs and tissues have these receptors designed to work properly *only when activated by estradiol.*

Our scientific understanding of women's hormones and their many receptors has expanded greatly. How is it that I "find" these connections when other physicians have not? I think part of the answer lies in one's mindset.

Most physicians still don't think through all the physiological hormone connections linking symptoms that appear to be separate, such as fatigue, headaches, moodiness, and loss of sex drive. Doctors still think each symptom has a **separate** cause and needs a **separate** evaluation, and a **separate** medication. The more medications used, the more likely there will be side effects and drug interactions that will complicate the picture.

Another mistaken, but common, mindset is that such a cluster of symptoms could "only" be linked with a diagnosis of depression.

In addition to the mindset of the physician, there is also the time it takes for new research to become incorporated into office-based clinical practice.

Hormone receptor research and the hormone effects on every organ system in the body are widely discussed in major medical journals today, it is new information that is not often filtering down and finding it's way into the practicing physician's office as quickly as we would like to think.

Research publications often have little information on *how* to put these new findings into practice, or give few practical guidelines on how these new findings affect women's body systems and produce the clinical problems women describe to their doctors. It takes creative thinking, sometimes "outside the box," to connect the dots between various research findings in a variety of specialty field with how the body works, patterns of symptoms, lab results, and what to *do* to solve clinical problems.

It takes time, patience, and give-and-take relationship with one's patients. Today's insurance-dictated 5-minute office visits for most doctors have undermined their ability to engage in creative thinking and the "art" of medicine. Doctors have been forced to focus simply on established protocols and standard approaches.

Estrogen Receptors:
- brain
- bladder
- bones
- muscles
- blood vessels
- skin
- breasts
- uterus
- eyes
- heart
- colon

Amazing
Estradiol is a powerful and very active hormone! It has many functions and complex interactions.

But WAIT!
A 2001 government survey found that it takes an average of *17 years* for new research to become commonly accepted in the average doctor's clinical practice.

Dr. Vliet's Guide to the
Body Changes Affected By The Menstrual Cycle

Body temperature	basal metabolism rate
blood glucose regulation, bladder/bowel function	estrogen levels in blood and urinary metabolites
breast size, texture, skin/nipple color	progesterone levels in blood and urinary metabolites
energy levels and sleep patterns	levels of brain hormones and neurotransmitters
neurotransmitter production	bile pigments (to digest fat)
thyroid and adrenal hormone production	blood levels of adrenalin
red and white blood cell counts	body weight
fluid balance	GSR (galvanic skin resistance)
Skin color, texture, permeability	pulmonary (lung) vital capacity
respiration functions: CO2 O2	blood protein levels and amounts
blood pH	vaginal mucus characteristics
memory and concentration	vaginal cytology (cell types)
citric acid (Vitamin C) content of mucus	visual , auditory, olfactory acuity
brain wave (EEG) patterns	serum bicarbonate
heart rate and rhythm	pain threshold
balance, fine motor coordination	feeling state and behavior
ESR ("sed rate") measure of Inflammation	Concentrations of vitamins A, C, E, and B group
pupil size and reactivity	cervix changes: size, color, position
platelet counts	urine volume, pH, specific gravity

©Elizabeth Lee Vliet MD 1995, revised 2001–2007

Migraine headaches? Take Imitrex. Insomnia? Take Ambien. Depressed mood? Take Prozac. PMS? Take Zoloft.

A hormone connection between all of these? "It's too expensive to check hormone levels." So doctors don't do it. As a result, they miss the fact that all of these seemingly different problems could be caused by low estradiol.

Over the years of working with women, I found these connections because I *looked for them* and *checked hormone levels.*

Time after time, I found that if I restored the estradiol to more optimal ranges, my patients would come back and tell me that they no longer had trouble sleeping and had stopped sleeping pills, or their mood was so much better, they no longer needed the antidepressant.

There are other ways our new understanding of hormone receptor action and specificity determines medical approaches for individual women. I use the analogy of hormone being "keys" that fit into their special receptor like a "lock," switching that receptor "on" or "off." In reality, it is much more complicated, but this visual image is still helpful in understanding why the right molecular key is important. If the molecular "key" is not exactly right, it may fit in the lock but not turn, so it can't "open" the action of that cell or pathway.

For example, when we replace estrogen when a young woman has her ovaries removed, it becomes important *what* type of molecular makeup the substitute estrogen has. *17-beta estradiol* is the naturally-occurring, human, primary estrogen made by the ovary before menopause.

If a young woman has her ovaries removed before menopause, she would likely want to replace what was lost and just use just 17-beta estradiol. Make sense?

Do you want an exact duplicate molecule of what your body used to make, or would you settle for a mixture that gives you many more, and many different molecules…some of which your body has never made and doesn't quite know how to use?

This second option has been offered to most women in this country in the form of Premarin for the last 50 years, even though it may not have been the best choice for optimal energy and well being.

In common
I try to find a unifying explanation, rather than separate causes and multiple diagnoses.

"Creative" thinking
That is what we call the "art" of medicine.

Discovery
Science has shown that the docking of a hormone at its receptor is greatly affected by having just the right molecule size and shape.

Square pegs

Differently shaped molecules may actually block or interfere with proper hormone action. It's like a square peg trying to fit into a round hole.

Horse urine?

Small changes in the molecule can make a big difference in the way a particular estrogen works in your body, and especially, in your brain.

Natural?

Women taking Premarin say they feel different, and not "back to my normal self."

Premarin is a group of horse estrogens and not an exact molecular copy of the hormones your body used to make. It is derived from **preg**nant **mar**e's ur**ine** and contains mostly horse estrogens (*equilin estrogens*).

Equilin estrogens are actually many compounds that are foreign to our bodies and have various chemical additions on their molecules that make them very different from own 17-beta estradiol. The equilin estrogens don't fit the body's receptor sites exactly the same way. Their effects can be very different.

This is one reason that women taking Premarin often say their memory isn't as good, or they don't sleep as well, or they gain weight or they don't have their usual energy.

This same concept will be important as we look at ways the molecules of endocrine disrupting environmental chemicals can mimic, block, or intensify hormone actions in your body.

There are other important differences from our own natural 17-beta estradiol. Equilin estrogens attach very strongly to the estrogen receptors and can block or interfere with the attachment and action of our own body's estradiol.

This is especially true in the breast, where the equilin estrogens are very strongly attached to the receptors and build up over time the longer you take Premarin.

It also takes much longer for the body to metabolize the equilin estrogens because our body doesn't have the enzymes necessary to break them down. This means they last a lot longer in the body than our estradiol does.

The mixture of equilin estrogens in Premarin provides a high level of total estrogens, but does not provide enough of the human 17-beta estradiol that most women need to feel their best.

Typically, with a standard dose of Premarin, even though the overall horse estrogen levels are so high, the *critical 17-beta estradiol levels* may only get to the 30–50 pg/ml range.

This is a long ways away from the 100 to 200 pg/ml range typical circulating estradiol over a healthy menstrual cycle. Estradiol patches or pills easily provide levels of 100–200 pg/ml to restore what has been lost.

Hormone Power: Incredible Potency from Your Ovaries

These are powerful hormones: Many hormones are measured in as little as a billionth of a gram, called a nanogram. Estradiol, for example, is measured in picograms, or one *trillionth* of a gram.

In her beautifully written book, *Woman: An Intimate Geography*, Natalie Angier paints this amazing visual image: to get *one teaspoonful of estradiol* you would need to drain *all* the blood from the bodies of 250,000 premenopausal women. Each of those bodies also contains approximately a teaspoonful of sugar and two tablespoons of salt. To get a teaspoonful of estrogen you'd have to deal with a hill of sugar and a mountain of salt. And they try to tell us testosterone is the "power" hormone!

We think of estrogen as the quintessential female hormone, but "it" is really 50 or more different types of compounds, some more potent than others. Our primary human estrogens are *estrone* (E1), *estradiol* (E2) made by the ovary and body fat, and *estriol* (E3) manufactured by the placenta during pregnancy. A newly-discovered estrogen, *estetrol* (E4), is made only by the fetus during pregnancy.

Many of the other estrogenic compounds in that 50+ group come from metabolism of our three major estrogens as they are broken down into a variety of compounds. Some are inactive, and others are still hormonally very active.

It can get quite involved, so I decided it would be much more practical to focus on E1, E2, and E3. They differ in their (1) chemical makeup, (2) when they play a role in a women's life, (3) the primary site where they are synthesized, and (4) what they do in our bodies.

Estrone (E1): Estrone was the first human estrogen identified in 1929 when scientists were doing a random search of pregnant women's urine looking for the hormones of pregnancy.

It is made in the ovary, body fat and liver; it is called E1 because it has only one (1) oxygen-hydrogen group attached (estradiol has two (2), estriol has three (3).

Estrone is important to us as a reservoir source of estrogen. It is known as the *postmenopausal* estrogen because it can be made from and stored in body fat with the help of an enzyme called *aromatase*.

Shocking! If you take Premarin and then stop, it may take 2–3 months for all the horse estrogens to be cleared from your body.

However— If you use 17-beta estradiol and stop, your body's metabolism clears it away in only a day or so.

Estrone

A major reason women's bodies look so different, and have different health risks, after menopause: estrone does not have the same effects that estradiol does.

Aromatase converts androgens (DHEA, testosterone, and androstenedione) to estrone, and then to estradiol. Estrone plays a role, along with androgens, in the change in our body shape from pear to apple. It is the only remaining source of estrogen after menopause if women are not taking estrogen therapy.

While estrone provides at least some estrogen effect, it doesn't have exactly the same actions and benefits we see before menopause with estradiol.

Estradiol (E2): Is our primary and most active estrogen from puberty to menopause. Estradiol is made primarily in the ovary, via the *aromatase* pathway, so when we run out of our follicles or our ovaries are removed, we no longer have a way to make adequate amounts of estradiol.

The body makes smaller amounts of estradiol in other areas of the body via the same aromatase enzyme pathway I described above, and it uses estradiol nearly everywhere.

Estradiol

affects over 400 functions in our body and receptors are located in virtually every organ of the body.

For example, research has shown that our bones make small amounts of estradiol critical for a healthy, strong skeleton. Our blood vessels make and use estradiol, the brain makes and uses estradiol, and even muscle tissue also makes both estrone and estradiol by the aromatase pathway. Women who are physically active and have more muscle mass often have better estradiol levels than less active women with less muscle mass. Clearly, there are many ways the body makes and uses estradiol to keep all our systems humming along efficiently.

Earlier, I described the levels of estradiol that correspond with feeling your best. In pregnancy, both progesterone and estradiol levels rise rapidly in the first trimester. Then progesterone decreases sharply at the sixth to eighth week, while estradiol continues to rise and remain high throughout pregnancy. Progesterone does not rise again until about the 34th week of gestation just in time to prepare the body for delivery. Estradiol is rising from early pregnancy until the very end, peaking in the range of about 20,000 pg/ml for the last few weeks before delivery.

Estriol

Estriol does not appear to play a significant role at times other than pregnancy.

If you have been pregnant, think about how you felt the last six weeks compared to the beginning and middle months. When did you feel your best? That will give you a clue as to which hormone affects you with the most positive feelings, physically and emotionally.

If you pay attention to the changes in how you feel based during your cycle, you can again see some of the physical and psychological differences between estrogen and progesterone.

Estriol (E3): Is a much weaker form of estrogen made by the placenta during pregnancy. E3 receptors are primarily concentrated in the vagina, hair follicles, and skin, and may help to account for the skin and hair "glow" that women often notice during pregnancy.

Hundreds of studies over the last fifty years have found that estriol has very little estrogenic action at bone, brain, heart, and other critical sites where estradiol plays crucial roles and has multiple actions. Estriol does not "protect" against breast cancer, contrary to a popular myth.

The balance of estrogen shifts from about 1:1 estradiol to estrone *before* menopause to far more estrone present after menopause. The ovaries no longer make estradiol, and our body fat is now making more estrone.

After menopause, women have a greater than 1 to 1 estrone to estradiol ratio, unless they are *taking* estradiol. The more overweight a woman is, the higher this ratio of estrone becomes, because another interesting aspect is that, as we get older, aromatase becomes more efficient in making estrone from conversion of androstenedione in fat tissue.

Women with PCOS or Syndrome X, due to excess body fat, will have an even greater estrone dominance long before menopause.

 In case you wondered, men make estrone in their fat tissue by the same aromatase pathway as in women. This is why as men get older, they have less of the active testosterone: they have higher estrone as they gain body fat.

Progesterone

Progesterone is another major ovarian hormone. The name means pregnancy-promoting, or *"pro-gestation"* hormone. It was first identified in the 1920s, in the yellow-bodied corpus luteum of the ovary by researchers seeking to identify the hormones made by the ovary.

More and more
The more body fat women have the more aromatase, and the more estrone is made.

Vital
This is important because higher estrone levels are a risk factor for high blood pressure, diabetes, endometrial and breast cancers in women.

How?

Progesterone is made primarily after ovulation by the corpus luteum, from the "building block" molecule cholesterol.

Mother Nature

You have to eat more if you are going to be pregnant. So progesterone makes you hungry!

Slowed down

Progesterone and its metabolites have a tranquilizing effect on the brain, much like our current antianxiety medications.

Until ovulation, progesterone blood levels are typically less than 1 ng/ml. After ovulation, progesterone rises to about 8–25 ng/ml by the peak, about day 20 of your cycle.

If there is no ovulation, there is no corpus luteum to make progesterone, so there is no rise in progesterone. That is the reason *you may not have typical PMS symptoms if you don't ovulate.*

The rise in progesterone in the second half of your cycle prepares for metabolic changes the body will need to support a pregnancy: *increased appetite, increased thirst, breast engorgement and more rapid proliferation of the breast cells, suppression of the immune system, and many other effects.*

Progesterone also triggers insulin to shift toward more fat storage for the fuel needs of a growing baby. The progesterone effects on the insulin-glucose pathways trigger more "blood sugar swings" and reactive hypoglycemia in the luteal phase. This is why you have more sweet cravings in your premenstrual week.

Researchers at Tufts University found a 12 percent increase in appetite and metabolic rate in the high progesterone phase of the cycle. You are not imagining it—you really are hungrier then.

Progesterone also relaxes the smooth muscles of the intestinal tract, so that the waves of contractions (*peristalsis*) are decreased. This slows the movement of food through the GI tract. The metabolic effect is that the digestive system has more time to work on breaking down foods and is able to absorb maximum nutrient value for mother and baby.

The low fiber content of our typical American diet, on average about 10 grams of fiber daily, rather than the 30 grams we need, makes the progesterone effects of premenstrual bloating and constipation even worse.

We feel sluggish and fat. Other common complaints when progesterone is high, are feeling headachy, lethargic, depressed, irritable...and having no sex drive! These same feelings can occur in your own cycle, or when you take high amounts of progestins in birth control pills or HRT or progesterone in hormone therapy after menopause.

For some women, progesterone feels like a sedative and they don't like the groggy feeling. For other women, the "slowing down" effect of progesterone feels "wonderful," "soothing," "relaxed," or "more centered."

Other women on progesterone have a full-blown "depression," severe fatigue, or lethargy. They say, "I don't have any get up and go." "I withdraw." "I can't get out of bed." "I don't have any energy."

You can see how a hormone that calms and tranquilizes might be an evolutionary advantage in the early stages of pregnancy. Being calmer at the time the egg is implanted, helps to prevent it from being jostled out of the uterus. This facilitates early development of the embryo.

However, If not pregnant many women don't like feeling sedated and slowed down.

There is much misleading information claiming progesterone is the "mother" hormone because it comes at the beginning of a chemical pathway, and is the one from which all of the other hormones, including testosterone and estradiol, are made by the body.

This is a sales pitch urging you to buy progesterone creams to treat PMS and other problems. Many women's health books do not accurately portray what is going on in your body, or where and when these reactions take place.

First of all, most of the conversion of progesterone to the end products of testosterone and estradiol *require the presence of enzymes in fully functioning ovaries.*

Problem If your ovaries aren't functioning normally, or if you have reached menopause, then you are not able to convert a load of progesterone into estradiol and testosterone.

If you had a hysterectomy with the ovaries removed, it is obvious you no longer have these ovarian "converting" enzymes.

If you are menopausal, the ovaries don't convert progesterone to other hormones, so you end up getting much more progesterone than you need, and not enough of the others. This leads to all kinds of adverse effects on metabolism, brain and immune function, to name a few. You can't assume that simply loading up on one building block at the beginning of the process will end up making all the same molecules the body makes when your ovaries are working optimally.

This metaphor may help to explain: Think about the many stages of growth and development that have to occur for a baby to become a child, then an adolescent, and then an adult.

Think of progesterone as the "baby" in our hormone development process. It can't carry out all the functions of the "adult" hormones, estradiol and testosterone, until it has been shaped and altered by the changes of this *entire* series of chemical reactions.

Bottom line
Progesterone will not replace the symptoms and problems accompanying declining estradiol or testosterone levels. Period.

Warning
Our bodies, do not have the enzymes needed to change the plant building blocks into the same molecules our bodies make. Eating lots of soy or yams will not supply your body with the identical molecules of hormones you need.

Absolutely
Just as men require estrogen in their system to function, women also require testosterone.

Progesterone can't be made into testosterone or estradiol directly; it *has* to undergo further changes to become the building blocks for testosterone and then estradiol.

This is just like our life process: we can't fully function as an adult until we have gone through the life stages (infancy, childhood, adolescence) that shape and equip us to be an adult.

Without our ovaries to facilitate this "development" of the "baby" progesterone into "adult" testosterone and estradiol, we are stuck with a molecule that doesn't have the specific shape to activate the receptors for normal function. Each of these molecules acts like a different "key" in various receptor "locks" throughout the body, so the proper shape to the molecule key is crucial to create the desired effects in various parts and organs of our body.

Scientists have discovered ways to make various estrogens and testosterone, as well as the synthetic progestins, in the laboratory, from plant compounds.

Today, all of the pharmaceutical grade estradiol, testosterone, and progesterone come from precursor molecules in wild yams and soy that are then chemically converted in the laboratory to make bioidentical hormones.

One of the major problems in finding a way to prescribe "natural" progesterone is that when taken orally it is quickly deactivated by stomach acid. A process called *micronization*, developed in the 1960s, made these large hormone molecules tiny enough to be absorbed before being broken down by stomach acid. But, by the time the technology had solved the problem, physicians had become accustomed to using Provera, which was cheaper and also reliable.

Micronized progesterone was widely used in Europe, but not much in this country, except by compounding pharmacies for PMS and other special needs. It was not until Prometrium and Crinone, and later Prochieve, were FDA approved in 1998 that there was wider acceptance of the micronized progesterone over the synthetic progestins like Provera.

Testosterone

The third primary hormone of the ovaries is what is popularly referred to as the *"male hormone," testosterone*. This hormone is part of a larger group of hormones called *androgens* that bind at androgen receptors throughout the brain and body.

Dr. Vliet's Guide to Progesterone and Progestins

Progestogen is a general term that describes any chemical substance that has the metabolic effects in the body to *sustain a pregnancy* and *activate the progesterone receptor*. There are number of types that fall into this category:

Progesterone is a biologically natural pregnancy-sustaining hormone (progestogen), produced by many species. In women, progesterone is made by the corpus luteum after ovulation, although a very small amount is also produced by the adrenal gland, and by the ovary. It's primary role is to stimulate the metabolic, functional and structural changes needed for a woman's body to adapt to, and sustain, a pregnancy as well as undergo delivery.

Progestins are man-made chemicals that are more potent than progesterone because of a different chemical structure. Some actions are similar to progesterone, and some are different actions. Progestins may be ***derived from progesterone***, called *progestational* progestins, such as Provera; or they may be **derived from testosterone**, called *androgenic* progestins, such as norethindrone (common brands are Aygestin, Nor-QD or Micronor). Progestins in the Provera group are more likely than testosterone-based progestins to cause depression, weight gain, headaches, and low libido. Progestins have many important medical uses, such as contraception or suppression of endometriosis and fibroids. The lower potency of progesterone cannot do these functions as reliably.

Progesterone USP is a chemical molecule made in the laboratory to be *identical* in all respects to the natural hormone make by the ovary. It begins as building blocks found in soybeans and wild yams, then is purified, and processed through a series of chemical changes that require enzymes we don't have in our bodies. It has been available in injectable form since the 1940's, and is now available as a tablet (**Prometrium**), or a vaginal gel (**Prochieve**). Progesterone USP is also used by compounding pharmacists to make individualized prescriptions in many forms, including tablets, suppositories, and creams. Because it is identical to the natural molecule, many women find that it has fewer unpleasant side effects than progestins such as Provera. Some women, however, feel terrible on natural progesterone and prefer the synthetic progestins.

© 2001–2007 Elizabeth Lee Vliet, M.D.

Fact
During our years from puberty to menopause women have higher testosterone than estradiol!

Balance is key
You need to have the right balance of estradiol with your testosterone to see all the positives and not so many negatives.

A Shock!
Hysterectomy and removal of the ovaries before the age of natural menopause causes a rapid drop in testosterone and estradiol.

All androgens are made also from cholesterol by the female ovary, the male testes, and some by the adrenal glands. They are also made in limited quantity by body-fat tissue, muscle, the liver, skin, and brain, using precursor molecules made in the ovaries and adrenals.

Men's optimal testosterone levels are about 600–1000 ng/dl, or even more, while an optimal testosterone range for women is 40–60 ng/dl (the units we usually use).

For an interesting and surprising comparison, however, 40–60 ng/dl would actually be 400–600 pg/ml if we use the same units as we use for estradiol. For the rest of the book, I will stick with the conventional units ng/dl used in the U.S.

Testosterone has many benefits. It helps you keep and build your muscle mass, which burns more calories than fat tissue. It helps you build bone and prevent osteoporosis.

Women lose approximately 50% of their testosterone production by the time their ovaries decline at menopause, and the adrenal glands have also begun to reduce their testosterone and DHEA output. I don't know of many men who would like a 50% reduction of their testosterone.

Testosterone activates the brain's sexual circuits in both men and women. Just as it is hard to light a campfire using wet matches, it is hard to arouse the sexual circuits in the brain without the metabolic fuel they need in testosterone.

Your sexuality is an important dimension of your life, and many of my patients ask, 'How do I get my libido back?' If your doctor suggests seeing a sex therapist, have your hormone levels tested first! You need your hormones functioning properly before psychological and relationship therapies can be effective.

Other causes of ovarian damage can also lead to loss of testosterone, although not as abruptly as the loss that occurs when the ovaries are removed surgically. Even if your ovaries were not removed, you still have a decrease in your hormone levels within just a few years after hysterectomy. This decline doesn't "wait" until you reach that magic age of natural menopause, as doctors have mistakenly thought. I explain how this occurs in Chapter 8.

If you take oral estrogen after a hysterectomy, the amount of free active testosterone falls even further because of the increase in SHBG. Then many women lose interest in sex, and have lower energy levels. It is not due to depression, or the effects of the surgery. *It is the loss of your key hormones.* You may not need an anti-depressant, as doctors commonly recommend. Anti-depressants also further reduce your sex drive.

Taking DHEA supplements won't help increase your testosterone, since it is in the ovary where most of the enzymes and pathways exist to convert it to testosterone or estradiol.

When the ratio of estradiol to testosterone falls during perimenopause, the usual androgen effects are unmasked: *facial hair, thinning scalp hair, deepening voice, the male pattern of middle body fat distribution.*

There are even more adverse body changes: increase in blood pressure and total cholesterol, decrease in HDL ("good") cholesterol and increase in LDL ("bad") cholesterol. Up go your risks of heart disease, hypertension and diabetes.

The Hormone Cycle of Your Breasts

One of the often overlooked aspects of the menstrual cycle is the way hormonal fluctuations cause many changes in the breast. Some are visible and you feel them, others are microscopic, so you are not aware of the changes. There are estrogen receptors in the tissue of the breast that respond to rising hormone levels to stimulate both growth of the ducts and the breast connective tissue.

Most women notice that their breasts change each month during their cycle. The significant difference comes in the luteal phase, when your breasts feel larger and full or swollen. The rise in progesterone at this time of the cycle causes increased fluid retention, as well as more growth, or proliferation, of the breast lobular tissue, in preparation for a possible pregnancy.

These changes cause the breasts to increase in volume and become sensitive, or at times, even painful. These same changes also occur in the early stages of pregnancy, when the progesterone and estrogen levels also rise rapidly.

Estradiol in the first half of the menstrual cycle causes growth of breast cells, but the rise in progesterone in the second half of the menstrual cycle triggers *even more rapid and greater proliferation* of the breast than estradiol does.

Power failure! Without optimal testosterone, you lose sex drive, energy, and muscle strength.

Dragging... You may feel depressed, have achy joints, or an overall loss of your sense of well being.

Essential The right balance of estradiol and testosterone is a key to feeling your best.

This is one reason that you now hear more concern about increased risk in breast cancer when *combination* hormones are given. Doctors and health writers seem to only focus on "estrogen," overlooking the physiology of progesterone and its negative effects on the breasts, as well as other body systems.

There are also a number of women who experience more intense breast pain, called *mastalgia*, which can vary from discomfort to a debilitating level. The best research points to an imbalance in the ratio of progesterone to estradiol, and/or an excess of prolactin, a pituitary hormone that stimulates lactation.

Studies also show that breast pain changes in a pattern that follows hormonal changes in your life, by age, by stress level, and for some women by diet. We know that much of this goes away with menopause, when hormone levels fall significantly.

I often explain to women on Hormone Therapy (HT) that they can tell when their estrogen or progesterone levels are too high, because their breasts will become too tender as a result of excess amounts of *either* hormone.

If you have any concerns about breast pain and a possible relationship to other problems, you should consult your physician. If the pain is in one breast only, or non-cyclical, I also recommend you have this checked.

In menopause the loss of estradiol results in a decrease in breast tissue, and an increase in the fat cells. The breasts become less dense because of the increase in fat, and they are softer and flatter. For women on HT, breasts are denser and fuller.

Hormone Cycles and Your Body

There are many ways that the hormonal changes of your menstrual cycle may contribute to symptoms and changes in your health.

For example, falling estradiol can trigger migraine headaches, regardless of your age. Falling estradiol at your period's start can cause a spasm of the arteries that serve the heart, called *coronary vasospasm*. Falling estradiol can cause major mood swings. Women are uninformed about these hormonal connections,.

One patient, *Linda*, age 23, had a history of three serious, and nearly fatal suicide attempts, each time at the onset of her menstrual period. Although various physicians and psychiatrists had evaluated her, no one had ever asked where she was in her cycle when these self-destructive feelings hit her.

No one had thought to do simple blood tests at the key times of her menstrual cycle to see if her hormone levels dropped precipitously when she had these difficulties.

During her last hospitalization, physicians told Linda's parents that she had permanent brain and liver damage from the drug overdoses and the loss of oxygen during the coma that followed. Her parents were devastated.

Clue #1
The biggest clue for the therapist and Linda, was the connection between the suicide attempts and the onset of her menstrual bleeding.

Finally, a *non-medical* therapist recognized the menstrual cycle connection, and recommended a consultation with me to see if this young woman's hormones were a factor.

When I evaluated her, I carefully went over her history of both the mood and physical symptoms. I checked her hormone levels, and found that she had a form of exercise-induced premature ovarian failure, a result of her strenuous training as a dancer and her constant dieting.

Several years later, she is alive and healthy on a steady hormone regimen to restore her ovarian hormones and provide stability from the terrible mood swings and suicidal "crashes" each month. She is no longer on antidepressants.

She has returned to the dancing she loves, and has achieved a healthy balance in her training schedule. She now understands what her rigorous training and inadequate nutrition did to her ovaries and is beginning to rebuild the bone she lost earlier.

Clue #2
She did not have such suicidal thoughts at any other time of her cycle.

Brain and liver damage? Based on current test results, these problems have been resolved. She says, "*My mind feels sharp and clear again. I have my energy back.*" She went on to graduate school and is now working full-time.

A Guide to Your Other Hormones

The brain and body are interconnected by an incredible array of chemical and electrical circuits, each one interacting with and affecting others. The brain has a multitude of ways to direct the orchestra of the body. In women's bodies, the entire process is even more complex, with the menstrual cycle changes causing brain-body systems to continuously adapt to the internal and external environments.

Men have it "easy"
Their bodies have a steady production of testosterone 24/7, women don't.

While men have a fairly steady production (*tonic* pattern) of testosterone all month, women's brain and body are designed to work with our *cyclic* pattern of ovarian hormone rise and fall.

Since we will be talking throughout this book about other hormone systems, and their interactions with the ovaries, the following table lists our other hormones and their key roles.

In Summary

Our wondrous, at times infuriating, hormonal ebb and flow occurs every month and has widespread effects on brain-body processes and on our psyche.

Perfect Design
From an evolutionary standpoint these hormonal actions make sense, for the tasks they govern in our body, and for sustaining our survival as a species.

Every cell participates in the flow of our menstrual rhythm. Cyclic changes occur in almost all body functions as the levels of female hormones rise and fall. All of these physiological changes then affect how we respond to the external world and the impact of external stresses on our brain-body pathways.

Science is discovering at an amazing rate how these hormonal shifts interact with the endocrine, immune, metabolic, cardio-vascular, respiratory, musculoskeletal, reproductive, urinary, and nervous systems.

The specific effects and roles of each of the primary female hormones show how beautifully orchestrated the female endocrine system is for creating and sustaining new life.

We are not at the mercy of our hormones. If we understand what is happening, we can learn to "go with the flow," in positive ways, rather than making things worse with uninformed or misinformed lifestyle choices. I want us to better understand women's physiological changes, and *not confuse the physiological with the psychological*, so that we can effectively manage our complicated lives in a body that is more complex than a man's.

No limits!
Our hormonal cycles are *not* limits for what we can do with our lives.

What limits us is that most doctors don't fully use the available medical research on hormonal cycles to address our unique health needs. It is often easier to prescribe an antidepressant than to measure and interpret women's hormone levels, and then design an individualized treatment approach. And drug companies spend billions of dollars on ads convincing doctors and consumers that we need a different pill for every symptom.

Let's continue the journey to discover more about your marvelous ovarian hormones!

Dr. Vliet's Guide: A Look at Key Hormones And What They Do

Primary Actions

I. Steroids

- **Cortisol**—many metabolic actions, especially to store more body fat; produced in higher amounts under stress and suppresses normal immune function due to anti-inflammatory actions;

- **Aldosterone**—regulates fluid balance by stimulating kidney to retain sodium and water and excrete potassium; contributes to excess *water* weight gain when progesterone levels are high in second half of menstrual cycle and stimulate more aldosterone secretion.

- **Androgens** (DHEA, others)—enhances sex drive, produces male features in women (e.g. facial hair, male body shape), stimulates appetite, contributes to middle body, and waistline fat gain when levels too high

- **Estrogens** (three)—female secondary sex characteristics; key role in menstruation, pregnancy, over 400 other crucial functions throughout the body and brain, including increased metabolic rate, improved insulin sensitivity and carbohydrate tolerance, role in body temperature regulation

- **Progesterone**—helps maintain pregnancy, many metabolic effects including increased appetite, increased fat storage, and reduced sensitivity to insulin; high levels give sedative, analgesic effects at brain; may produce depressed mood, decreased libido

- **Testosterone**—produces male secondary sex patterns; triggers sex drive and arousal in both males and females, many metabolic effects (bone and muscle growth, increased metabolic rate, etc.), also enhances mood and energy level.

II. Amines

- **Thyroid hormones: Thyroxine (T4), Triiodothyronine (T3)**—stimulate body metabolism by increasing cell energy release; increasing heart rate, heat production, and brain activity. Helps maintain normal regulation of metabolic pathways, normal growth and function of nervous, musculoskeletal systems

- **"Adrenaline" hormones: Norepinephrine (NE) and Epinephrine**—"fight or flight" (stress) hormones, prepare body for emergencies by increasing heart rate; act on brain to lift mood (or in excess, cause anxiety) increase alertness; dilate arteries to key organs to provide more oxygen, glucose, and nutrients

Dr. Vliet's Guide: A Look at Key Hormones And What They Do

III. Peptides And Proteins

- **Insulin**—lowers blood sugar (moves glucose into cells to be used for fuel in muscle or stored in fat cells), stimulates fat storage and protein synthesis
- **Glucagon**—raises blood glucose (glycogen breakdown and glucose release from liver, gluconeogenesis)
- **Somatostatin**—mild effect to raise blood glucose
- **Parathyroid (PTH)**—major role: increase blood calcium levels by   stimulating bone breakdown, calcium release
- **Calcitonin**—involved in regulating blood calcium levels by inhibiting bone breakdown, calcium release
- **Thymosin** (thymus gland)—major role in development of immune system
- **ACTH**—Adrenocorticotropin Hormone; stimulates part of the adrenal gland to make cortisol
- **FSH**—stimulates ovaries, activates and promotes follicle growth to produce estrogen
- **LH**— triggers ovulation, formation of the corpus luteum, secretion of progesterone, estrogen
- **Growth Hormone (GH)**—oversees entire process of normal body growth; stimulates formation of more muscle and less body fat; declines during menopause with loss of estradiol; improved with estrogen therapy.
- **TSH**—stimulates the thyroid gland to release T3, T4; TSH will be *high* in low, or *hypo*thyroid conditions, and *low* in *hyper*thyroid conditions
- **Prolactin**—stimulates breast enlargement during pregnancy and regulates milk production after delivery; increases appetite and body fat to support nursing; often elevated in PCOS.
- **Anti-Diuretic Hormone (ADH)**—prevents dehydration by stimulating kidneys to increase resorption and retain water
- **Oxytocin**—stimulates uterine contractions during labor, helps trigger milk release after delivery.
- **Melatonin** (pineal gland)—regulation of sleep cycles, body rhythms; promotes fat storage by increasing appetite, especially for carbohydrate foods (example: to prepare for winter hibernation); plays a role in winter depression (SADS) syndromes that are characterized by low energy, weight gain, daytime sleepiness, depressed mood.

Chapter 3
Your Ovaries and Their Life Cycle

Our ovaries travel a remarkable journey from gestation to the waning days of our lives. There are a number of important stages during their life cycle. The dietary excitotoxins and chemical endocrine disruptors (See Chapters 4 and 5) can act at *any* of these stages to damage our ovaries and our overall health.

Illness, lifestyle habits, and surgical interventions can also have a critical impact. Knowing what is happening at each stage will help you to understand how the "disruptors" decrease your hormones, and what you can do to avoid problems.

Before Puberty

By puberty you will probably have about 300,000 follicles or so left to start your periods. A number of follicles are "recruited" each cycle, of which one or two are used. The other follicles die, leading to a decrease in follicles with every menstrual cycle. Today, more women are delaying children until their thirties and forties, and having fewer children and more menstrual cycles. By forty, the average woman has only 5,000 to 10,000 follicles remaining.

Many factors, such as illness, environment, and stress also contribute to the loss of follicles. If you are not trying to get pregnant, what is the problem with losing follicles?

Follicles and maturing eggs produce estradiol, the most active form of estrogen. As you lose follicles, estradiol levels decline erratically, causing disruptions and problems throughout your body.

Rule #1

You are born with all the eggs/ follicles you will ever make.

Declining estradiol brings on many of the classical symptoms of menopause. Usually, menopause is only associated with *older* women. That's why younger women experiencing these problems are often undiagnosed.

Too young?
No. Menopausal symptoms can occur in younger women, if follicles are damaged or prematurely lose the ability to produce adequate amounts of estradiol.

Think about your body now and the changes you have experienced. These are your clues for checking hormone levels. The good news is that there are simple blood hormone tests to measure and diagnose premature hormone decline.

Puberty: The Awakening of Our Ovaries

American girls generally enter puberty between age nine and fourteen. If puberty occurs earlier than this, it is called *premature (or precocious) puberty*.

The first stage of puberty is called **thelarche**, with the beginning of breast development.

This stage is followed by **adrenarche**, so called because it is triggered by the release of adrenal androgens, with the appearance of *pubic hair, axillary hair, oily skin, and acne.*

Menarche is the beginning of menstrual periods. The first menses usually occur when the breasts are more defined, typically around the age 11.5 to 13.

From 1850 to 1950, the average age of menarche decreased approximately 3 months every decade, due to better nutrition. The average age of 12.8 years held fairly steady until the 1990s, when we began seeing girls develop breasts and menstruating at much younger ages.

Onset of menses
The average time span from the first stage of puberty to the first menses runs about four years.

Menstrual onset also varies due to race, diet, weight, percentage of body fat, light exposure, and the presence of certain diseases. There is also a genetic clock that sets in motion the chain of events.

African-American and Hispanic girls tend to start menstruating earlier than Caucasians. Girls with diabetes tend to have a delayed menarche. Blind girls, who do not have significant light stimulation of brain centers, tend to have an earlier menarche than girls with normal vision.

Puberty is triggered by a series of hormone reactions. It starts with the hypothalamus increasing secretions that cause the pituitary gland to release increased amounts of *gonadotrophins* into the bloodstream.

Gonadotrophins are hormones that stimulate activity in the gonads (ovaries in females, testes in males). This causes the ovaries to produce elevated levels of estradiol, which leads to visible signs of maturing, such as developing breasts, pubic hair, underarm hair, and often a change in the timbre of the voice.

These secondary sex characteristics are typically followed by a growth spurt. Such changes usually occur two years earlier in girls than boys and are why girls at this age are often taller.

Internal changes are also occurring due to the influence of pubescent hormones. The walls of the vagina become thicker, and the uterus becomes larger and more muscular. The pH of the vagina also changes from alkaline to acidic due to estrogen effects and to the increase in vaginal and cervical secretions.

Early in puberty, menstrual flow is usually very light, and comes with little warning. Periods may be irregular at first but *usually become regular within the first two years*. The ability to conceive and bear children (fertility) occurs when ovulation begins.

It is difficult for many adolescent girls to know when they are fertile since both ovulation and the menstrual cycle can be erratic. This is one reason (among many) for accidental pregnancies, so it is important to always use some form of contraception if you are sexually active.

You can even get pregnant, although it is less likely, if you have sexual intercourse on the bleeding days of your cycle or have missed periods due to stress, illness, eating habits, or intensive athletic training.

Most of the physical changes occur during the early years of puberty. Prior to puberty, the body's growth focuses on becoming taller and stronger. With puberty, the hormone changes in women and men prepare the body to reproduce. These physical changes are a portion of the complex process of growing up. Behavioral changes and social expectations dramatically change throughout adolescence.

Adolescence is a time for psychological and psychosocial growth, when social adjustment and maturation are added to our physical changes. These emotional and social transitions

Findings
Recent research suggests it may be more the ratio of body fat to weight, rather than just weight.

Again
Thin girls tend to get their periods later than heavier girls.

Hormone "Roller Coaster"
Unpredictability leads to the "turbulent teens."

It's natural
Your menstrual cycle is a normal process of being a woman and there is no reason to curtail your normal activities during your period.

are less defined and less orderly than the physical ones. Thankfully, we eventually transition into a mature young adult.

It is helpful to pay attention to your monthly cycles and patterns of physical and emotional changes such as headaches, bloating, tiredness, changes in mood, body aches, food cravings, acne or minor breakouts, cramps, tender breasts, constipation, cold sores, and even nosebleeds.

Paying attention to your body signals and understanding your unique responses during your cycle will help you recognize changes triggered by hormone shifts.

Keeping a menstrual response calendar can be helpful in understanding your patterns, which in turn will help you head off more severe symptoms.

It is important to have regular exams after periods have begun. A pediatrician or primary care physician will probably do these during the adolescent years.

Too fast, too soon
We have a whole generation of girls who are hormonally accelerated.

If you become sexually active, it is especially important to have a pelvic exam and begin annual Pap tests and get tested for STDs. This may be the time to establish care with a gynecologist.

Take your menstrual tracking records, or a calendar if you have one, to your doctor. This is an important component of your medical record, and your doctor should appreciate this information.

I have described the more "typical" onset and stages of puberty. But what about girls who enter puberty far ahead of the average age? Why should we be concerned about early puberty? Why is it happening?

Shocking!
50% of African-American girls now reach puberty by *age 8*; another 15–20% have hit puberty by *age 7*.

Premature Puberty: Health Risks When Puberty Comes Too Soon

Look around at malls and schools and your community. More girls today are entering into puberty at younger ages. Girls only 5, 6, and 7 are developing breasts.

During the 1800s, girls on average began to menstruate at about age 17. By the mid-1990s, however, about 1 in 5 Caucasian girls *by age* 8 were showing breast buds and pubic hair, the beginning signs of puberty. ***This is a staggering change.***

Hispanic girls show patterns of early puberty closer to those of African–American girls. What future health problems lie ahead for girls who enter puberty so young?

Premature Puberty—A Myriad of Health Issues

Physical:

Researchers worldwide are looking at these important issues. Premature puberty also increases the likelihood of becoming sexually active at younger ages, with increased risk of sexually transmitted diseases and unplanned pregnancy. We see an ominous trend with girls 10–12 becoming pregnant and even younger girls with sexually transmitted diseases (STDs).

Dr. Dimartino-Nardi at Montefiore Medical Center in New York evaluated African–American and Caribbean–Hispanic girls with premature increases in adrenal androgens, and found that both ethnic groups were obese, had high insulin levels with insulin resistance, elevated androgens, and subtle decreases in their "good" cholesterol (HDL). Many of these girls also had a strong family history of type 2 diabetes mellitus.

Dr. Dimartino-Nardi found that girls with premature adrenarche who *remain* obese are at risk of developing Polycystic Ovary Syndrome (PCOS) as they go through puberty. They develop classic symptoms of PCOS related to the high androgens and insulin: irregular menses, excess facial and body hair, and severe acne. This sets up a lifetime of health problems. See Chapter 13.

Premature adrenarche and early puberty can be a risk factor for continued obesity for certain girls, and an early stage in the progression to the adult metabolic disorder we call Syndrome X. This also increases diabetes and heart disease risk.

A recent study found that levels of Growth Hormone Binding Protein (GHBP) are significantly higher in girls with premature puberty and middle-body fat. Less muscle mass creates a vicious cycle of more body fat, followed by more insulin resistance, that in turn helps store more body fat, and then even less free growth hormone to build bone and muscle. This is another reason overweight children get even fatter.

Early puberty and a high percent of body fat work together to increase a girl's risk of later developing breast cancer through

Risks due to early puberty
PCOS, diabetes, obesity, breast cancer, STDs

Danger
The girls with elevated androgens and insulin resistance before puberty continue to have obesity, insulin resistance, and high androgens after puberty.

High GHBP
Leads to less free, active Growth Hormone to stimulate building bone and muscle.

The "C" word

The longer the breast is exposed to abnormal hormone ratios, especially if insulin is high, the higher the risk of breast cancer.

exposure to estrogens, particularly estrone, at an earlier, critical window of time in development. Early puberty and being fat is even more of a concern when you add the increase in breast cancer risk as a result of high insulin and environmental exposure to hormone-like chemicals (See Chapter 5).

London researchers, Stoll and colleagues said in 1994,

> *"Earlier onset of menarche and tallness in adult women are mainly confirmed as risk markers for breast cancer. Recent…studies have reported abdominal-type obesity and higher circulating levels of insulin, testosterone, and insulin-like growth factor 1, to be further risk markers for breast cancer. There is evidence that abdominal-type obesity is recognizable in girls even before puberty, and disparate studies have shown it to be correlated with earlier onset of menarche, insulin resistance leading to hyperinsulinemia, and an abnormal sex steroid profile."*

Latency

Girls hate those "creepy" boys and boys think all girls have "cooties."

Psychological:

Girls (and boys) between ages 6–10 enter the psychological stage we call *latency*. This is a stage when both sexes retreat into their own world, avoiding the other sex almost like the plague.

This is a critical developmental stage for both sexes. Girls especially need these years to develop confidence and a strong sense of self, separate from a role defined by boys or men. They need this phase of their lives to develop close friendships with other girls, to develop social skills and a sense of mastery in school and activities—especially sports—that help them successfully navigate the turbulent years of puberty.

Trouble

If the physical changes of puberty come too early, their body is attracting boys like flies to honey, but their psyche is still in latency, not wanting anything to do with boys.

Our society already pressures children to grow up too fast. When the body too is filling out and accelerating into puberty *before* the psychological "work" of latency has been completed, it can wreak havoc with later psychological, social, and academic adjustment. The body may *look* like a young woman, but the mind is still a child.

If girls don't have enough time in the latency years to develop an adequate sense of self before they are pulled into relationships with boys, they have difficulty defining their sense of independent identity.

They become further defined by how they *look*, rather than who they *are*. It becomes more and more difficult to develop positive self-esteem.

Many social pressures already make it difficult for today's kids to feel good about themselves, so the psychological consequences of early puberty compound an already serious problem. These social issues contribute to the *medical consequences* of early puberty.

Sociological-cultural:

Girls whose sexual development comes too early also get teased by boys their age but get more sexual overtures from older boys.

Girls who look 17, but are really 12, are under much more pressure from older boys to engage in risky behaviors like smoking cigarettes or pot, drinking alcohol, and experimenting with street drugs. Younger teens are even more susceptible to all this because of the taunts from boys their own age. The dangers of all of these cultural pressures are quite real.

Theories about Causes of Premature Puberty

What is happening to cause this widespread problem of premature puberty? Doctors across the country see this in their offices daily. Let's look at some of the culprits.

Environmental Chemicals

The problem is not limited to the United States. Studies done in numerous countries have found that children's normal progression of sexual and reproductive development is being affected by exposure to the hormone-disrupting chemicals that permeate our food chain and water supplies worldwide.

These hormone-mimicking compounds or *persistent organic pollutants* (POPs) are *everywhere*. Chemical contaminants from the environment make it into our water and foods. Many of these compounds also pass through the placental barrier and expose the developing baby in the mother's womb.

POPs are concentrated in our body fat and breast milk because of its high fat content, and are then passed to infants during nursing. This is a primary reason that various studies show earlier onset of puberty in breast-fed children.

Most scientists think the benefits of breast milk for the baby outweigh the risk of exposure to these environmental chemicals, but no one can say with certainty because these issues are just beginning to be studied more aggressively.

Danger! Girls who are sexually developed too early experience more sexual harassment, increased risk of date rape, and risk of accidental pregnancy.

Caution Late teens and twenties are a time when one third of sexually active individuals will contract a sexually transmitted disease (STD), so use protection.

Ominous These chemicals have known adverse effects for the onset of puberty.

PCB Poisoning

Damaged skin, eyes, immune and reproductive function.

Obesity

Junk food and lack of exercise—only the tip of the iceberg!

Apocalypse

We are sitting on a time bomb that is beginning to explode on this current generation of children.

These chemicals—DDE, PCBs, Bisphenol A and a host of others—have profound effects on the brain centers that regulate everything from sexual development to metabolism and body weight. They have known adverse effects on development of puberty in animals.

Ominous findings are now being seen in humans as well, confirmed by studies worldwide. Early puberty is one risk.

The number of these endocrine disruptors is increasing rapidly, and they are not limited to just pesticides. Several different compounds used in the food industry, in plasticizers, and in dental restorations, are also estrogenic. (See the complete references listed in the Appendix.)

We are still learning sad lessons from the 1968 accidental poisoning of 2000 people in Japan. Rice oil was contaminated with PCBs leading to a condition called "Yusho" disease. A similar PCB poisoning in Taiwan was named "Yu Cheng" disease. Both of these conditions had many damaging effects on skin and eyes, but researchers also found symptoms of endocrine disruption: altered menstrual cycles and abnormal immune function.

A May 2001 summary of the consequences of these poisonings said "The most tragic aspect of Yusho and Yu-Cheng diseases was the exposure of children to PCBs. In the case of Yu-Cheng, children exposed to PCBs in utero and (in breast milk) were reported to have poor cognitive development. Intellectual impairment was also observed in children born to women who had eaten fish contaminated with PCBs in the United States."

How does PCB exposure do all this damage? Some PCBs cause the thymus gland to shrivel, and also adversely affect androgen metabolism. Animal studies show exposure to PCBs during fetal development causes profound disruptions in thyroid hormones along with other changes, including abnormalities in brain development, that appear to lead to the higher incidence of learning and attention disorders in the children.

There is strong scientific evidence that these same chemicals are altering critical metabolic pathways that can clearly add to the existing problem of childhood obesity. (See Chapter 5.)

Any chemical exposure that damages the thyroid and its hormone functions during development in the womb or during breastfeeding will have profound impacts on children's ability to maintain normal body weight as they grow. Dietary excess with the junk food so prevalent in our culture is a huge factor in the epidemic of obesity among children. But, I don't think *all the blame rests there.*

We can no longer afford such simplistic explanations for obesity in children by saying they are fat because they eat too much and don't exercise enough. The rest of the story lies in the profound degree of chemical pollutants in everyday life that disrupt critical thyroid and sex hormone pathways and functions in our body.

No longer rare
Premature puberty is no longer only a rare case seen in specialty centers for pediatric endocrine problems.

We may not yet have the final "proof," but the evidence is staggering. We can no longer afford to ignore the warnings that we see in animal populations all over the world. Like the canary in the mine, the animal population is giving us warnings we would do well to heed before we sacrifice an entire generation of children.

For the health of your children, as well as your own, I recommend that you read: *"Children's Environmental Health Risks: A State-of-the-Art Conference."* (See review in March–April 2001, Archives of Environmental Health).

Dietary Excess

We live in the age of "super-sizing," not only food and beverage portions but our bodies too. We live in a culture of *excess everything*: excess calories, excess fat, excess sugars and simple carbs that promote more fat, and excess "couch-potato" time in front of TVs and computers. How does this contribute to earlier onset of puberty?

We have known for a very long time that reaching a certain amount of body fat for girls plays an important role in signaling the brain to begin menstrual cycles. Overweight girls tend to begin to menstruate at younger ages, while girls who are very thin or anorexic have later onset of menstrual periods—many times as late at 17–18 years of age.

Sociological Pressures

Sexualized messages and images besiege girls and boys at younger and younger ages. Such immersion in provocative, often erotic, images may also contribute to changes in brain chemistry that trigger the onset of puberty signals in the pituitary.

For all of us, seeing things around us will trigger physiological changes in the brain and body. We also know that women who live together—in families, in college dorms, in residential high schools, etc. will typically begin to menstruate together. This phenomenon has been described for centuries, as in *The Red Tent,* by Anita Diamant (St. Martin's Press, 1997), a story of Jacob's wives and their experiences in the menstrual tent in Biblical times.

This menstrual synchrony seems to occur from a variety of olfactory and environmental cues that stimulate the brain-ovarian pathways to entrain, or synchronize, menstrual cycles.

It may not be so far-fetched to think that constant exposure to visual sexual images contributes to brain changes that accelerate sexual development.

The Ovary Life Cycle Continues: Our Fertile Years

Your menstrual cycle tends to regulate itself by late teens or early twenties and you can generally count on it to be a regular length throughout your twenties and into your early thirties.

By twenty-five, we have usually reached the peak of our fertility and the peak function of our circulatory, respiratory, and digestive systems to meet the demands of pregnancy with the least stress on our body. Hormone production is more predictable, helping keep the cycles regular.

Estradiol levels are high in the first half of the cycle, fall around ovulation, and then rise slightly in the second half of the cycle when progesterone production dominates. Testosterone levels remain fairly constant throughout the cycle.

Stages

Estradiol is the first ovarian hormone to decline and the imbalance in the estrogen/ progesterone ratio may cause PMS symptoms.

By your mid-thirties, you may begin experiencing a small change in your menstrual flow. By your late thirties or early forties flow may become noticeably lighter and last for fewer days. Your cycle length may become either longer or shorter.

This is a time when women notice more pronounced premenstrual mood, energy, and appetite changes that we know as premenstrual syndrome (PMS), or as more severe cases are called, *premenstrual dysphoric disorder* (PMDD).

At this stage, we are often experiencing the wide variety of effects of estradiol decline: worsening migraines, fibromyalgia, bladder problems, vulvodynia, loss of lean tissue, increasing fat stores, and other annoying symptoms that worsen as we enter our pre and perimenopausal years.

Women in this first phase of ovarian decline typically still have normal ovulatory progesterone levels even though estradiol typically is lower than it should be. Current studies in reproductive medicine worldwide discount theories that a *decline* in progesterone precipitated PMS.

Premenopause: The Waning of Our Ovaries

The "climacteric" has recognized stages of premenopause and perimenopause.

This decline in estradiol and progesterone commonly begins between the ages of 35 to 40, as the number and/or quality of remaining follicles decrease. It begins much earlier in some women.

New Insights on Stages of Ovarian Decline

The standard medical teaching is that *premenopause* begins with anovulatory cycles (a cycle which does not produce an egg), and loss of progesterone rather than estrogen.

It is difficult to "observe" if there is no egg being produced each month, so this is why most doctors don't have a good understanding of what is happening to your *actual hormone production.* I have been tracking and checking cycle-specific hormone levels for many years, in thousands of women, and then correlating them with symptoms. The objective data shows how incorrect our standard teaching can be.

In the women I have tested, I find significant decrease in estradiol levels that **precede** the onset of anovulatory cycles and loss of progesterone.

I have discussed my observations with many reproductive endocrinologists trying to help infertile women become pregnant. They do regular checks of ovarian hormone levels to achieve pregnancy, and see the same patterns of estradiol decline I find in my patients.

Infertility specialists do not address the types of problems I see in my practice as effects of waning ovarian hormones because their focus, appropriately so, is on helping women get pregnant. But many women who struggle with infertility also experience some of the problems I see in my patients as a result of lower estradiol and testosterone: increasing PMS, headaches, muscle-joint pain, fatigue, weight gain, insulin resistance, bone loss, immune prob-

The climacteric
Decline in hormone production that takes us from full reproductive capability to menopause

Try testing?
Standard "wisdom" is primarily based on observations of women's menstrual patterns, however, not on actual systematic hormone levels

lems, low sex drive, bladder and vaginal problems, and a host of others.

In the chart that follows, I divided our current standard definition of "premenopause" into Stage 1 and Stage 2 of ovarian decline that come before perimenopause.

Dr. Vliet's Model: Stages of Ovarian Decline

Premenopause

Stage 1: Declining Estradiol, normal cycles

- FSH and LH are within normal ranges
- Estradiol (E2) level is beginning to decrease
- Testosterone may be starting to decrease
- Progesterone is within normal range but may be out of balance with your estradiol making PMS worse
- Menstrual cycles are still regular and most are ovulatory
- Beginning of restless sleep, fuzzy thinking, memory loss, mood swings, fatigue, muscle/joint pain, headaches, allergies, bladder or vulva pain and other symptoms of low E2.

Stage 2: Beginning of Anovulatory Cycles

- FSH and LH are within normal ranges, still less than 10
- Estradiol level continues to decline, hot flashes typically begin at times of the cycle when estradiol is falling (menses, ovulation)
- Testosterone is typically decreasing
- Fewer ovulatory cycles mean progesterone (P) does not rise second half of cycle. PMS doesn't typically occur if there is no ovulation and no rise in progesterone (don't load up on progesterone cream!)
- Menses becoming irregular
- Insomnia, memory loss, depression and pain syndromes get worse, low libido, leaking urine, vaginal dryness, and loss of energy are common

© 1996, revised 2001–2007 Elizabeth Lee Vliet, M.D.

Timeline

My contention is that we have estradiol decline as the first step toward menopause.

Stage 1—Declining Estradiol

I call this stage Premature Ovarian Decline or POD. This occurs when your estradiol level begins to decrease, but you *still have normal menstrual cycles*. In what we call the "normal" or usual time frame, this stage would generally begin in our late thirties or early forties.

One of the first symptoms of lower estradiol is multiple awakening during the night, with difficulty getting back to sleep. Our dreaming phase (REM sleep) is altered and you may notice that you don't dream as much as you used to. Because sleep is now more restless, you wake up feeling tired.

Other early signs may include *fuzzy thinking, memory loss, mood swings, fatigue, muscle and joint pain, headaches, increasing allergies, more sensitivity to strong smells, vulvar pain, loss of sex drive,* and others.

In this phase, progesterone is generally within normal ovulatory ranges, but estradiol has declined below optimal levels, which makes PMS symptoms worse.

Women are usually able to recognize these as hormonally related changes because of the way they come and go with the menstrual cycle. Often doctors say "You are "too young" to have hormone problems," or "you're still menstruating, so your hormones are fine." Not so!

Here is where I find so many women are under-diagnosed, undertreated, and are seeking answers in the alternative medical field because their symptoms are not recognized by most doctors.

Most of my supposedly "premenopausal" patients are still having regular periods, and yet their estradiol levels are far lower than what we now know from menopause research is needed to preserve bone and maintain healthy brain function.

But my detective work to find out *why* my younger patients have these menopause-type symptoms shows that *bleeding patterns are not an accurate marker of hormone levels.*

Any of you who struggle with infertility know: you can have regular periods, yet still not get pregnant. You have to *measure* the ovarian hormones at specific times of the menstrual cycle to see if there are healthy amounts of all these crucial hormones, and in the optimal balance. Women with menstrually-related symptoms deserve the same attention to lab tests that we give other health problems.

Stage 2—Beginning of Anovulatory Cycles

This is the beginning of classically defined *premenopause*. In our "normal" model, this phase would generally begin in our midforties, but like all the other phases, can occur much earlier.

There will be cycles when ovulation does not occur, because follicles don't develop properly and estradiol is not produced normally in the first half of the cycle.

Rethinking
I propose that we "reclassify" these stages, based on patterns shown by systematic hormone testing.

Wrong!
Doctors are taught that women who are still menstruating must have "normal" hormone levels. They may not!

No progesterone = No PMS
PMS doesn't usually occur if there is no ovulation to cause a rise in progesterone.

Oops!

With cycle irregularity and erratic ovulation at this phase of life, you could find yourself with an unexpected pregnancy.

This means progesterone doesn't rise as expected in the second half of the cycle. Levels of FSH and LH are typically still low and haven't risen to the menopausal range.

Fewer ovulatory cycles result in estradiol levels continuing to decline, and this is the time you may experience hot flashes and night sweats, especially with the drop in estradiol when your period starts. Your periods typically become irregular, or may skip.

Often common symptoms, from mild to more severe, include insomnia, further memory loss, inability to concentrate or focus, feeling depressed or anxious for no clear reason, pain syndromes get worse (such as phase of life, you could find yourself with an leakage or feelings of urgently having to go to the bathroom, vaginal dryness, painful sex, and feeling that your "get-up-and-go" got up and went.

Dr. Vliet's Model: Stages of Ovarian Decline

Stage 3: "Perimenopause"

- FSH and LH are beginning to rise, typically in the range of 10–20
- Estradiol much lower now over the entire menstrual cycle
- Loss of ovulatory cycles, Progesterone decreases further
- Testosterone continues to decline, affecting libido, mood, energy level, muscle and bone mass
- Periods become much more erratic, cycles are skipped, there may be more bleeding problems due to the changing balance of estradiol and progesterone
- Hot flashes, restless sleep and fuzzy thinking become more pronounced and disruptive,
- Other symptoms develop or become magnified—you may feel an alien has taken over your body!

Stage 4: MENOPAUSE

- FSH and LH have risen to levels above 20, (the level that defines menopause)
- Menses no longer occur
- Estradiol level is decreased to levels typically below 30-40 pg/ml
- Progesterone levels remain low since no further ovulation occurs
- Testosterone levels decline further, often less than 20 ng/dl
- Brain symptoms (insomnia, hot flashes, memory loss, pain, etc.) increase as estradiol declines. Many other changes occur with loss of estradiol, such as bone loss, elevated blood pressure, decrease in HDL cholesterol, waistline weight gain, hair loss, dry skin, dry eyes, crawly skin, incontinence, difficulty reaching orgasm, loss of sexual interest, and many others.

© 1996, revised 2001–2007 Elizabeth Lee Vliet, M.D.

Perimenopause

This stage is classically defined by rising FSH and LH levels as the brain struggles to stimulate the failing ovaries to increase the falling hormones. The amount of estrone, produced primarily by body fat tissue, is rising relative to decreasing estradiol.

Since it doesn't act quite the same way as estradiol does, estrone doesn't keep your body functioning at your previous level. This is why you may notice more "brain fog" and mood changes, as well as more fat around your waist. Blood pressure may also go up.

You will still have periods but they now become more erratic and most cycles will likely be anovulatory. You may skip periods now as well. The color of your flow changes too; it is more likely to be brown rather than a healthy, bright red.

Bleeding is typically lighter, and shorter in duration, but it can also become heavier, and longer in duration some months. You may also notice worsening menstrual cramps. Simply said, at this phase of your ovary life cycle, your periods will most likely be erratic, with changing bleeding patterns. If menses come more often than every three weeks, or if you have heavy bleeding, you should talk with your gynecologist to discuss options. Hysterectomy is recommended for many women, although there are a number of non-surgical options to help control or prevent many of these problems. (See Chapter 16.)

If pregnancy is not desired, then you still need to use contraception until you are clearly menopausal with an FSH greater than 20.

Menopausal Stage

This final stage brings our ovary life cycle to completion. The average age in the United States for natural menopause is between 48 and 52 years of age, but this is just an *average*.

Approximately 10–13 percent of women experience true menopause between age 40 and 47. When menopause comes so early, it can come as quite a shock. It is a physical shock to your body to lose these important metabolically active ovarian hormones at too young an age, not just an emotional blow of feeling old before your time and feeling the loss of your fertility.

We no longer menstruate because our follicle supply has been depleted and we can't make the hormones that trigger our menstrual cycles. The brain senses the decrease in estradiol, and sends out more FSH and LH to stimulate the ovaries to

Perimeno
- rising FSH
- low E2
- low testo
- erratic cycles

Peri problems
- worsening cramps
- more fibroids
- more ovarian cysts

What sex?
Lower levels of both estradiol and testosterone can rob you of your sexual drive and makes it much harder to have an orgasm as clitoral nerve endings are less sensitive with loss of hormone effects.

"Official Menopause"
- FSH>20
- no menses for one year

produce more hormones. But the extra push is useless because there are no follicles to produce estradiol and progesterone. The low levels of ovarian hormones are now present in steady, non-cycling patterns

Low Fuel

☙ Almost all estradiol is gone

☙ Half of testosterone is lost

With menopause, we lose almost *all* of our 17-beta estradiol production, with levels typically below 30–40 pg/ml. That's a lot lower than the average 100–500 pg/ml of a menstrual cycle, so it isn't surprising you feel so many body and brain changes!

Progesterone levels remain low because there is no ovulation, no corpus luteum, and progesterone is no longer needed to sustain a pregnancy.

The ovary still produces testosterone and other androgens, though at lower levels, but it is no longer producing adequate estradiol to balance these male hormones.

The uneven balance of estradiol and testosterone causes some of the unwanted changes in skin, facial hair, and distribution of body fat. The "pear" shape female (gynecoid) fat pattern around the hips and buttocks suddenly begins moving up toward the middle of the body to become the "apple" shape (male or android pattern), as shown in the diagram.

It could be

Part of your loss of energy may be due to declining testosterone levels as well as the loss of estradiol.

In official "medicalese," menopause is defined as *one year from* the "last menstrual period," which may seem a little strange that we identify it so long after the fact. The problem is that our periods get more irregular at the end, so we never know which period is the last one for a number of months. We can then look back and realize "that was it."

Many of the earlier described symptoms get more noticeable and bothersome with lower menopausal hormone levels. Women often notice a *marked worsening of brain symptoms* such as insomnia, memory loss, foggy or slowed thinking and pain symptoms. Hot flashes may still occur and get worse with lower estradiol levels.

Changes in appearance also become more noticeable: skin becomes more dry and "crawly," and loses its elasticity leading to more wrinkles. Hair gets thinner and more brittle and you may start losing large amounts.

You may notice more facial hair as well as loss of hair on your legs and arms. There is typically more weight gain around the waist, and your breasts become less firm.

It can be confusing to determine what changes occur as a result of the loss of our ovarian hormones and what changes occur as a result of just getting older. Hormone levels help sort this out.

Some women experience no major physical symptoms at all; they stop menstruating and that's that. Others have a few irksome symptoms, but aren't significantly bothered by these changes.

Still other women have a very difficult time in the years leading up to menopause with symptoms and health risks that profoundly disrupt quality of life and ability to function well each day. This latter group often describes serious declines in energy level, mental sharpness, sex drive, quality of sleep, and overall well-being. Many will develop chronic debilitating diseases, such as diabetes or osteoporosis, that further sabotage quality of life.

A Shock! 1% will undergo complete menopause, or premature ovarian failure, before age 40.

Risk of diabetes, colon cancer, osteoporosis, and Alzheimer's disease all increase after menopause as you lose the critical estradiol. Blood pressure and cholesterol rise in menopausal women, similar to the pattern in men because testosterone effects become more pronounced as estradiol is lost.

There is a decrease in the good "HDL" cholesterol, and a rise in LDL and triglycerides. These changes combine to increase risk of cardiovascular disease (CVD). Previous gender *differences* now become gender *similarities*. For example, CVD risk for menopausal women is now similar to the risk for men. This happens from being menopausal, regardless of your age when it occurs, and regardless of the cause.

Risks Breast cancer risk also increases after menopause *even if you never take any hormone replacement therapy.*

The rate of CVD increases as estradiol levels decline relative to testosterone levels, as we see in younger women with PCOS. Since cardiovascular disease is the number one killer of women, it is critical to measure ovarian hormone levels in order to assess your risk of CVD, particularly if you notice body changes that suggest hormone imbalance, regardless of how old you are.

Menopause involves all dimensions of our being: physical, emotional, and spiritual. The biological process will happen sooner or later to all women who live long enough. Psychological and spiritual changes are more variable, and include learning to see our later years as fulfilling and meaningful, taking stock of our lives and what we want to accomplish in the years ahead, changing priorities for how we spend our time, and exploring our spiritual beliefs. While there may be a sense of loss over no longer being able to bear children, there is also the opportunity for the years after menopause to have a sense of freedom that is equally gratifying.

Mystery explained
Hot flashes may decrease as estradiol becomes steady, instead of fluctuating as much as it does in perimeno-pause.

Symptoms of hormonal decline can occur at any age. When I describe the ovaries' "normal" aging process, I am only giving you age ranges for a relative idea of when these changes can occur.

Each woman's body marches to its own drummer. Each woman has slightly different experiences along the way, just as it was with puberty and pregnancy.

The stage of life when you notice changes and symptoms, as well as the symptoms themselves, is not necessarily going to be the same as your friends. You may be perimenopausal in your early thirties or you could even be endocrinologically menopausal in your twenties. I have many patients in both categories.

Whatever age these changes occur, the stages and body markers, or symptoms, are similar and we may use some of the same treatments. The key is to recognize what is going on at any age, understand why it is happening, and have the knowledge to make informed health decisions that meet your needs.

In my practice, I primarily see women who feel terrible and want ways to regain their energy and vitality. As one woman said so succinctly: *"I don't like this foggy-brained feeling, I want my brain back!"*

Double Whammy
The effects of age and hormone loss combine to produce many of our body changes.

I help women achieve their goals and desires, based on working together to assess what causes such disruption in their quality of life. I want to find ways for them to have a smoother transition. I want to avoid the pitfalls and uncomfortable symptoms that can become even more pronounced if untreated or *mistreated* with wrong doses of hormones or other medications.

Since women are now living 30 to 40 years after menopause, our ultimate goal is to find healthy, safe, effective ways to maintain vitality and zest for those years ahead.

The Sixties and Beyond: Postmenopausal Stage

We have seen an impressive increase in the average life span for both men and women in the last century. Thanks to medical technology, new medications, a more plentiful and varied food supply, and better knowledge of disease prevention and lifestyle risk reduction, we are living longer than ever before.

While most of us view this as a good thing, it also presents a whole new set of challenges. Women today may live thirty to fifty years beyond menopause.

You don't need to fear your years after menopause if you integrate healthy lifestyle changes with information from the rapidly advancing science about how our bodies change, and incorporate common sense treatments outlined later.

Hormones may be one of those options to help you feel your best. There are many ways to improve your health and vitality, reduce disease risks, and enjoy a better quality of life for all the years you live.

Premature Ovarian Decline

Now that we have talked about a "normal" progression through the life cycle, let's explore the term "premature ovarian *decline* (POD)."

This is a stage of your life when you are transitioning from optimal fertile hormone levels to less optimal levels. It is not the same as true premature ovarian *failure* (POF) because you still have follicles and menstrual periods.

POD simply means that your ovaries are not producing ovarian hormones at levels sufficient to maintain "optimal" metabolic function throughout the body, even though your FSH still remains in the premenopausal range.

You are too young for this, so no one is really looking for it and it is blamed on something else.

That "something" is usually labeled psychological, or just "stress," and young women are told to take an antidepressant. The consequences throughout your body can be dramatic, as you will see in later chapters.

Early onset of menopause has many causes, which we'll discuss later. Certainly our genetic makeup is one factor: studies of women around the world have shown that heredity is major determinant of when we will reach menopause. It helps to find out when your mother and grandmothers reached natural menopause, (unless they had a hysterectomy that created an artificial menopause) to give you an idea of what you might expect.

Looong The entire process of ovarian decline may take fifteen years or more, or it can be a fairly rapid fall, occurring at nearly any age.

Outwitting Mother Nature

Only in the last four generations have large numbers of women lived long enough past menopause to see the brain-body effects of declining ovarian hormones.

One caveat for younger women who are athletes: intensive training may cause you to stop having periods, but you are not classically considered to be "menopausal" because your FSH is *suppressed* by exercise and you still have ovarian follicles. Once you decrease the intensity of your workouts, periods are likely to begin again.

Medical studies show that women who go through premature menopause have a shorter life span. To some extent, these same risks can be increased in women who are experience the early *decline* in estradiol as well, although definitive studies are lacking.

Perhaps because the body has less time with the full benefits of estradiol, including its immune system effects; or it may be that these women have earlier onset of the diseases and conditions such as osteoporosis, diabetes, cardiovascular disease, Alzheimer's disease, and colon cancer, as a result of the absence of the critical 17-beta estradiol.

There are many clues to declining estradiol. Some of the common ones I see in patients are in the chart on the following page.

It is obvious from this list that estradiol affects many body functions. In women with POD, loss of estradiol can sometimes be sudden, but more often, it is a subtle, gradual change usually occurring over several years.

Your mind and body make adjustments, similar to the way the body adjusts to a gradual loss of hemoglobin in an early anemia, but gradually, you begin to notice you just don't feel like your usual self. Eventually, the decline in estradiol changes the balance of estradiol in ratio to testosterone, DHEA, and progesterone to lead to a wide variety of physical and psychological experiences. Some of these may occur for the first time, or take a turn for the worse as the hormone balance changes.

There are many known causes and contributors to early ovarian decline, and even more that we don't fully understand yet. Some of these we can control, some we can't. Good lifestyle habits will certainly help slow and ease the aging process. But when it comes to our ovaries, this is not always enough and women may need hormonal support.

The following table lists many of the potential causes of POD. Note how varied they are. In later chapters, I will explore these in more depth.

Dr. Vliet's Guide to Overlooked Causes of Premature Ovarian Decline

- Chronic dieting, eating disorders (anorexia, bulimia) that suppresses hypothalamus regulation of ovarian function
- Compulsive exercise for weight loss, or the intensive training schedules of competitive athletes that interferes with ovulation and release of follicle and thereby estrogen production
- Cigarette smoking which damages ovarian follicles
- Tubal ligation which interrupts normal ovarian blood flow
- Hysterectomy without removal of the ovaries which also interrupts ovarian blood flow
- Thyroid disorders which interferes both with brain regulation of ovaries as well as ovarian hormone production and function
- Polycystic ovary syndrome which leads to excessive production of testosterone and insulin that prevents normal ovulation with normal production of estradiol and progesterone
- Viral oophoritis, a viral infiltration that may damage the ovary just as happens with the thyroid and pancreas glands
- Post-partum phase, in which high prolactin levels during nursing suppresses the normal menstrual cycle hormone production and ovulation; with older age at pregnancy, ovaries may not come back into full normal cycles after nursing ends
- Cessation of birth control pills after long term use, especially high progestin pills
- Toxic exposures: examples of this in my practice include black widow spider bites, Lyme disease, pesticides, mononucleosis
- Hypothalamic dysfunction or suppression due to excessive exercise, chronic dieting, high intake of soy, high intake of excitatory amino acids (such as glutamate, MSG, aspartate, Nutrasweet)

Other Potential Risk Factors For POD:

- Mother had early onset of menopause
- Body weight—thinner women have earlier onset
- Vegetarian diet due to lower amounts of protein, fat and generally higher intake of soy products and lower body weight and fat composition
- Malnutrition
- Living at high altitudes
- Never having been pregnant (more pregnancies leads to later menopause)

© 2001–2007 Elizabeth Lee Vliet, MD

Dr. Vliet's Guide to Clues to Declining Estradiol

- ❧ Worsening PMS
- ❧ Restless sleep, difficulty sleeping especially prior to menses, multiple awakenings during the night
- ❧ Loss of energy, feeling too tired to get through the day
- ❧ Mood swings, episodic tearfulness for no reason, irritability, angry outbursts, and spells of feeling depressed especially premenstrually
- ❧ Worsening allergies, sensitivities to chemicals, perfumes
- ❧ Palpitations, especially those that get worse a few days prior to menses and during bleeding days when estradiol is low or falling
- ❧ Anxiety attacks, worse around menses Premenstrual migraines, more frequent migraines
- ❧ Increase in tension headaches
- ❧ Aching joints
- ❧ Muscle soreness, stiffness, fibromyalgia pain syndrome
- ❧ Memory and concentration problems that are worse before menses
- ❧ "Spiking" blood pressure, higher blood pressure than normal
- ❧ More "irritable bowel" problems prior to menses and during menses
- ❧ Dry eyes occurs early; later, as women lose their estradiol, risk of macular degeneration, cataracts, and glaucoma increases
- ❧ Hair gets thinner, more scalp hair loss
- ❧ Nails are dry and brittle
- ❧ Facial hair increases
- ❧ Skin becomes dry, crawly, and looser, less elastic due to decline in collagen, wrinkles start to appear
- ❧ Vaginal dryness, pain with sex, vulva pain
- ❧ Loss of sex drive, difficulty having orgasm
- ❧ Bladder changes: more infections, pain on urination, more frequent urination, urinary leakage
- ❧ Posture becomes more slumped as bone is lost from spine
- ❧ "Spare" tire around middle—abdominal fat gain
- ❧ Food cravings
- ❧ Difficulty losing weight, even with diet and exercise

© 1995–2007 Elizabeth Lee Vliet, M.D.

Summary

Your hormones can be both marvelous *and* maddening: marvelous when they allow us to create new life and function at our best, maddening when they are out of balance or declining.

But ovarian hormones are more than just for creating new life; our female hormones are at the core of our being, fundamental to every part and function of our body, mind and spirit.

The patterns of physiological changes that occur each month and throughout the ovaries' lifecycle give us observable phenomena that help us to then "connect the dots" and see the hormonal triggers related to physical and mood symptoms.

We need to look for these patterns, track them, and then find ways to communicate our observations to physicians.

The "life cycle" of ovaries refers to overall stages of our lives rather than the monthly menstrual cycle we discussed in Chapter 2, one affects the other.

As our ovaries age and we approach menopause, or undergo surgery, or experience other problems, our menstrual cycles change too.

Is everything supposed to be downhill from now on? Is this just part of life we must accept? I don't think so. As the woman below said so eloquently:

"It was about 14 years ago that I had my hysterectomy for severe PMS, and they also found endometriosis. I was better after the surgery and managed for a few years, but for the last several, I started having really horrible menopausal symptoms even though I was taking estrogen daily. After reading your books, I finally insisted on getting my hormone levels checked and they found my estrogen was too low... but they added testosterone! It is so frustrating... I have learned a lot from all my reading because I had to in order to help myself! But doctors don't seem to want to listen to what I know, even when it is my own body. Every time I try to do something I am up against obstacles, but I keep fighting because I know it isn't right and I stand up for what I need."

When you don't feel well over a long period of time and have sought help from multiple doctors only to be told there is nothing wrong, it can leave you doubting yourself physically as well as psychologically.

You are YOU! Your ovaries are as individual as you are and may not follow the "typical" timeline outlined.

Why? It isn't a matter of "medicalizing" menopause when we replace what is lost to restore hormone balance.

Slowly— The change in hormone production may be so gradual that it is virtually unrecognized as you go along, day by day.

Hidden issues

I know it is difficult to convince doctors of something that they can't see—hormone problems are not visible like a broken leg.

Please! Listen to me

Many of my patients tell me it is often hard to get their physicians to listen to their observations and pay attention to these hormone-related issues.

You feel battered, frustrated, and alone. You suspect it is your hormones, yet no one takes you seriously. Many of my patients have done so much research to educate themselves, they often know more about these issues than many doctors!

There are ways to help you get what you need when dealing with health care professionals. I encourage you to be assertive about getting checked for these potential hormone connections. I urge you to get answers that make sense. There are too many health consequences if you don't.

While there are no easy solutions for changing the health care system to be more responsive to women's observations and insights, I do have some suggestions you may consider.

Many women depend on their gynecologist for primary care as well as annual pelvic exams. But you may find, as have many of my patients, that family medicine or internal medicine physicians are more open to the idea of checking hormone levels than are many gynecologists. I think this is related to the fact that medical specialists are more accustomed to using laboratory tests both to evaluate health problems and to monitor response to medications.

You may also find that internists and family physicians are likely to be responsive to your written summary of the patterns you notice in relation to your menstrual cycle. It facilitates communication with your physicians if you bring any journals you have keep to track your symptoms as you go through your menstrual cycle.

Don't focus on just treating or "getting through" symptoms. That's a lot like just putting a band-aid on an abscess instead of treating the cause of the infection.

Look for the underlying causes and make decisions based on what you need for overall vitality and health for many years to come.

It is *your* body, *your* health, and *your* life.

Chapter 4
Ovaries At Risk—Surprising Toxins in Your Diet

I see so many more women today suffering from serious health problems, including infertility, arising from premature ovarian hormone decline.

Are we overlooking a crucial connection that lurks "innocently" in the foods we are eating and the soft drinks we are collectively consuming, literally by the gallon, every day?

I think the answer is YES.

Endocrine saboteurs MSG, HVP, additives, soft drinks and more. Pay attention!

Many women I see for consults have one thing in common: ovaries have been damaged by subtle, insidious dietary and environmental "hormone disruptors." The ovaries aren't making optimal levels of the ovarian hormones they need to effectively "run" the cellular engines making up every organ in their bodies (See Chapter 5 on environmental disruptors).

Some of these hormone disruptors are in common everyday things in our lives—such as soft drinks and flavor enhancers like MSG. We would never dream that they could wreak such havoc with our ovaries and our hormones.

Soft drinks? "Impossible," you say. *MSG* in all those foods? "Couldn't be in a million years."

This chapter may shock you. You may not think it is real. But I am describing *worldwide* research showing adverse effects on men and women and animals and fish and birds and insects and reptiles—from all over the planet. Dietary toxins are *very serious* problems, and can affect many aspects of your health, from future cancer risk to your fertility now.

Let's first explore some surprising "ovary damagers" that lie in some unsuspecting foods and beverages you probably eat or drink every day.

Heads up!
This is your
call to action.

The Soft Drink–Fast Food Menace: Excitotoxins and Hormone Health

How can soft drinks and foods affect our ovaries? The answer may be more astounding, more macabre, and more insidious, than the twists of a horror movie. Truth is sometimes stranger than fiction. Here's the truth we know about certain types of food additives and sweeteners that fall into a group of chemicals called *excitotoxins*.

Basically, excitotoxins stimulate such intense and rapid firing of the nerve endings that the cells run out of their chemical messengers, and then die a few hours later.

Fact
Excitotoxins,
or
neurotoxicants,
are chemicals
that cause
damage or
death to
nerve cells.

The nerve cells in the *hypothalamus*, our master hormone regulator, are some of the most sensitive neurons in our body to this excitatory damage and death.

While we are still quietly developing in our mother's womb, our brain cells in the hypothalamus can be damaged by these excitotoxins, but the impact doesn't show up until many years later when our menstrual cycles begin.

As children, we typically consume large amounts of these excitotoxins in soft drinks and other processed foods. The damage to the hypothalamus accumulates each day and each year, and we don't realize what is happening. The damage shows up later on in our reproductive years, when "hormone problems" can begin in earnest.

What Are Excitotoxins and Where Are They Found

Some excitotoxins are amino acid compounds that occur in nature: *glutamate*, *aspartate*, and *cysteine* which are the building blocks of proteins.

Some excitotoxins are man-made chemicals and are even more potent. One example is MSG; the well-known chemical culprit that causes "Chinese-restaurant headache" syndrome.

MSG, or monosodium glutamate, is a flavor-enhancer first synthesized in the 1920s. It is widely used in making all kinds of processed foods to improve taste and make us want to eat more, and more!

MSG is made by adding sodium to the amino acid glutamate, and *it is the glutamate part of the molecule that does the excitatory damage to nerve cells.*

MSG-induced damage to the brain has been studied and written about for at least *forty* years. The food manufacturing industry has effectively managed to keep this research from broader public awareness, so you may not know about it.

In spite of continuing research showing more damage than first thought, concerns about the over-use of glutamate have not been heeded. Problems have only intensified with the addition of even more MSG-related compounds to an ever-increasing array of foods and beverages.

MSG makes foods taste better, by causing a chemical reaction in our mouth to keep us coming back for "just one more." We eat more and buy more…a manufacturer's dream. No wonder it is added to all kinds of foods. Manufacturers are not likely to stop using these additives anytime soon—the prepared foods market is too lucrative.

George R. Schwartz, M.D. described this critical problem in his excellent book, *In Bad Taste: The MSG Syndrome,* *(Health Press, 1999).* You may want to read his book for more details.

In Bad Taste focuses on the role of MSG in learning and behavioral disorders in children, as well as degenerative neurological syndromes that occur later in life, but it didn't address the damage to women's hormonal systems that leads to the health problems I describe.

I am taking this extensive MSG research to a new level: daily use of MSG and other excitotoxins can adversely affect women's health and reproductive system via their effects on our brain.

Manufacturers won't tell you this, and most doctors don't know it.

Another man-made excitotoxin is *HVP* or *hydrolyzed vegetable protein* (sometimes shown on food labels simply as vegetable protein or plant protein).

Warning
Excitotoxins can be naturally-occurring or man-made. Even "natural" ones are damaging.

Shameful!
The FDA has failed to warn us of the dangers of these hidden additives in our foods.

Duh…
MSG and "flavor enhancers" make us want to eat more… and more… Then we wonder why we are a nation of *obese* kids and adults?

HVP is derived from plants that aren't fit to eat, but are high in the excitatory amino acids such as glutamate or aspartate. The plants are processed with acid and caustic soda, dried, and made into a concentrated powder that contains *a potent mix of the same three known excitotoxins—glutamate, aspartate, and cystoic acid.*

Just do it!
It is up to you to eliminate these damaging additives from your diet.

In spite of the known adverse brain effects, it is almost hard to find something that doesn't have HVP! It is in protein drinks (an obvious place), but also finds its way into cereals, frozen dinners, diet meals (without it, these meals would taste like cardboard), sauce mixes, soups, salad dressings, diet drink powders you mix with milk or water, to name a few.

The research about adverse effects is compelling, but the food industry has fought to keep this hidden from the general public.

Even babies weren't spared getting dosed with MSG. Manufacturers add flavor enhancers to intensify the flavor of baby foods and stimulate babies to eat more. MSG consumption in infancy and childhood makes kids eat more and also alters brain pathways.

It wasn't until 1970 that adding MSG to baby foods was finally stopped as an outgrowth of brain research by Dr. John W. Olney. Dr. Olney showed that the amount of MSG in even one jar of baby food was enough to cause permanent cell death in crucial areas of the retina and brain during development. Damage to the ultra-sensitive hypothalamus was especially severe.

Be Aware
MSG and HVP are found in so much of what you eat today.

Dr. Olney's studies showed that high dose exposure to MSG in mice caused the pituitary glands and ovaries or testicles to *shrink* (*hypoplasia*). That's not exactly what you need!

High dose MSG also caused a major loss of the pituitary secretion of Luteinizing Hormone (LH), and Growth Hormone (GH). But even more alarming, *low doses* that were well *below* toxic levels, caused abnormally *high* LH and loss of the normal bursts of GH secretion.

As a result, "MSG babies," were short in stature, obese and had difficulty reproducing. Reduced GH explained the short stature and obesity. Abnormal levels of LH explained the infertility. These same body changes are seen in girls with PCOS, a serious neuroendocrine disorder in young women that causes infertility. (See Chapter 13.)

The reproductive disruptions and infertility found in all the animal studies are strikingly parallel to what I see in patients.

The combined evidence suggests that excitatory amino acids cause damage to the hypothalamus so that the hypothalamus–pituitary–ovarian pathways can't work properly. This in turn contributes to the many endocrine abnormalities seen in PCOS and other reproductive disorders as women reach puberty.

I am convinced that excitotoxins hitting the brain in the womb, in infancy and childhood play an insidious role in the development of ovarian dysfunction, including PCOS and other "hormone havoc" syndromes I see in women.

Scientists have also discovered that a *human* infant's brain is *far more sensitive to damage* from excitotoxins than the brains in all other species studied. Unlike animals, human brains have additional development during infancy and childhood, not just while in our mother's womb.

The data became so overwhelming about this hidden health hazard to babies that researchers raised the alarm to Congress, which banned MSG additives to baby foods.

This was too late for the generation of children born in the 40s, 50s, and 60s (actually, many of the baby boomers, including me) who ate baby food laced with large amounts of this additive.

I am certain that this is another factor for the high incidence of reproductive disorders and subtle forms of "learning disorders" in adults now between the ages of 30 to 60. These are the *same* kinds of learning and abnormal hormone effects seen in all the animal species exposed to MSG in studies.

It is more frightening to realize excitotoxins are still added to baby foods today, in spite of the ban, as *caseinate, beef or chicken broth,* and *"natural flavorings"—all of which may be made from sources high in these excitatory amino acids.*

Scientists think that the rise in learning disorders, impulse control disorders, behavioral problems, and premature puberty is triggered, in part, by these additional excitatory amino acid additives.

Liquid forms of excitotoxins are much more toxic to the brain than dry because they are absorbed faster and produce higher blood levels than when ingested in solid foods. Since their damage primarily hits the hypothalamus and "learning and memory" centers, the effects aren't seen until you are much older, so you don't realize they are a problem.

Caution
MSG banned from baby foods has now morphed into other chemicals that consumers don't recognize.

Warning
Why are *diet* soft drinks a problem? They contain MSG or aspartate, found in the Nutrasweet used to sweeten them.

Adults are hit with damaging effects of excitotoxins. Studies link the rising rate of degenerative diseases in older people to a lifetime of excitotoxin consumption in food and soft drinks.

Danger
When you look at how many soft drinks an average American drinks every week, you can see there is a serious potential for causing hormonal chaos.

Diseases, like Parkinson's, ALS (Amyotrophic Lateral Sclerosis, or Lou Gehrig's disease), Alzheimer's, MS, and other less common debilitating nervous system disorders, may have additional primary causes, but the evidence is strong that excitotoxins increase brain damage and younger onset of symptoms.

These links are described in detail in an excellent book by neurosurgeon Russell L. Blaylock, MD, called *Excitotoxins: The Taste That Kills* (Health Press, Santa Fe, NM, 1994.)

Common neurological disorders—such as migraine headaches, some forms of daily "tension" headaches, strokes, and seizures (particularly the more subtle types, such as complex partial, absence-type and petit mal seizures) are also linked to these same excitotoxins.

I am suspicious that there is also a link between high intake of dietary excitatory amino acids and damage to the pituitary-ovarian hormone production in young women who develop the mysterious "Chronic Fatigue Syndrome" and diffuse muscle pain syndromes. We lack research to confirm this.

We do know, however, that dietary excitatory amino cause subtle nerve cell damage in hormone-governing centers. This can lead to premature decline in your ovarian hormones!

Brain Basics: Your Body's Chief Executive Officer and Chief Operating Officer

Our hormones affect our brain directly, and our brain regulates hormone production by endocrine glands throughout the body. Our brain is far too complex for me to find a perfect metaphor for its function.

Clever
Think of a CEO and COO of a multi-trillion dollar, global company.

Your CEO brain has to oversee incredibly complex actions, interactions, ramifications, repercussions, and constantly changing information bombarding it from thousands of sources constantly 24 hours a day, 365 days a year.

Your brain has to organize, analyze, direct, execute, evaluate, delegate and coordinate—all day long, and all night long.

The Brain's Communicators

Nerve cells have to "talk" to each other for our brain and body to work as a coordinated whole. They connect to each other by branches we call *axons* and *dendrites*.

Chemical messengers called *neurotransmitters* travel back and forth across gaps (*synapses*) between the nerve endings to pass messages from one nerve to another.

Hormones also act as messengers, helping nerve cells carry their messages. Our hormones also "talk" to nerve cells and to neurotransmitters like serotonin by way of special "docking sites" that we call *receptors*, specific for each type of molecule.

Neurotransmitters and our hormones also have docking sites on the cells of the immune system, as well as our endocrine glands, the intestinal tract, and other organs all over the body.

There are many chemical messengers in the body, but I want to focus on those most critical to the interactions between our hormones and the brain: *serotonin* (5-HT), *norepinephrine* (NE), *dopamine* (DA), *acetylcholine* (ACh), *gamma aminobutyric acid* (GABA), *glutamate*, *N-acetylaspartate* (NAA). These neurotransmitters scurry throughout our brain and body, day in and day out, relaying and modulating information between cells in different parts of the body. **These same chemical messengers and pathways are** *ones that are seriously disrupted by excitotoxins.*

We make these information-carrying molecules from "building blocks" called *amino acids,* found in the food we eat. We need various vitamins and minerals as catalysts and cofactors for the synthesizing enzymes to make the neurotransmitters.

If you don't eat a healthy, balanced diet, your body can't make neurotransmitters *or* hormones, or make them work properly.

When you drink a lot of soft drinks, the *excitotoxins* cause even more damage by *interfering with your ability to absorb vitamins and minerals.*

Your brain's chemical messengers have incredibly diverse roles and functions. Serotonin, for example, turns out to be involved in many behavioral dimensions of our lives, including aspects we previously thought were caused by "psychological conflicts."

Pain, sleep, anxiety, and eating are all regulated by serotonin. We need the right balance: insomnia, anxiety, and overeating can

Connect

Our hormones work as chemical communicators that facilitate connections and help brain functions run smoothly.

Critical Communicators

5-HT
NE
DA
GABA
ACh
NAA

Dr. Vliet's Guide: Major Brain Areas and What They Do

- **Cerebral Cortex:** our master "thinker," and overseer for integrating information between the body and the outside world; it is made up of the brain's frontal, temporal, parietal and occipital lobes.

- **Limbic System:** Deep in the brain, in what we call the "sub-cortical" area, lie several structures that regulate many functions we called the human "drives" (appetite, thirst, sex, aggression, sleep-wake cycles). The limbic system is crucial to our discussion in this chapter because it encompasses our body's master hormone regulators, the *hypothalamus* and *pituitary,* that oversee endocrine regulation, memory processing, mood and emotion, alertness, focus, movement coordination, and helps integrate sensory information, including pain. Pain-carrying signals from the body relating to *chronic* pain come through the limbic center, while *acute* pain pathways bypass the limbic system and go directly to the higher brain centers. This is one reason that chronic pain shatters the stability of our mood and sleep governing centers, and causes more insomnia and depression along with the pain. People suffering acute pain usually do not have such depression or severe sleep disturbances .

- **The Cerebellum** lies below the cortex and to the back of our head. Its major role is to coordinate movement (with the cortex), balance, and fine-motor control. For example, imbalance seen with alcohol intoxication and the abnormal movements seen in Parkinson's disease result from damage to these movement-control pathways.

- **The Brainstem (Midbrain, Pons, Medulla):** This group of structures regulate our "survival functions," such as respiration, heart rate, and blood pressure in response to all the information it receives from multiple connections in the brain and spinal cord.

- **The Spinal Cord:** This is a thick band of nerve fibers that connects to the brain at the base of the skull and travels the length of our spine to the low back. It carries all the nerve tracts and the constant flow of chemical messengers from the body to the brain and from the brain back to the body so that our brain and body functions can be properly coordinated.

© 2001-2007 Elizabeth Lee Vliet, M.D.

each occur when serotonin is either too low or too high. Serotonin imbalances may also cause other behavioral problems, from compulsive shoplifting and gambling, to compulsive sexual behaviors, compulsive hand washing, and hair-pulling (*trichotillomania*).

The *balance of* brain chemical messengers also helps regulates mood: Mania can result from excessive levels of norepinephrine and dopamine. Depression can occur when serotonin, dopamine, and/or norepinephrine are either produced in inadequate amounts or the receptor sites are not functioning properly.

Depression of this type is a *biological* disorder occurring as a direct result of marked changes in these chemical messengers and an alteration in the receptor numbers and sensitivity. It is *not* a "character" problem or lack of willpower.

Attention deficit disorders are also affected by the balance between serotonin and norepinephrine and affected by the decline in estradiol and testosterone as women grow older.

Abnormal dopamine production and function appear to be the primary disturbances causing schizophrenia and Parkinson's disease. Loss of acetylcholine, accentuated by loss of estradiol, is a primary deficiency leading to Alzheimer's dementia.

Irritable bowel syndrome and fibromyalgia are two of many so-called "vague" medical problems aggravated, if not caused by, serotonin and norepinephrine imbalances also aggravated by low estradiol or excess progesterone.

Glutamate is another widespread chemical messenger in the brain, along with its acidic amino acid relatives such as N-acetylaspartate (NAA). Glutamate is an *excitatory neurotransmitter* that is used by about 40% of the brain's nerve junctions.

Remember, excitatory amino acids stimulate nerve cells to fire. *Inhibitory* amino acids, like GABA, described below, *slow down* nerve cell activity. Glutamate plays a key role in learning and memory formation, among other functions. "Learning" results in an immediate release of glutamate, followed later by another release of glutamate during memory processing. We seem to require this increase in glutamate outside the nerve cells in order to properly consolidate, or "store," long-term memory.

When glutamate is released from nerve cells, it is then taken up by special cells called *astrocytes* and converted to *glutamine*,

Vital
They link our emotional and physical health.

Fact
Ovarian, thyroid, and adrenal hormones influences the balance of these neurotransmitters. Tiny molecules have powerful effects!

Fact
Excitatory amino acids are stimulants like cocaine. Inhibiting amino acids are depressants like Valium.

Scary
Concentrated glutamine, glutamate, glutamic acid-herbal mixtures sold in health food stores as memory "boosters" can actually damage memory pathways.

Caution
Many different types of glutamate receptors explain why many diseases can result from this one compound.

Injury
Brain injury such as a concussion, releases high levels of glutamate from nerve cells in the area of injury.

which is returned to the neurons that require it for their function. Glutamine is then used again to make more glutamate.

The *balance* of glutamate delivered to nerve cells appears to be critical in how well they can function. If *too much glutamate* is delivered at one time, short-term memory can be disrupted. *Memory loss* can occur when the extra glutamate causes over-excitation, or activation, of nerve cells.

I strongly recommend you avoid such supplements, especially since there is already such widespread presence of glutamate and aspartate in foods and beverages today. Taking these memory boosters delivers a large dose all at once, which disrupts the normal functioning of the memory pathways.

L-aspartic acid, another amino acid in this group, can also block glutamate uptake into nerve cells and interfere with memory processing. Other substances can also damage memory processing if they interfere with either the production of glutamate or with action of glutamate receptors.

Glycine is another amino acid that affects both normal action and the toxicity of glutamate and aspartate. The amount of glycine in the diet or in supplements contributes to glutamate damage.

There is also evidence that continued over-excitation of glutamate-regulated channels in the brain is one cause of nerve damage and cell death in a number of neurodegenerative disorders such as ALS, Parkinson's, Alzheimer's, and subtle types of seizure disorders, among others.

Concussions, or blows to the head that do not cause a skull fracture, can cause significant short-term memory loss because brain damage from the blow leads to high levels of glutamate in the hippocampus, our primary memory center.

Strokes, seizures and high blood pressure also cause extremely high levels of glutamate release in areas of injury as well as a breakdown in the protective blood-brain barrier.

People who have had brain injuries should be even more careful to avoid excitatory amino acids in foods and beverages because these chemicals cause even more brain damage.

N-acetylaspartate (NAA, for short) is the second most abundant amino acid in our brain, found mostly in the nerve cells. NAA itself hasn't been found to have specific neurotransmitter effects but it is important to our discussion of excitotoxins because of what it does, and because of how it can be affected by the amount of aspartate, glutamate, and cysteine in our diets.

The NAA balance available to nerve cell seems to be critical. *Low* levels of NAA have been found in the brains of people with such severe degenerative neurological disorders as Alzheimer's or Huntington's disease.

Awash High levels of offending chemicals in the bloodstream can bathe the hypo-thalamus directly.

Excessively high levels of NAA, on the other hand, actually disrupt the formation of myelin, a protective fatty sheath around nerves that helps conduct of nerve impulses. Multiple sclerosis is a disease in which myelin is lost and leads to progressive loss of nerve function. I am not aware of any research investigating levels of NAA in MS patients, but clearly this needs to be done.

Chemicals in our environment and in our diet can disrupt *any* of our hormones and chemical messengers and cause depression, anxiety, insomnia and other brain symptoms.

In spite of what current advertisements want you (and your doctor) to believe, depression is not just a "serotonin deficiency." Nor is it always "psychiatric" in the usual sense. Many causes are "medical," physical-endocrine-metabolic changes that affect the physical function of brain pathways overseeing our moods. See the chart below for some of these diverse, common causes.

The Many Triggers of Mood and Anxiety Problems

- *Hormonal changes:* loss or decline of estradiol and testosterone, imbalance of estradiol and progesterone (especially excess progesterone relative to low estradiol), thyroid too low or too high, excess or deficiency of cortisol.
- *Nutritional factors:* deficiencies of key vitamins and minerals, excess or deficiency of amino acids, imbalance of protein, carbohydrate and fat.
- *Metabolic imbalances:* abnormal glucose regulation, such as rapid rises or falls in blood glucose, or levels that are too low or too high;, sodium-potassium imbalances, and iron deficiency.
- *Infectious organisms:* viruses and bacteria that damage the brain directly or have indirect effects via damage to the thyroid and ovary hormones that in turn affect our moods.
- Environmental exposures: food additives, pesticides, xenobiotics, heavy metals, molds, and other chemicals. Many of these can disrupt formation or action of neurotransmitters and hormones. (For more details, see Chapter 5).

© 2001-2007 Elizabeth Lee Vliet, M.D.

How Do Excitotoxins Affect the Pituitary and Ovaries?

Let's look at just how excitotoxins wreak so much havoc in our brain and our hormone balance.

Sensitive Sites, Hardest Hit

The **hypothalamus**, as I mentioned earlier, is the master controller for our hormone systems, body temperature, appetite regulation, body weight, sleep cycles, and a host of other critical functions. It is a brain area extremely sensitive to excitatory amino acid damage.

The hypothalamus is so vulnerable because, even in adults, *it lacks the protective blood-brain barrier* found in the rest of the brain. This is one reason that Dr. Olney and other brain researchers have been so concerned about the increasing *use* of MSG, HVP, cysteine, and aspartate as food additives.

Dr. Ralph Dawson showed that even low doses of MSG produced profound alterations in sex hormone release via the hypothalamus that it caused marked abnormalities in the onset of female puberty.

Mice (remember, they are less sensitive than humans) given low doses of MSG had decreased estrogen binding at the hypothalamic receptors, abnormal patterns of LH and LHRH release, delayed vaginal opening, and disturbances in sexual behavior.

Even *subtoxic* doses of MSG can cause severe abnormal changes to the hypothalamus and thereby disrupt our entire endocrine "control center."

I wonder if these food additives might be yet another reason I see some young women that need much higher than usual blood levels of estradiol to maintain their sense of normal mood, sleep and memory. A lifetime of soft drinks and "flavor-enhanced" foods act in your brain to change the way the estrogen receptors respond, much like a computer virus disrupts computer functions. More estradiol is then needed to counteract the effects of these excitatory amino acids that have disrupted hypothalamus pathways.

With what I know now, I shudder to think about all the MSG I added to foods when I was a teenager, and all the hundreds of "diet" soft drinks I consumed in high school, college, and medical school. I quit drinking them in 1983, and doubt that

I've had more than a half dozen in the last 20 years. But the damage was probably already done.

I had no way of knowing then, but I suspect this was a factor in some of the ovarian hormone imbalances and weight gain I have had since my mid-twenties. It was in college and the 10 years afterwards that I really guzzled those diet sodas. That was about the time I really started having menstrual irregularities and weight gain similar to that seen with PCOS.

I hate to admit this, but I also smoked cigarettes in college and for a couple of years afterwards. Boy, was that dumb. I finally got smart and quit before I was 25. Cigarettes had these same flavor-enhancer chemicals added, unbeknownst to us consumers. Toxicity of cigarette smoke caused an even greater neurotoxic effect with the EAAs in foods and soft drinks (See Chapter 6). So I was getting an overload of these chemicals that damaged the hypothalamus, and I didn't realize it.

Unfortunately, the damage is not limited to the hypothalamus. Two other hormones, thyroid and cortisol, are adversely affected by glutamate. This can lead to weight gain and also interfere with the normal function of ovaries.

MSG causes both *"miswiring"* of nerve pathways and *"misfiring"* of nerve signals during brain development, which affects *all* the endocrine glands the brain oversees. This explains why thyroid and adrenal gland hormones, as well as the ovaries, are altered.

Dose Effects: Animals and Humans, Infants, and Adults

Human infant brains are many times more sensitive to damage by excitotoxins like MSG and aspartate than the brains of animals used in *all* the studies. This really shouldn't surprise us, since the human brain is one of the most complex and highly organized in all the animal kingdom.

Dr. Olney's studies showed that *human* children get a 20-fold increase of glutamate in blood levels while the same dose causes only a 4-fold increase in mice. *That's a huge difference.* This fact is overlooked by people who dismiss the toxicity concerns of MSG and aspartate based on the studies in mice.

The human brain continues to develop throughout childhood, not just while in the womb, unlike mice. The foods we eat and

Warning

Getting EAAs in liquid form from soft drinks is far more damaging than solid food because they are more readily absorbed and reach higher levels in the blood.

File Not Found

The brain on too much MSG is like having a computer virus take over you computer's operating system and change all the settings.

Caution

MSG causes both *"miswiring"* of nerve pathways and *"misfiring"* of nerve signals during brain development.

the chemicals we are exposed to during infancy and childhood have additional potential for harm.

Dr. Olney found that human children often get MSG doses in the range of 100–150 mg per kilogram of body weight just by eating manufactured foods containing these flavor-enhancers and hydrolyzed vegetable protein, and his work was done forty years ago *when 12 oz. cans of soft drinks were all we had.*

Today's prevalent 32 and 64 oz. super-jumbo drinks were non-existent then. Parents have no clue what subtle brain damage is occurring with all the soft drinks kids have.

Timing of exposure is critical. Mother nature has carefully choreographed the complex process of egg and sperm uniting and then dividing and dividing to ultimately become an embryo, then a recognizable human infant in the womb. Each day of gestation is important, with certain developmental events unfolding in sequence. Disrupt one step and another cannot occur properly.

Excitatory amino acids and environmental endocrine disruptors are so incredibly damaging to the brain—they interrupt this normal developmental sequence.

Day 56

The momentous day of human gestation when a female is transformed into a male —IF the Y chromosome is activated with the right amount of testosterone.

That's also why the endocrine disruptors you will read about in the next chapter are often called *"gender-benders."* Tiny amounts of these chemicals are so powerful they can completely derail the process of gender development, preventing the full complement of male or female characteristics from being displayed at puberty, adolescence, and adulthood.

We are all genetically programmed to be female, and have a female cyclic brain pattern of response. Unless the embryo gets the proper signal at the proper time to trigger the testes to start pumping out testosterone.

If the embryo gets the signal activating a gene on the Y chromosome at just the right time, then testicular testosterone begins to be produced and changes the basic primordial female brain pattern into a *male one.* The brain pattern is programmed to steady testosterone levels (*tonic* pattern) throughout life rather than the cyclic pattern of sex hormones women have. Fetal tissue that would have become ovaries, uterus, and vagina develops as penis, testicles, and prostate.

When does this momentous event occur? **Day 56.** If *anything* interferes with the activation of this Y chromosome gene on day 56, it can alter this exquisitely timed sequence of hormone messages and permanently skew the male pattern of brain, body, and hormone development.

If environmental or dietary chemicals interfere with mother nature's plan on day 56 in human gestation, a genetic male embryo can be left in a bizarre "limbo" state—genetically male, but with his male body and hormone patterns not operating normally for the rest of his life.

Chuckle
Don't you know men will love finding out they *really* started out as female!

This is one explanation for the rising incidence reported in the last two decades of stunted penises, undescended testicles and lower sperm counts in male children, findings reported from around the world. Countries still using pesticides banned in the United States (but still exported by U.S. companies that manufacture them) have the highest incidence of these male abnormalities.

Studies on women lag behind. There are similar disruptive effects in female embryos and developing babies, but these are harder to quantify because the changes are more subtle changes, such as endometriosis and "unexplained" infertility. Women's internal reproductive organs are more difficult to directly observe and quantify, unlike males where the penis is visible.

Other Diet Risks for Your Ovaries: Excess Fats and Sugars

Sometimes we really don't want to know everything we are eating. We enjoy a particular food, we want it, we buy it, it tastes good and we play ostrich to what might really be there and what it "may" do to us later.

DRAT!
It isn't just fat that makes you fatter. So does excess sugar.

If you consider the role diet plays in disrupting optimal ovarian function, it's time to take your head out of the sand.

Excess body fat (as in obesity) as well as too little body fat (as in anorexia) can *both* cause irregular menstrual cycles, abnormal ovulation, infertility and a variety of other hormone problems.

We have an epidemic of obesity in children today, not to mention the staggering rise in obesity-induced diabetes in elementary school age children. Fertility problems lurk in the future.

Girls are particularly hard hit: childhood obesity leads to premature puberty, increased risk of PCOS and endometriosis, increased risk of infertility, a later risk of diabetes, and a higher risk of developing breast cancer, even before menopause.

Excess Fats and Your Ovaries: What's The Connection?

Most women don't realize that the average American diet is about 45% fat, a culprit in many health problems that affect your ovaries, and your overall health.

Heads up!
If you want to be around to "worry" about menopause, pay better attention to what you are eating now in your younger years.

The *Persistent Organic Pollutants* (POPs) accumulate in fat tissues because they don't dissolve well in water (See Chapter 5).

That means the fat of animals and fish, the fats your food is fried in, and even your own body fat, become the depository for all these POPs that subtly, but persistently, permeate your body systems and damage important hormone pathways. The more fat in your diet, the higher your exposure to these endocrine disruptors. The fatter you get from the fat in your diet, the more your body becomes a storehouse for these toxic chemicals.

Most women have heard *ad nauseum* about saturated fats that increase the risk of heart disease. Long before that happens, however, you may inadvertently sabotage your fertility or make endometriosis or PCOS worse by eating a lot of fats. High saturated fat causes increased body fat which increases your load of estrone, which helps the growth of both endometriosis and fibroids.

What's the message?
Be careful what you eat or drink (or smoke or inhale or spray into and around your body) during these critical early days of pregnancy

The more you eat, the more likely you are to develop early onset of insulin resistance, and then diabetes. As you get older, the more saturated fats you have eaten over your lifetime, the greater your risk of heart and blood vessel disease, and the greater your risk of developing breast, colon and/or uterine cancer.

What are some of the fat shockers lurking in those tasty foods we enjoy? Getting this list on the previous pages together even makes me feel guilty for enjoying some of them! Most of us don't think about the damage we can do in just a few minutes of indulgence.

Sugars in Soft Drinks and Everywhere Else

Sugars in these soft drink beverages add further to the neuron damage of excitotoxins by making you fatter and increasing your risk of insulin resistance. Excess intake of sugars leads to a type of cell-damagers called AGEs, or *advanced glycosylation end-products*. These AGEs literally *age* your cells at the same time they fill you with empty calories that make you gain weight.

A recent study at Boston Children's Hospital confirmed the obvious: consumption of sugar-sweetened drinks in childhood leads to obesity in children!

Ratchet down your sweet tooth. Be wary of these "no fat" but high sugar "diet" snacks cookies and frozen desserts. Your brain and body will feel better and work better for you—and so will your ovaries.

Vegetarian Diets: Benefits to Your Body, Pitfalls for Ovarian Health

Low B12
Vegetarian diets are also notoriously low in B12 because the richest sources of this vitamin are animal foods.

I am not against vegetarian diets per se, but I think they have been excessively glorified in the media. Most women don't realize the potential pitfalls of vegetarian diets or how carefully you must plan vegetarian meals in order to make certain you are getting complete proteins, adequate vitamins, and minerals.

If a vegetarian diet isn't properly balanced, you end up with subtle deficits of essential amino acids, vitamins and minerals that can lead to increased problems with infertility, earlier ovarian decline, increased fatigue, muscle pain syndromes, and other "vague" problems.

What are some of the *well-documented nutritional deficits of vegetarian diets*, especially with a true *vegan* diet that has no meat, fish, dairy, or eggs?

Vegetarians have been found to have *low levels of three crucial minerals: iron, zinc, and magnesium*, in part because the plant sources provide less than optimal amounts of iron and also a type (non-heme iron) that is not as well absorbed. High fiber and phytate content of a plant-based diet also impairs absorption of these minerals.

Magnesium, in particular, is a crucial mineral to help defend against the cell damage from the excitotoxins you read about earlier.

Depending on the soil content where vegetables and grains are grown, vegetarian diets may be deficient in *iodine* as well, which in turn impairs thyroid function, another factor in infertility.

Many vegetarians also have *inadequate protein intake*, substantiated in many studies from different cultures. This is one of the reasons more vegetarian women have menstrual irregularities.

Many grains and vegetables have high levels of estrogen-like compounds (*phytoestrogens*) that attach to the body's estrogen

Caution

In younger women, phyto-estrogens in soy can also suppress the menstrual cycle and decrease hormone production, which then impairs fertility.

receptors and impair the ovaries' hormone production. This is another reason for the menstrual irregularities and higher incidence of infertility in vegetarians.

Cassidy and colleagues in the UK analyzed the influence of a soy-based diet on the hormonal status and menstrual cycle in premenopausal women with regular ovulatory cycles. 60 grams of soy protein containing 45 mg isoflavones was given daily for 1 month. This caused a significant increase in length of the follicular phase and delayed menstruation.

We see similar responses with tamoxifen, an anti-estrogen. These effects are due to non-steroidal isoflavones and phytoestrogens that sometimes behave as estrogen "boosters" (*agonists*) and sometimes function as estrogen "blockers" (*antagonists*).

Soy foods in modest amounts may have some potential benefit with respect to later risk factor of breast cancer and high cholesterol. Studies have shown, and the media has reported, that "eating vegetarian" has cardiovascular benefits due to a lower intake of saturated fats. That's true.

Too low

Low fat diets mean you can develop symptoms of low estrogen at unexpectedly early ages.

But for younger women who may be trying to become pregnant, too *little* fat means less of the building blocks to make ovarian hormones, which in turn increases the risk of infertility.

It's trendy to eat vegetarian these days. If this is what you want to do, then pay careful attention to getting adequate protein, combining foods properly to get all of the essential amino acids, and eating the right balance of foods to insure adequate levels of key vitamins and minerals critical for the body's production of hormones and other chemical messengers. Your brain and body deserve it.

Caution

A vegetarian diet is one you can't approach haphazardly and expect to stay healthy.

In Summary

These are serious health issues that haven't adequately made it into mainstream medicine. Start now to eliminate as many of the sources of excitotoxins in your diet as possible.

The bottom line is that excitatory amino acids in your foods disrupt function of the hypothalamus that oversees the pituitary, which in turn regulates ovary cycles and other endocrine organs that produce hormones. It is *your* brain and body that is getting messed up.

As far as we know with certainty, you only have one life to live. Don't let it—and your health—slide away in a slurp of soda and fat. I hope these shocking facts will make you think twice about what you're eating and drinking when you decide to skip breakfast and have a soft drink. Or grab a Big Mac and fries for lunch. Or have your daily indulgence with one of these ubiquitous "fun foods." I am not saying don't ever eat these things, but stay aware of the pitfalls.

When you think about the collective impact on our *neuro-endocrine* system, you can see why premature puberty, PMS, PCOS and POD are all on the rise.

Watch how often you have the unhealthy foods, and control your portion size—you really don't have to eat the whole thing all at once.

Don't just unconsciously reach for what's easiest or quickest.

Stop and ask yourself:

- ₰ "Do I really want this? Will something else satisfy me?"
- ₰ Consider other options that are a better use of your daily calorie and fat allowance.
- ₰ Cut out the diet soft drinks and the flavor-enhanced snack foods—the excitotoxin load builds up every day of your life, reaching critical levels of damage.
- ₰ Drink water or seltzer instead of soft drinks…they are really much better for you!
- ₰ *You* make a positive difference each time you make a *healthy* choice.

Culprits
Excitatory amino acids. Excitotoxins. Hypothalamic damage. Hormone disruption.

Start now
Each positive change you make is a step toward better hormone balance and a healthier body.

Dr. Vliet's Guide: Sticker Shock: A High Cost to Your Hormone Health

One regular soft drink (12 ounces) = 10 teaspoons of sugar (40 grams!), 140 calories and most of you drink more than one a day. Soft drinks also give you high levels of sodium and phosphates that leach calcium from your body, causing bone loss.

One movie-theater popcorn with "butter" (medium, not jumbo) = 8 potatoes, 910 calories, 75 grams of fat. The carbs in this popcorn are equal to *8 whole potatoes!* With all these calories, and the average rate of burning about 100 calories per mile of walking, you'd have to park about **9 miles** away from the theater to walk off all those extra calories!

One Big Mac and large fries (McDonald's) = the fat content of 1 cup of Crisco (Yuk! Is that what you meant to eat?) Most of us would feel repulsed to think about eating a cup of lard or Crisco. But that's what you are doing here: a Big Mac is 590 calories and 34 grams of fat; if you add this to 26 grams of fat and 540 calories in the fries, you get 60 grams of fat, and over 1130 calories, about the fat equivalent of one cup (2 ounces) of Crisco...plus almost your entire day's worth of calories. Try a grilled chicken <u>without</u> the mayo, and just hold the fries.

One bag of potato chips (15 ounces) = 1 cup of oil (150 grams of fat!), 1400 calories. They are also loaded with "flavor enhancers," those EAAs I described earlier… and FAT. This is more than your whole day's allowance of fat—not to mention almost your entire day's calories—all easily consumed by "couch potatoes" in about 15 minutes! The calories and fat add up fast and you don't even feel all that full, so you don't realize how much you've eaten.

1 pint of Haagen-Dazs ice cream (plain vanilla!) = 2/3 stick of butter It can't be too bad, right? WRONG. At 1080 calories and 72 grams of fat, you'll be sorry when you get on the scale again. Not to mention the 82 grams of sugar…not exactly a "sweet nothing" for your body.

1 Bagel with Cream Cheese = 2½ slices of pepperoni pizza Bagels from specialty stores, at 4 ounces and 350 to 500 calories on average, have twice the size and calories of a traditional bagel. A normal serving of cream cheese is about two tablespoons or 75 calories. But most bagel specialty stores and delis pile on as much as *half a cup* of cream cheese, bumping the calorie count up to 400! Don't do it!

© 2001–2007 Elizabeth Lee Vliet, M.D.

Chapter 5

Ovaries At Risk:
Gender-Benders and Endocrine Disruptors Around You

For years, I have been exploring the links between environmental chemicals and their effects on our endocrine system.

These synthetic, man-made, hormone-like chemicals called **xenoestrogens**, chemicals that interact with the estrogen receptors in our body, sabotage our hormones and increase our long-term risk of diseases like breast cancer.

There are also *xenoandrogens*, and *xenoprogestins*, and some of these chemicals have mixed effects, acting at all of our hormone receptors. Since we now have found that most chemical pollutants disrupt more hormone pathways and receptors than just our sex hormones, they are more appropriately called *endocrine or hormone disruptors*.

These synthetic chemicals have been found in the body fat and breast milk of humans throughout the world, as well as mammals on land and in the oceans, fish, birds, reptiles and amphibians.

Many of these chemicals, such as dioxin, the pesticide DDT and its breakdown product DDE, polychlorinated biphenyls (PCBs) and others have been linked with increasing rates of breast, prostate, testicular and bladder cancers, and endometriosis. But the issues are even broader.

Exposure to these chemicals contributes to the alarming rise in female infertility, ovarian cysts, PCOS, hormone-triggered depression and anxiety, premature ovarian decline or failure, and immune disorders.

Dr. Rachel Carson wrote eloquently in *Silent Spring* of the reproductive damage from the pesticide DDT. DDT use was later banned in the United States but it is still manufactured

Scary
There are ominous indications that xenoestrogens also seriously damage our ovarian function.

Hormone Chaos
You will see why they are called "gender-benders." Their damage is found in studies of all species tested to date.

here for export to countries around the world where it is still in widespread use.

DDT then comes back to us on the winds, oceans, rain and imported foods to continue its dirty work in our bodies. Since *Silent Spring*, the problem has *not* gone away.

Signals
One of the earliest warnings came from Rachel Carson in her classic book *Silent Spring*, first published in 1962

To the contrary, the problem has gotten worse and more ominous today. Creative chemists have exponentially increased the problem by creating even more deadly and persistent chemicals in thousands of common products used daily. We unknowingly are insidiously poisoning our hormone and reproductive systems.

Xenos is a Greek word meaning foreign or different. Our bodies do not have the ability to readily metabolize these chemicals, making them long-lasting and more damaging to our bodies.

Some are known carcinogens; some don't seem to cause cancer, but *all can damage endocrine pathways*. Most have never been studied to determine any *cancer*-causing effects, much less toxicity to reproductive, brain and hormone function.

We are destroying ourselves
We are the only species with a brain creative enough to make chemicals capable of wiping out our entire race.

Although these chemicals may have *estrogenic* or *androgenic* effects, their effects are *consistently negative*. They disrupt our body systems because they are not the same as the hormones produced by our bodies.

Let's look at the way these environmental chemicals put your ovaries, fertility, brain, and long-term health at significant risk. This is a complicated area, but it is critical for you to understand because there are profound implications for you as a woman, and for your daughters and sons.

What Are Endocrine Disruptors and What Do They Do?

These man-made chemicals belong to a group of environmental pollutants that are part of a larger class of both naturally occurring and synthetic molecules that can act like hormones in the body, although they are not really true hormones.

Because these man-made compounds, unlike natural ones, persist for decades or even *centuries* in the environment without being broken down, they are also called *persistent organic pollutants*, abbreviated POPs.

POPs pack a whollop to our endocrine system and hence our bodies: they may accentuate or *disrupt*, or completely *alter* or even *block* actions of multiple body hormones, not just estrogen.

These compounds may mimic or block testosterone, thyroid, insulin or other hormones, so POPs fit under the broader category *endocrine disruptors* and can affect everything in our body that is governed by our hormones—which means just about our entire body!

The number of chemicals with this endocrine-disrupting effect seems to grow almost daily; at this writing we know of several hundred, but that's just the ones that have been studied. There are potentially thousands more. The toxicology studies done before these compounds are put on the market focus only on cancer-causing effects. Chemical manufacturers do not look into *toxic effects* on all these *other* body systems such as killing ovarian hormones.

If your follicles are killed prematurely, it may mean decreased fertility or premature menopause. You then have symptoms like those I have listed in the Introduction that occur when we lose the ovarian hormones our follicles produce.

The endocrine disruptors affect the ovarian pathways in another way: *many of them cause profound damage to the thyroid*, our master metabolic regulator that affects the function of just about everything in the body. Some interfere with iodine metabolism, which can cause hypothyroidism as well as breast and ovarian cysts.

Beyond the ovarian and other endocrine pathways, these toxic chemicals are linked to the rising rates of autism, lower IQ, learning disorders, behavioral disorders, lowered sperm counts in males, and rising rates of testicular cancer.

For example, men in cultures around the world have been found with sperm counts as much as 50% lower than men had just 30 years ago, before there was such widespread use of these toxic chemicals.

From the increase in young women with symptoms of ovarian failure that I see in my practice, and from the worldwide studies, it is clear women are affected too.

Xenobiotics

A whole group of chemical compounds that are man-made, foreign to the body and have generally toxic or damaging biological effects to living organisms.

Technically speaking

Many of these chemicals kill ovarian follicles: the medical term is *follicular toxicants.*

"Egg counts" are hard to determine. We don't have good statistics about the early death of ovarian follicles from these chemicals.

Why now? None of these organic compounds existed before the 1930s.

Unsafe These chemicals made up an alphabet soup far less healthy than the food variety. DDT, DDE, DES, TCDD, BHA, PCB, PBB, PAH, CCA

I do not have the space here to go into all the years of world-wide animal studies that raised the red flags for humans, or the history of how we got in such a mess with chemicals that pollute and sabotage our fertility and survival.

If you are interested in the fascinating detective work done by scientists to identify these health effects in animals and humans, I encourage you to read two outstanding and well-researched books: *Our Stolen Future* by scientist Theo Colborn and her team of Dianne Dumanoski, and John Peterson Myers, and *Living Downstream* by ecologist Sandra Steingraber. Let their descriptions of the animals' plight and their urgent alarm call to humans be your health wake up call.

Why Is This Such a Problem NOW?

Pre-1930s people simply were not exposed to such an incredible array of synthetic chemicals. Most have been invented in the "chemical age" that started just prior to World War II. The 1940s and 1950s are when the world's living beings were first exposed to these pesticides and industrial chemicals on a wide scale. During the period from roughly 1970 through the 1990s, the *first human generation ever* exposed to DDT and other POPs during fetal life began reaching their own reproductive age. Subtle perturbations and disruptions began to appear. We are now seeing the higher cancer rates and health problems in people exposed to these chemicals since the 1940s.

Who are the Players in this Hormone-disrupting Drama?

There are hundreds more in this huge group of chemicals not normally found in nature and are potently toxic for living organisms. The man-made ones are consistently damaging, with serious, widespread toxic effects. Many are known carcinogens.

Their longer names are all listed in the chart that follows on pages 120–121, grouped by categories of where found, type of action, and types of damage they cause.

I want you to have this information available at home so you can check product ingredient labels on foods, cleaning compounds, cosmetics, household "pest" killers, dog and cat flea collars, lawn care products and so on.

Chronology: Development of and Human Exposure to Synthetic Endocrine Disruptors (POPs)

1929: Polychlorinated biphenyls (PCBs) developed

1930s: "nerve gases" developed in Germany, later Used by the Nazis in World War II (1939–1945). Became basis for pesticides.

1938: DDT first synthesized and manufactured and DES synthesized, the first synthetic estrogenic compound

1940–1945: First widespread use of synthetic chemicals worldwide and wide scale exposure to living organisms

1940s–1950s: First human generation to be exposed in infancy

1940s–1970: DES in widespread Use during pregnancy; first human generations born who were exposed to a potent, synthetic estrogenic chemical in the womb

1950s–1970s: First human generations born who had been exposed to many pesticides and other industrial pollutants (POPs) in the womb

1970s–2000: DES daughters and sons health problems manifest

1970s–1990s: First human generation exposed to POPs in the womb now reaching reproductive age when effect of hormone disruptions become more pronounced and noticeable—for women, infertility, endometriosis, PCOS, premature ovarian decline, thyroid disorders, and others.

2000—Second generation DES sons and daughters now old enough for adverse health effects to become manifest

© 2001–2007 Elizabeth Lee Vliet, M.D.

Then there are the *naturally-occurring endocrine-disrupting compounds*, such as the *phytoestrogenic isoflavones of soy, grains and clover*. Heavy metals are found in soils and water. Even though all may have significant "endocrine disrupting" effects, a few of the naturally occurring ones have modest positive effects—such as lower cholesterol seen from a diet higher in phytoestrogens.

But they may also disrupt the menstrual cycle and impair fertility, as seen in cattle feeding on red clover, rich in isoflavones. Others in the naturally occurring group, such as genistein found in soy, have mixed effects: beneficial at some concentrations, and showing adverse effects at other concentrations.

Where Are The Chemical Endocrine Disruptors Found?

Where are they?

POPs are NOW everywhere! Food, air, water, in our homes…

Simply put, *they are now everywhere*. Man-made endocrine disruptors, the persistent organic pollutants —POPs—may be found in the water we drink, the food we eat, the air we breathe, the objects we touch around our homes, workplaces and recreational areas.

They are found in the plastic linings of canned foods and plastic food wrappers. They are found in common chemicals probably sitting under your bathroom and kitchen sinks or in your laundry room and garage.

They are found in cigarette smoke, plastics, detergents, pesticides, herbicides, fungicides, hair dyes, paints, solvents, dry cleaning solutions, cosmetics, food additives and preservatives, fabric coatings, wall coverings, carpets, playground equipment, and vehicle exhaust—just to name a few of the sources we encounter daily.

We also unwittingly add these chemicals into the environment: you may not realize that all the things you flush down the toilet or rinse down the kitchen sink can end up in our water supply, bubbling up in rivers and streams!

A US Geological Survey on 140 waterways in 30 states tracked 95 different pollutants, with these surprising results: 74% of the samples contained insect repellants, 48% contained antibiotics, 40% contained reproductive hormones (e.g. birth control pill estrogens and progestins), 32% contained other prescription drugs, and 27% were found to have chemical compounds used for *fragrances*.

Don't!

Stop and think before you flush old prescriptions, such as birth control pills and antibiotics, or old perfumes or household cleaners, down the toilet.

Animals—and humans—at the top of the food chain accumulate the most POPs in body fat because each step in the series adds a little more of the pollutants to the fatty tissues.

Birds that eat fish from toxic waters every day build up more concentrated levels than are in each fish. Larger prey that eat the birds get a little more, and so on up the food chain.

Polar bears have very high levels of DDT, DDE, PCBs and other chemicals in their body fat because they eat high-fat seals that have eaten contaminated fish.

For human women, the fact that these toxic chemicals build up in fat carries a special risk: we have more overall body fat than do men, and the primarily fatty tissue of our breasts actively store these estrogenic compounds.

Nursing babies then get the full brunt of the mother's chemical storehouse, particularly the first nursing child. As nursing depletes the mother's breast stores of chemicals, subsequent babies receive smaller amounts.

DDT wasn't banned in the U.S. until 1972. All of us born prior to 1972 were exposed to DDT in our diet because the pesticide was commonly found in dairy products and meats as well as on vegetables sprayed with DDT for pest control. If you were born after 1972, you were exposed to DDT from residues in your mother's body fat that flowed across the placenta. As an infant you were getting DDT residues in either human breast or cows milk, since cattle that had eaten grains and grasses with DDT residues would have the persistent chemical in their body fat to then leach into their milk, just as in human breast milk.

In the body, DDT is metabolized to a compound called DDE. Recent research shows that DDE is an *antiandrogen* that blocks testosterone from activating its receptor complex. This receptor blockade causes undescended testicles in young boys, shorter stature, obesity, and less muscle development.

In adult men, DDE causes lowered sperm counts, smaller testicles, and increased testicular cancer. We don't know all the potential adverse reproductive effects DDE has in women. I suspect we will find that it leads to abnormal testosterone production and action in women.

Even though these chemicals are banned in this country, we are still exposed to them everyday because most are still manufactured for export to countries whose laws are less strict. Winds that blow across the ocean to our West Coast carry chemical residues from countries where they are still in use. Besides, banning their use doesn't help much because these chemicals are so long lasting.

Aldrin, a termite killer, is converted to dieldrin in body tissues and in the soil, where it remains for years. Dieldrin suppresses the immune system and causes abnormal brain waves in mammals. Although banned in 1975 in the U.S., Aldrin was allowed as a termite killer until 1987, so people were still exposed to it.

Pregnant women exposed to Aldrin would have daughters in their teens and twenties about now, just about the age we start seeing the reproductive damages, such as endometriosis, PCOS, severe PMS, irregular cycles, immune problems and mood-behavioral difficulties.

POPs
POPs are fat-soluble, they become concentrated in the fat tissues of fish, animals, and humans.

Breast damage
The breasts and breast milk concentrate these chemicals to a significant degree over our lifetime.

Dr. Vliet's Guide to Endocrine-disrupting Chemicals

1. General categories:

A. Man-made chemicals

- industrial and household products, such as pesticides, cleaners, plasticizers, solvents (ex. DDT, DDE, PCB, PBB, PAH, TCDD, dioxins, DEHA, toluene, xylene, perchloroethylene, etc.), triazine herbicides
- Pharmaceuticals like DES (diethylstilbestrol), cyclophosphamide (anticancer drug)
- Dietary supplements and food additives, such as MSG, glutamate, aspartate, cysteine, BHT, BHA (butylated hydroxyanisole)

B. Naturally-occurring compounds

- phytoestrogens in plants
- phthalate esters
- heavy metals (neurotoxins): lead, mercury, arsenic, cadmium, gallium

2. Examples based on types of actions:

Estrogenic

- o,p'-DDT, Methoxychlor, Lindane (organochlorine pesticides), Endosulfan, Dieldrin, Toxaphene
- Kepone (estrogenic effects in male factory workers)
- Nonylphenols (also weak androgen agonist*)
- Bisphenol-A
- DES
- Benzylbutylphthalate, dibutylphthalate
- Genistein, other isoflavones found in soy, clover, grains

Estrogen Blockers (Antiestrogenic)

- PCBs—(polychlorinated biphenyls)(isomers of DDT)
- Dioxin and related dibenzo-p-dioxins
- Dibenzofurans
- Compounds in cigarette smoke
- Genistein (both agonist and antagonist actions, depending on concentration), other isoflavones

Androgen Blockers (Antiandrogenic)

- P,p'-DDE (metabolite of DDT), also DDT*
- Vinclozolin
- Atrazine
- Bisphenol A*
- Butyl benzyl phthalate*

*based on recent data from Sohoni (see references)

© 2001–2007 Elizabeth Lee Vliet, M.D.

Dr. Vliet's Guide to Endocrine-disrupting Chemicals

Act By Other Mechanisms:

- Cyclophosphamide
- Benzo(a)pyrene, anthracenes
- Solvents-toluene, xylene, perchloroethylene)
- Methoxychlor
- Nitrous oxide ("laughing gas" anesthesia)
- Ethylene oxide
- Butadiene
- 4-vinyl cyclohexene
- Alkylphenols
- Phthalate esters
- Triazine herbicides (atrazine, simazine, cyanazine)
- Fungicides (Chlorothalonil, Maneb, Metiram, Thiram, Zineb, Ziram)
- Excitatory amino acids (glutamate, MSG, aspartate, etc.)

3. Examples Based on Type of Damage in Women

These are not all of the types of damages caused. I have listed the ones most relevant to the issue of ovaries at risk, the primary subject of this book.

Health Impact	Chemicals Found to Cause**
Breast Cancer	DDT, DDE, lindane, methoxychlor, PCB, TCDD, possibly DES, triazine herbicides (atrazine, simazine, cyanazine), others likely
Ovarian Cancer	DES, DDE, PCB triazine herbicides (most data is on atrazine), possibly many others
Infertility/impaired fertility	aromatic hydrocarbons in cigarette smoke, Isoflavones (soy, red clover), coumestrol, cyclophosphamide, PCB, TCDD, PAH, organochlorines (DDT, DDE, Lindane,etc.) organic solvents, heavy metals, nitrous oxide, ethylene oxide, 4-vinyl cyclohexene butadiene, DES, glutamate, aspartate
Menstrual irregularity	DDT, DDE, Lindane, heavy metals, PCB, Isoflavones (soy, red clover), coumestrol, PAH, solvents, TCDD, DES, atrazine, glutamate, aspartate
Increased miscarriages	solvents, nitrous oxide, ethylene oxide, DES isoflavones (soy, red clover), coumestrol
Early menopause	PAH, cigarette smoke, butadiene, DES 4-vinyl cyclohexene, phytoestrogens, possibly many others
Endometriosis	Dioxins (many types), TCDD, PCB, DES

Dr. Vliet's Guide to
Endocrine-disrupting Chemicals

Health Impact	Chemicals Found to Cause**
Reduced Lactation	DDE, DES, others not well studied
Osteopenia/Osteoporosis	Cadmium, lead, cigarette smoke chemicals
Thyroid Damage	PCB, organochlorine insecticides (DDT, DDE, Lindane, others), isoflavones (soy, red clover, others), phytates, iodine deficiency (iodine metabolism disrupted by a number of these compounds), MSG, glutamate, aspartate
Immune Damage	PCB, dioxins; dieldrin, may be others. Greater adverse impact on infant with immature immune system when chemicals passed in breast milk
Hypothalamic-	heavy metals, PCB, DES, excitatory amino acids (glutamate, aspartate, cystoic acid, MSG), triazine herbicides (atrazine, etc.)

** Based on studies in animals, humans or both   © *2001–2007 Elizabeth Lee Vliet, M.D.*

You too
Most Americans alive today carry some DDT residues because it is stored in the environment and the body for decades.

Others like chlorpyrifos (Dursban or Lorsban), are still infiltrating our lives and health. It is the active ingredient in over 1,000 products surrounding us daily—from flea and tick collars for pets, and roach and ant sprays under your kitchen counter to the sprays used on crops we eat.

Another group of POPs, called *triazine herbicides* (atrazine, cyanazine, simazine), are water soluble rather than dissolved in fat. They are widely used across the U.S. from the cornfields of the Midwest to the fruit groves of Florida and California. When sprayed on vegetable and fruit crops to kill weeds, they are taken up from the soil into *all* the plants and leach from the soil into the groundwater as well.

We ingest them via produce we eat and in our drinking water. We also get them in meat, poultry, milk and eggs because POPs contaminate corn feeds for cattle and chickens.

Tragic!
No research on DDE has been done on women.

Links between the herbicide triazine and ovarian cancer have been found for women farmers in Italy. These compounds have been in use since the 1950s and yet little has been done to study their link to risk of breast and ovarian cancers, much less investigate the degree of their adverse effects on fertility, reproductive disorders such as endometriosis and PCOS, or hypothalamic-pituitary regulation of our other endocrine systems.

Organohalogens

You may frequently see the term **Organohalogens** Used, and this refers to the following groups of chemicals that have added chlorine (organochlorines) or bromine atoms (organobromines) atoms, which enhances their actions, and their toxicity:

- ⮞ dichlorodiphenyl dichloroethene (DDE)
- ⮞ polychlorinated biphenyls (PCBs)
- ⮞ Polybrominated biphenyls (PBBs)

© 2001–2007 Elizabeth Lee Vliet, M.D.

What Are Gender-bending Endocrine Disruptors Doing To You?

Many of the endocrine disrupters used as pesticides for the last 50 years were actually the chemical descendants, only slightly tamed, of the terrifying organophosphate nerve gases tabun and sarin developed in Germany and used during World War I.

Both the early "nerve gases" and ones developed in recent decades for chemical weapons kill by blocking the critical enzyme cholinesterase so that nerve impulses can't be transmitted and the nervous system can't function to regulate the basic functions of life, such as breathing.

The slightly tamer organophosphates developed since the 1950s for commercial use as pesticides work the same way: they block cholinesterase and paralyze the nervous systems of insects so they die.

Symptoms *people* develop when they have been exposed to these chemicals show how they work to *interfere with nerve function: blurred vision, nausea, shortness of breath, headaches, dizziness, restlessness, agitation, and even asphyxia.*

And those are only the immediate effects. There are delayed effects on your immune system and nerve function. Death of your developing ovarian follicles leads to delayed effects of loss of your ovarian, and thyroid hormones and the resulting damage to body tissues. What about the ways these chemicals work in your body long term to accomplish their wicked tricks on the estrogen receptors? Or the ways they make breast cancer cells grow faster? They are pretty scary!

POPs on your table

Fish, vegetables, and fruits from other parts of the world are imported and bring chemical residues.

Breast Poison

All of these compounds are possible carcinogens, and atrazine is a known endocrine-disruptor linked to breast and ovarian cancers

How Do They Work To Disrupt Our Own Hormones?

Fact
Atrazine inhibits the ability to make testosterone and alters pituitary response to the hormones that oversee ovulation.

There are *many* ways these chemicals disrupt our normal body hormone pathways and damage different body systems. The chart summarizes ways they work to disrupt our endocrine systems.

False Reassurances, Hidden Dangers

The really sad part of the women's health story is that researchers and health care professionals have thought, until very recently, that these chemicals were harmless, in spite of *forty* years of serious reproductive damage in multiple animal populations around the world.

We were lulled into a false sense of security about POPs because there were a number of misconceptions and misunderstandings floating around scientific circles about how they worked.

For example, the estrogenic POPs, and their residues on foods or in water supplies, are present in much lower concentrations in the body than our own body estrogen, so researchers thought there were not enough to do damage. *As we are finding out, this has turned out to be seriously wrong.*

Gulf War Syndrome
Chemicals like this are ones involved in the "strange" symptoms experienced by veterans of the Gulf War.

Researchers also falsely assumed that estrogenic POPs had a chemical structure different enough from our own body estradiol that these molecules could not function as "keys" to unlock or activate at the human estrogen receptor complex.

This was *another profound mistake*, because they *do activate it.*

Lab analyzes have shown POPs to be less potent than our own body estrogens, in some cases a few thousands times weaker, so researchers thought they didn't have much effect in our bodies. *We now know this is also wrong.*

Many weaker estrogenic compounds, including many plant foods we normally eat (soy is a good example), are loaded with compounds that can interfere with normal function of our hormone pathways.

The Emerging Truth

Newer studies reveal a frightening picture far more alarming than many scientists ever realized. The following table gives more detail about these dangerous effects.

I hope this summary helps you see why I am concerned about all the fear focused on hormone therapy when everyone seems to be ignoring the more serious estrogenic threats all around us that wreak insidious havoc with our bodies.

Let's look at the POPs and breast cancer connections and then explore crucial lessons from the DES experience.

Estrogenic Subverters: POPs Wicked Tricks

1. The Human Estrogen Receptor (HER) turns out not to be as difficult to activate as once thought. HER *works best* with the identical estradiol key our ovary makes, but doesn't *require only* this "identical" key for activation. HER is, unfortunately, rather promiscuous—it will *accept many* molecular "keys" of different sizes and shapes and be activated to some degree by all of them.

   That doesn't mean, however, that all of these different "keys" will work the same way or have the same effects in the body, as I have described in detail in my earlier books. In addition, different types of estrogenic "keys" may have *adverse effects over time*, including increased likelihood of cell mutations leading to breast or ovarian cancers.

2. Estrogenic POPs are far more common than researchers realized. Many different compounds and chemicals we use every day at home or in the workplace fall into this category.

   Many organic compounds, such as pesticides, plastics, paints, chemical fragrances, chemical air fresheners, detergents and many others, can trigger estrogenic effects even if their molecules don't look anything at all like estradiol!

3. For even more damage, estrogenic POPs gang up on us, acting *together* to create even worse effects than any one compound alone. In medicine, we refer to this as a *synergistic* effect. In this case, $1 + 1 + 1$ does NOT equal 3, it may equal 300, or 3000, instead!

   Profound carcinogenic effects have been found when more than one of these compounds is present, even if each one is present in a very low concentration. Dr. Abou-Donia at Duke University showed that the pesticide *chlorpyrifos* when combined with another organophosphate *propetamphos*, caused catastrophic destruction of the nervous system in doses *lower* than chlorpyrifos would alone.

4. Even though estrogenic POPs are *less potent* on laboratory

Here's how…
POPs and excitotoxins are able to wreak havoc with the brain's central command centers that direct the function of our entire endocrine system.

Lies, lies and damned lies
Lab analyzes showed POPs to be less potent than our own body estrogens, so researchers thought they didn't have much effect in our bodies. *Wrong*!

Sad truth

The true picture is not as simple or as innocuous and reassuring as researchers once thought.

measures than the estrogens our bodies make, they make up for their lower potency by sneaking around the body enzymes that break down hormones, and thereby escape the normal metabolism that our bodies use to deactivate our natural hormones.

DDT is a good example. Although banned in the United States in 1972, women today, over thirty years later, *still* have measurable DDT residues in their body fat and breast tissue from earlier environmental exposure.

Our natural hormones are broken down in metabolism in a few hours.

For example, if you take off an estradiol patch, the blood levels drop down within about 12 hours. If you take a tablet of estradiol, it is metabolized to less active or inactive compounds in just a few hours, a very short duration of effect.

5. POPs have another trick to overcome their lower concentration and lower potency. Our own hormones (ovarian, thyroid and adrenal) are attached to carrier, or transport, proteins in the bloodstream called sex hormone binding globulin (SHBG), thyroid binding globulin, corticotropin binding globulin, and albumin. The binding proteins hold on to the hormones, and slow down the rate hormones leave the blood to enter cells. This controls the rate that our hormones activate cell receptors.

Wicked!

POPs have some wicked tricks that turn them into serious, insidious weapons and subtle poisons that affect our bodies in terrible ways, especially our ovaries, breasts and brain.

But POPs are different. They don't attach as tightly to these transport proteins as our own sex hormones do. This means POPs are more easily and quickly released from the carriers. Many pesticides behave like this in the body.

6. POPs don't just *mimic* actions of our own estrogens; if they did, they wouldn't be so dangerous. POPs compounds can also *intensify* the effects of our own body estrogens to create new, undesirable effects such as increased risk of cell growth and changes that may lead to cancers.

7. Many different POPs actually block the healthy functions of our own estrogens, making us even sicker from the loss of the beneficial effects of our own body's natural 17-beta estradiol. I have seen this clinically in daughters of mothers who took DES in pregnancy.

8. Some POPs stimulate the body to make more estrogen receptors, which means more sites for estrogen actions, but not always in desirable ways. It also means more different types

Dr. Vliet's Guide to
How Endocrine Disruptors Work

Environmental chemicals that mimic hormones may act in several different ways to disrupt our normal body functions:

- *Duplicate* normal hormone responses, but produce slightly different variations since their molecules are different from our own hormones
- *Block* normal hormone function (much like the drug Tamoxifen does) by interacting with receptors.
- *Interact* with receptors to produce an abnormal response. The exaggerated androgen and insulin production in women with PCOS is an example of this type of effect.
- *Interact* with hormones and/or receptors to produce an additive or synergistic response, leading to exaggerated hormone effect. We think this is one way that these chemicals increase risk for ovarian and breast cancers.
- *Interrupt* normal signaling mechanisms that control making our body's proteins, enzymes and other hormones.
- *Alter genes* that control activation or inactivation of critical pathways. A good example is the Y chromosome gene I described in chapter 4 that has to be activated exactly on day 56 of human gestation to turn on the testicle of a male embryo to make testosterone and convert the "unisex" brain to a male one. If one of these "endocrine disruptors" blocks that gene from turning on at the right time, a genetic male embryo is destined to live out his life in a hormonal and physical "limbo-land, " medically called "inter-sex." I'll tell you more about this problem later in the chapter.
- *Interfere with neurotransmitters* (MAO, ST, NE, DA, ACh, etc.) that oversee the manufacture and release of GnRH, the hormone in the hypothalamus that regulates the pituitary hormones (FSH, LH) regulating the ovaries. The result is disruption of the normal menstrual and reproductive cycles.
- *Direct toxic effects* on nerve cells in the pituitary
- *Direct toxic effects* on the ovaries and testes to disrupt production of sex hormones, kill hormone-producing cells
- *Bind* to hormone receptors on sperm and oocytes (cells that become "eggs") to cause abnormal function and impair fertility

© 2001–2007 Elizabeth Lee Vliet, M.D.

Multipliers
When several estrogenic POPs are present, they may have effects several hundred times, or even several thousand times, greater than any one alone.

Multiplying
This trick enables the estrogenic POPs to persist in the body much, much longer than our own ovarian hormones do

Example
Premarin, a mixture of horse estrogens takes about three months after the last dose to be cleared from the body.

of estrogenic substances can activate all these new receptors. Many researchers think this is one way that pesticides increase the growth of breast cancer cells.

9. Estrogenic POPs can change the way our body estrogens are broken down (metabolized). They push the process toward undesirable compounds that new research shows *increase* the risk for breast cancer.

Our normal healthy direction for estradiol metabolism is the 2-pathway in which it is broken down into "A ring" or catechol estrogens. The undesirable direction for estradiol breakdown is called the 16-pathway, or D-ring metabolites.

Current research on breast cancer shows that *shifting estradiol metabolism more toward the 2 (A ring) pathway actually lowers risk of breast cancer.* A shift the other way, into the 16 (D ring) pathway leads to an *increased risk of breast cancer.*

A number of pesticides like atrazine, benzene, DDT, endosulfan, and some PCBs all push our bodies to make more of the 16, D-ring types of estrogens. It is another insidious way that these chemicals turn our own natural estrogen into a potent chemical weapon. It is rather like a glitch in a torpedo's program that makes it turn back on the submarine that launched it, instead of heading out to its intended target.

Endocrine Disruptors and Breast Cancer

DDT, lindane, chlordane, dieldrin, aldrin, heptachlor, chlorpyrifos, toxaphene, endosulfan, and triazines —all are known or probable carcinogens. For example, toxaphene and endosulfan cause breast cancer cells in tissue culture to grow faster; DDT converts to DDE in the body, and both have been found in levels 50–60% higher in breast cancer patients than women without the cancer.

In 1993, Dr. Mary Wolff at Mt. Sinai School of Medicine in NY published a study showing that women who developed breast cancer had 35% *more DDE* in their blood than women who didn't. Dr. Wolff analyzed the blood specimens of 14,290 women and found that those with the highest DDE levels in their blood were *four times* more likely to have breast cancer than those with the lowest levels of DDE.

In 1990, researchers in Finland found that women with breast cancer had higher concentrations of lindane-like residues in their breasts. The combined blood from women with breast cancer was analyzed and had 50% *more* of this pesticide residue than the blood from women without breast cancer.

An analysis of Connecticut women published in 1992 showed similar trends: levels of PCB, DDE and DDT in the breast tissue of women with breast cancer were 50–60 % higher than in women without cancer.

So why is it that *all* you hear about in the news is the *slight* increase in risk of breast cancer that may occur with some types of estrogen therapy after menopause? There are many other aspects to this cancer link that are imperative to investigate, and more serious.

Similar epidemiological data from Israel links breast cancer rates with the pesticides DDT, lindane, and BHC. After twenty-five years of *rising* breast cancer rates there, two researchers noted that Israel was the only one of twenty-eight countries showing a *significant decrease* in breast cancer rates over the ten-year period that ended in 1986. Israel had allowed use of DDT, BHC, and lindane until the mid-1970s, when they were banned.

Prior to the ban, all three of these pesticides were found in dramatically high concentrations dairy milk, other dairy products, and human breast milk. Two years after the ban, studies of human breast milk from residents of Jerusalem, showed lindane levels dropped 90 percent, BHC levels decreased 98 percent, and DDT levels went down 43 percent.

In countries like Sweden, Germany, and Italy that banned use of DDT in the 1980s, the concentrations of DDE and PCBs in human breast milk have been slowly declining.

In addition to all of this damning evidence, epidemiological studies in the United States have clearly shown that certain occupational groups of women have significantly higher risks of breast cancer than the general public.

Breast cancer data from Hawaii suggests that the significant increase in breast cancer rates over the past few decades are related to endocrine disruption by environmental chemicals.

Agricultural chemicals, including endocrine disruptors, have been used intensively in Hawaii's island ecosystem over the past 40 years, leaching into groundwater, and leading to unusually widespread exposures.

Still here
Estrogenic POPS may remain for *many years* after the last exposure.

You are being poisoned
Women with the highest DDE levels are *four times* higher risk for breast cancer.

Dangerous directions
POPs alter the direction of estrogen metabolism towards more cancer-causing compounds, turning our natural estrogen into a chemical weapon.

Hawaii hazard
Increased breast cancers may be the ominous result of these agricultural chemicals.

Hawaiian women have been significantly exposed, in particular, to two endocrine-disrupting chemicals; chlordane-heptachlor and DBCP (1,2-dibromo-3-chloropropane), at levels that exceeded federal standards by several thousand times.

Specialists there do not think that the increased rates are due solely to improvements in screening and detection; they think this is the result of pesticide exposure.

Different mechanisms allow these environmental estrogenic pollutants to act in ways that increase breast cancer risk and spread the disease once it develops. They attach to the estrogen receptors and ramp up the effects of our own body estrogens, stimulating growth of new blood vessels (*angiogenesis*), altering our DNA, and triggering growth promoting changes in our body's estrogen target tissues.

Yet to date, the American Cancer Society and other U.S. cancer organizations have done little to explore this critical evidence of the role of environmental pollutants in breast and other cancers. *Instead they scare us about our own estrogen, and fuel fear about replenishing hormones after menopause.*

Wake up call!
Women with the highest lindane residues were 10 times more likely to have breast cancer than women with lower levels.

In my view, this ignores the far more serious issues that we face from insidious exposure to these incredibly damaging, known carcinogens in the environment. We've been steeping in them like a teabag in a teapot for most of our life, perhaps since conception. Why isn't the American Cancer Society focusing on what these estrogenic chemicals do to damage our estrogen receptors and make us more susceptible to female cancers?

The American Cancer Society also spends millions of dollars on ad campaigns exhorting us to clean up our lifestyle, change our diet and exercise more. The implication is that if we don't do those things and then get cancer, why it's our fault. Yes, a healthy diet is important, but this is not the only factor in who gets cancer.

Israel's Ban
Within 10 years of the ban on DDT and lindane, there was a drop of 30 percent in breast cancer deaths in women under age 44.

If girls begin menstruating earlier and also delay pregnancy until later, as is common today, there is a longer period of continuous excess estrogen stimulation during critical phases of breast development.

Our total estrogen exposure comes not only from natural body estrogens, but also from all the estrogenic chemicals in our environment, including those causing puberty to switch on too early. It creates a more serious problem for later life if there is too much stimulation of breast growth around puberty, especially if it comes from exposure to non-natural estrogenic chemicals found in POPs.

Most breast cancers in later life begin in the breast ducts. These ducts are formed during the phase of rapid breast growth at puberty just before your menstrual periods begin. Exposure to the environmental estrogens at this stage of development has the potential to cause much more damage than if such exposure comes later on.

The damage that occurs in puberty, however, won't likely appear until you are several decades later. Many scientists now think that exposure to the estrogenic chemicals in childhood and puberty combines with other known risk factors to increase risk of having breast cancer later in life.

Researchers are looking at these endocrine disruptors' effects on male reproductive function, such as lower sperm counts, but they have not yet systematically looked for similar reproductive effects in women.

Many pesticides also interfere with the synthesis of crucial mood-regulating chemical messengers. Dursban (chlorpyrifos) inhibits the conversion of tryptophan to serotonin, a critical neurotransmitter that functions in mood, pain, sleep, appetite, and thirst regulatory pathways.

Where do you find Dursban? It is a common ingredient in many pesticides used in our homes, schools, and workplaces.

If your ovarian hormones are also too low when you are exposed to Dursban, you have a triple whammy:

- ॐ low estradiol leads to loss of serotonin synthesis and function, and
- ॐ decreased absorption of the vitamin and mineral cofactors needed to make more serotonin, and
- ॐ you have the inhibitory, damaging effects from the Dursban.

No wonder women with low estrogen get hit especially hard by pesticides and potent synthetic chemicals. It isn't so surprising that *many women describe experiencing depression after exposure to pesticides and other POPs.*

Israel's Ban
Researchers could not identify any other change to account for these differences *except the prohibition against using the three pesticides.*

Occupational hazard
Women in the petroleum and chemical industries exposed daily to higher concentrations of these same chemicals have higher rates of breast cancer.

Synthetic Estrogenic Substances: What Have We Learned from DES?

Research
A wiser approach would be to use some of the advertising dollars to fund research on cancer links with persistent organic pollutants.

Hormone Havoc
Many of these pesticides also cause earlier onset of puberty.

Later risks
Rapid breast growth in puberty around the time your periods begin is an extremely important factor in your later breast cancer risk.

I have a number of women patients who were "DES babies." It strikes me as more than coincidence that these women have experienced "strange" hormonal problems since puberty. This is a complex problem with many connections. Just what is DES and why is it important in relation to endocrine disruptors?

Diethylstilbestrol, or DES, is a highly potent synthetic, non-steroidal estrogenic compound first synthesized in Britain in 1938. DES was subsequently used medically for over three decades in more than 5 million women in the United States, United Kingdom, Europe and Latin America.

Doctors gave DES to pregnant women thinking that it would prevent miscarriages. Later, DES was more widely used, even in women who had not had prior miscarriages, with the idea that it would create healthier pregnancies and stronger, healthier babies.

DES use was further expanded to include emergency "morning after" contraception, to suppress milk production after delivery in women who did not want to nurse, and for treatment of menopausal symptoms such as hot flashes.

Used in animal feed and hormone implants to fatten livestock, DES was even given to chickens to make them develop faster. Even if your mother was not given DES, you could have been exposed to it during your developmental years in foods your mother ate.

During the time DES was used in the 1940s to 1960s, doctors believed the placenta created a "safety barrier" so that drugs given to a pregnant mother did not harm the developing baby. **This was seriously flawed thinking.**

Many substances do cross the placenta and have profound impact on the developing baby, many of which are permanent and irreversible. Some everyday examples are caffeine, alcohol, cigarette smoke, cocaine, and even prescription medicines.

You are probably aware that developmental and learning difficulties occur in babies born to mothers using cocaine, tobacco, or alcohol. These drugs tend to produce effects that show up soon after birth.

What were the consequences of being exposed to DES? Daughters of mothers who took DES have high rates of a formerly rare type of vaginal cancer, called *adenocarcinoma*. This type of cancer is not only rare, but is usually is not seen in women younger than 50.

Late effects are harder to recognize. The rare form of vaginal cancer that developed in young women whose mothers had taken DES showed up years later in the daughter's late teens and 20s. Now we know that DES causes reproductive tract, immune system and brain abnormalities in all species studied, including humans, primates, rodents, and birds.

New research has also shown that amounts of drugs and other chemicals that don't cause damage or side effects in adult woman can have devastating effects on a developing embryo and fetus.

An example is thalidomide, safely used in the 1960s as a sleeping pill for women during pregnancy, but the drug caused profound deformities in arms and legs of a developing baby. Thalidomide effects showed up at birth and were quickly obvious to all.

An infant's brain and body, especially during key times of organ formation, can be critically and permanently injured in ways that may not show up for decades. This is exactly what occurred with DES. Infant girls and boys looked healthy and appeared to develop normally. But, the sabotage done by DES within those apparently normal bodies began to emerge years later.

To cause these effects later in life, the timing of DES exposure during the baby's development in the womb is more crucial than the amount. For example, female babies exposed before the 10th week of gestation have a higher incidence of the rare vaginal cancer. Those exposed after week 20 of gestation, however, did not develop the deformities of the reproductive tract. This pattern of a *"critical window" for exposure* is seen with other types of endocrine disruptors as well.

Vaginal cancers robbed women of fertility and even their lives. Now we know there are additional insidious ramifications of DES exposure. *DES also caused structural deformities of the uterus, fallopian tubes, and ovaries leading to ectopic pregnancies, miscarriages, and infertility.*

There is also a much higher than normal incidence of endometriosis and other reproductive problems in DES daughters.

Permanent
POPs appear to permanently damage the body's estrogen receptors.

DES Babies
Tend to have unusual responses to hormones—either exquisitely sensitive to small doses, or need higher doses than usual.

There is now disturbing evidence that the risks of DES exposure passed along to a second generation of children. DES grandchildren—many of you reading this book—may also have these risks to your health and fertility.

I have been suspicious that DES may also have altered brain response to our own body hormones and affected the way in which women responded to birth control pills and hormone therapy at menopause.

WHAT?
DES even became popular for a while as a way to stop growth if teenaged girls were becoming "too tall" to be attractive!

Interestingly, they have often needed higher than usual doses of estrogen to relieve menopausal symptoms. I believe this relates to a higher "set point" of the brain's estrogen receptors in the women exposed during fetal development to this highly potent synthetic estrogen.

Often, they do not respond as I would expect to testosterone replacement either. Nor do they experience an improvement in sex drive that I typically see in other women.

Another atypical response I see in some of my DES-exposed patients is that they are unusually sensitive to even small amounts of medicines, in particular hormones. It is as if their estrogen receptors have been altered to be overly responsive.

All of these adverse effects need to be explored, but to date, there is little research on these subtle types of hormone disruption from exposure to DES and other environmental hormone disruptors.

Effects
Environmental chemicals, even hormones like DES, cross the placenta to produce effects that show up many years or decades later.

There are clues *in studies on animals*, however, to support my concerns. Some of the same problems I described above in my patients have also been reported in medical articles. These include *increased ovarian inflammation, early depletion of follicles, abnormal follicles, increased number of cysts, absent or decreased number of corpora lutea* (normally present from ovulation), *thickened interstitial components, abnormal ratios of FSH and LH, elevated production of androgens, increased number of ovarian, breast and uterine tumors.* You don't see much about this possible connection in the writings on PCOS in human females, but I am convinced it is there.

Animal studies indicate DES acts on other body systems, such as the brain (especially the pituitary), the breast, and the immune system. But these DES effects have not been studied adequately in humans. In mice, DES causes suppression of two important components of the immune system: T-helper cells that oversee our body's total immune response, and the natural killer (NK) cells that patrol the body looking for abnormal cells to eradicate and prevent from spreading. If our NK cells aren't working optimally, we are not able to ward off other carcinogens very well, and become more likely to develop cancers as we age.

Women exposed to DES in the womb have later been found to have permanent, adverse changes in their T-helper and NK cells.

DES effects on brain development in the womb are far more difficult to tease out. Research has hardly begun to scratch the surface of potential health effects on brain pathways disrupted during development.

Beyond the Ovary: Endocrine Disruptors' Effects on the Thyroid

The endocrine disruptors I have been describing, especially polychlorinated biphenyls (PCB's) and dioxins, also seriously interfere with thyroid hormone action in addition to our ovarian hormones.

PCBs bear a striking structural resemblance to our body's active thyroid hormones and appear to fool the body's thyroid receptors, acting as agonists, antagonists, or partial agonists to thyroid hormones.

They may also increase the number of thyroid hormone receptors, which then means the brain and body will need even more hormones to function properly.

Our thyroid hormones play a major role in regulating metabolism of the body and brain, as well as modulating reproductive functions, including our ovarian cycles.

Exposure to synthetic chemicals that interferes with thyroid function as we develop in the womb has profound effects on brain function for the rest of our lives. Human brain development occurs at very specific windows of time throughout our time in the womb, and it is essential to have the proper levels of thyroid hormones during these critical windows.

If we don't have the thyroid hormones and iodine present in the proper amounts and balance during brain development, permanent brain damage occurs.

Wrong again
If there were no visible defects at birth, doctors did not think that a drug had other long-term adverse effects on the baby.

Tragic effects
DES daughters who developed vaginal cancer were hit in their teens and twenties. Some died at very young ages due to the aggressiveness of the DES-induced cancer.

Boys, too
DES sons have a greater incidence of malformations of the penis and testicles than in boys not exposed to DES.

Other DES Effects
Many of my patients whose mothers took DES have earlier menopause, severe PMS, atypical depressions, recurrent ovarian cysts, and uterine fibroids.

Links?
Abnormal changes in the ovary after DES exposure are strikingly similar to what is described for PCOS.

Mercury rising
"The toxic metal isn't just in seafood. It's showing up everywhere —and it's more dangerous than you think."
Time,
Sept. 11, 2006

The type of brain damage, and the symptoms that occur in childhood or later life, will depend on when and how much disruption occurs in the thyroid hormones. Thyroid hormone deficiency during brain development is one of the leading causes worldwide of learning and attention deficit disorders and other subtle types of neurological/cognitive dysfunction, as well as a severe form of mental retardation.

POPs may interfere with normal thyroid metabolism and hormone synthesis by a number of different mechanisms. The simplified flow chart below shows how POPs interfere with thyroid activity and how this cascade effect impacts the ovaries.

Healthy thyroid function is crucial for normal fertility and healthy ovarian hormone production, so POPs disruption of thyroid activity is another way that they disrupt fertility, as well as cause premature menopause. If you suspect you may have a thyroid disorder in addition to problems with your ovaries, I have described more about this in Chapter 7.

Heavy Metals and Menstrual Disturbances

I am sure you have heard the phrase *"Mad as a hatter."* This refers to a mental illness caused by mercury that manifested with *hallucinations, delusions* and *disordered thinking.* This type of illness occurred in hat-makers (hatters) in the 17th century, when mercury was used to tan animal hides.

The symptoms of psychosis were identical to what we see in the psychiatric disorder, schizophrenia, but here they were produced by toxic brain damage from the hatters' chronic exposure to a physical agent, mercury.

These metals can produce multiple neurological symptoms, even from exposure to low levels. I had a recent patient with a bizarre cluster of neurological symptoms that was quite a challenge to unravel.

After a lot of detective work, we were able to determine that she was unknowingly poisoned with low levels of arsenic, in addition to her other serious problems, including bone loss from her low estradiol and testosterone.

What were her symptoms? *Severe exhaustion, dizziness, lightheadedness, marked difficulty with word recall, concentration problems, dull headaches, vomiting and weight loss, among others.*

She had seen two neurologists, but all the neurological studies and brain imaging studies were normal. But I had several clues that her symptoms were not all due to her ovarian hormones.

First, her symptoms did not improve with estradiol the way I would have expected, and second, she was much sicker than I usually see from just from losing estradiol.

I decided to order a blood test for heavy metals and it showed the elevated arsenic levels.

As with other chronic heavy metal intoxication, arsenic exposure had caused damage to brain pathways, and it had also disrupted her menstrual cycle, leading to diminished production of ovarian hormones.

One group of researchers found that low levels of lead exposure over several years disrupted menstrual cycles in Rhesus monkeys. The monkeys were given drinking water that contained lead acetate daily for three 1-year exposures over a 5-year period. The monkeys had further lead intake for three additional consecutive years, providing additional time to observe the effects on menstrual cycles.

The lead acetate in the drinking water produced average circulating lead concentrations in the blood between 44 and 89 micrograms/100 ml and zinc protoporphyrin concentrations between 87 and 105 micrograms/100 ml. *These are not high concentrations, but menstrual cycles were significantly impaired even at these levels.*

Even though the lead-treated monkeys had completely normal menstrual cycles prior to the study, for the entire last two years of lead exposure their cycles decreased in frequency (called *oligomenorrhea*), and their cycles were longer with greater variability in intervals between bleeding.

The number of bleeding days also decreased compared to the monkeys who did not receive any lead (control group), which indicates a hormone imbalance. These changes were not due to differences in exposure to environmental influences such as light or diet because when the monkeys were no longer getting lead in their drinking water, their menstrual bleeding returned to normal duration.

Warning
Naturally-occurring heavy metals— lead, mercury, arsenic, cadmium and gallium— have long been known to cause nervous system damage.

And...
Women exposed to DES also have higher rates of several autoimmune disorders, such as Hashimoto's thyroiditis, Grave's disease, rheumatoid arthritis, and possibly Lupus.

Poisoned

The difficulty with arsenic and other heavy metal toxicity is that symptoms are so nonspecific, they can be caused by a hundred different things.

The other effects of lead exposure, however, remained for over a year after they stopped getting lead in their drinking water. This was troubling.

Even more worrisome was that the monkeys had none of the usual observable signs of lead toxicity, such as loss of appetite, weight loss or change blood counts such as hematocrit. For a woman, this means it could be difficult to recognize exposure to lead, or some other heavy metal.

Menstrual cycle disruptions due to prolonged lead or other heavy metal exposure may also lead to premature menopause. I wanted you to be aware of the subtle effects of these metals so that if your menstrual cycles change and you have symptoms like fatigue, low energy, "blah" mood, fuzzy thinking or other "vague" symptoms without apparent cause, or symptoms that don't respond to the usual treatments, you may want to consider asking for a screening test for heavy metal exposure. There are reliable blood tests for these metals.

Effects

In younger women, chronic heavy metal exposure can cause infertility.

In Summary

Silent Spring was an early warning that what happened in animal populations could affect all of us. Over forty years have passed since Rachel Carson published her alarm, yet we have even more reason for concern now.

More endocrine disrupting chemicals have been created. These chemicals are more potent than ever, and more persistent. We know that they cause significant perturbations in our exquisitely sensitive endocrine system. Check around your home, and eliminate products with chemicals included on this list in this chapter.

Danger

The level that disrupts the menstrual cycle may not produce any obvious or classic signs or symptoms of heavy metal toxicities.

Everything in this chapter should help you see how sensitive you are to the harmful effects of endocrine disruptor chemicals.

You can make a difference.

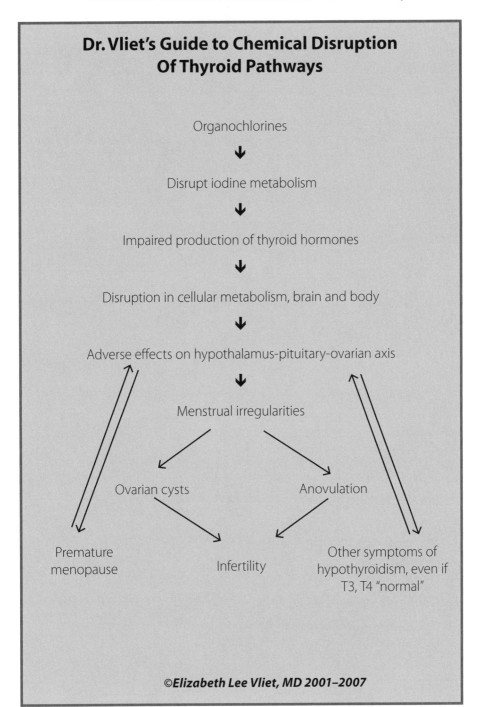

Dr. Vliet's Guide to Chemical Disruption Of Thyroid Pathways

Organochlorines

⬇

Disrupt iodine metabolism

⬇

Impaired production of thyroid hormones

⬇

Disruption in cellular metabolism, brain and body

⬇

Adverse effects on hypothalamus-pituitary-ovarian axis

⬇

Menstrual irregularities

Ovarian cysts   Anovulation

Premature menopause   Infertility   Other symptoms of hypothyroidism, even if T3, T4 "normal"

©Elizabeth Lee Vliet, MD 2001–2007

Chronology: The DES Time Line

1938: First synthesized in Britain

1940s and 1950s: widespread Use for millions of women--to prevent miscarriages, to help "support" a healthy pregnancy, for a "morning after" contraceptive, to treat menopausal symptoms, etc.

1952: Dr. William Dieckmann and colleagues at Univ. of Chicago published study of 2000 pregnant women, half given DES and half given placebo, to see the effect on miscarriage rate. Their conclusions were unequivocal: DES did NOT decrease either the number of miscarriages or the number of premature births. Later analysis of their data showed that there was an increase in miscarriages, increase in premature births, and increase in deaths of newborns in women given DES. In spite of these terrible findings, the FDA did not take any action to curb its use.

1952–1970s: Some doctors begin to cut back on DES use after the University of Chicago study is published, but hundreds of thousands of pregnant women are still given DES in the belief it would reduce miscarriages and lead to healthier babies

1966 –1969: specialists at Massachusetts General Hospital, affiliated with Harvard Medical School, had 7 cases of clear cell adenocarcinoma, all in the unusually young age range of 15 to 22. Normally this cancer isn't seen until after age 50, and even then, it is very rare.

4-22–1971: The MGH–Harvard researchers publish an article in the *New England Journal of Medicine* reporting that 7 of the 8 young women with the rare vaginal cancer had mothers who took DES in the first 3 months of pregnancy.

1970s, 1980s, 1990s: Researchers found other abnormalities in children of DES mothers: (see adjacent page)

© 2001–2007 Elizabeth Lee Vliet, M.D.

Dr. Vliet's Guide to Consequences of DES Exposure

DES Daughters:

- deformed uteruses that could not sustain pregnancy
- deformed Fallopian tubes and ovaries
- higher than normal rates of infertility
- increased rates of ectopic pregnancies and miscarriages
- increased rates of premature babies
- increased rates of endometriosis
- increased rates of uterine tumors, both benign (fibroids) and malignant (sarcomas and endometrial cancer)
- increased rates of both benign and malignant breast tumors
- increased frequency of ovarian cysts and abnormal follicles (also seen in PCOS)
- diminished formation of corpora lutea ("eggs")
- abnormal progesterone and estrogen production, abnormal receptor function
- increased incidence of prolactinomas (a benign pituitary tumor) and elevated blood levels of prolactin (also seen in PCOS).
- immune system problems
- abnormal glucose tolerance and decreased glucose utilization (also seen in PCOS)
- abnormal development of gender-specific sexual behavior in DES-offspring (males feminized, females masculinized), suggesting that DES caused abnormal sex differentiation of the hypothalamus during fetal development

DES Sons:

- increased genital defects
- undescended testicles
- stunted testicles and penises
- cysts in the epididymis
- low sperm counts
- abnormal sperm
- reduced fertility
- hypospadius (deformity of the penis)
- increased rates of testicular cancer at earlier ages than expected
- immune system problems
- abnormal glucose tolerance and glucose utilization
- abnormal development of male sexual behavior

1980s—present: Second generation of DES children reaching puberty and early adulthood and show similar problems as above

© 2001–2007 Elizabeth Lee Vliet, M.D.

Chapter 6

Ovaries At Risk:
Toxic Effects of Alcohol and Cigarettes, Marijuana and Other Drugs

Cigarette Smoking

You have heard a thousand times or more that smoking cigarettes is bad for you, and that it increases your risk of lung cancer, heart disease and stroke. Lung cancer deaths *in women* have increased more than 600% since 1950. At the same time, rates have been dropping in men as more have stopped smoking. Smoking is down overall about 40% since 1965.

22 million women now smoke; as result, women now make up over half of all the new cases of lung cancer each year. If you are like many young women who smoke, you probably aren't all that concerned about lung cancer or heart attacks if you are 15 or 25 or 39. I can hear you saying to yourself right now, "I'm young, so it really isn't a problem. It won't hurt me because I can stop any time I want to." If that's the case, why don't you? Could it be that you are more addicted than you think? The younger you start, the greater the risk of severe nicotine addiction.

New research has serious implications for *all women who smoke or live with someone who does.*

❦ Cigarette smoke, whether your own or second-hand from others, increases your risk of breast cancer.

❦ Cigarette smoke increases your risk of having one of several defective genes K-ras, GSTM1, and GRPR. Each of these genes create a much higher than average risk of developing lung cancer.

For example, the K-ras gene mutation, *three times more common in women*, enhances the growth of cancerous tumors. The GSTM1 gene normally functions to deactivate carcinogens in tobacco

Fact

At least 2 million adolescent girls in the U.S. smoke cigarettes, and nearly 4,000 teenagers a day become regular smokers.

smoke. Second-hand (environmental) smoke alters this gene so that it cannot detoxify the carcinogens.

Fact
Getting pregnant is more difficult for smokers, and smokers have much higher rates of infertility than non-smokers.

The more second-hand smoke you live and work with, the more likely you are to have this defective gene, and the greater your risk of lung cancer.

The GRPR gene, fueled by exposure to nicotine, helps lung cancers grow. This gene *is more common in the airways of women than men*, which is another reason that smoking is a greater cancer risk for women than men.

OK, so maybe you are blasé about lung cancer. But did you know that cigarette smoking can damage your ovaries, even if you are "only" a teenager? And what about when you want to have a child?

Did you know that smoking cigarettes can lead to infertility?

Did you know that women who smoke have more risk of endometriosis and ovarian cysts?

Did you know that cigarette smoking may lead to premature menopause in women as young as 30?

Yes, smoking has all these harmful effects.

Many components of cigarette smoke not only cause cancer, but are also *directly toxic* to the follicles in your ovaries. The more you smoke, the more follicles you kill off.

Fact
Women smokers who go through in-vitro fertilization and other assisted reproduction techniques have lower success rates than non-smokers.

And remember, unlike men who make more sperm throughout their lives, women are born with all the follicles we will ever have. When they are *gone*, they are *permanently gone*.

Without follicles, you lose your hormone-producing factories; that means lower estradiol levels, lower testosterone levels, and abnormal menstrual cycles.

Lower hormone levels also mean less energy, loss of sex drive, loss of mental sharpness, poor sleep, an immune system that doesn't work as well, and a host of other problems described earlier.

Multiple studies from many different countries over the past forty years have shown the relationship between smoking cigarettes and impaired fertility.

In one 1985 study, women who smoked cigarettes, compared to non-smokers, were 57–75% *less likely* to conceive, depending on how much they smoked. For those smokers who finally did get pregnant, it took over a year longer to conceive than it did for the non-smokers.

In addition, smokers are more likely to have significant fetal growth-retardation, creating smaller babies, more likely to be born prematurely. And the problems don't stop there.

Even female children born to mothers who smoked during pregnancy can later have more problems conceiving their own children, even if they do not smoke. Specialists think this occurs because *smoking during pregnancy actually kills some of the primordial follicles in the developing female baby.* Since she isn't born with the normal number of follicles, she has a harder time getting pregnant later.

Women who smoke regularly may go through menopause five to seven years sooner than nonsmokers. Many of my patients tell me that when they ask other physicians about a relationship between smoking and early menopause, their doctors say, "There isn't one. I never heard of this problem." **Yet, medical studies showing this connection were published over twenty-five years ago!** Even *before* periods completely stop, women who smoke cigarettes have significant *declines in their levels of estradiol for years before menopause.*

In my practice, I see smokers with multiple hormone-related health problems, and most of them also have muscle and joint pain syndromes. Pain regulation is one of estradiol's many functions. Estradiol also helps muscle metabolism and repair. So healthy levels of estradiol prevent pain from occurring, reduce pain when it strikes, and also helps (along with testosterone) to build healthy muscle tissue. So, if cigarette smoking has lowered your estradiol, you lose its pain-relieving properties.

So when you put all the pieces together, the picture for women who smoke is not pretty. Like hundreds of young women I have seen in my practice over the years, she thought she "wouldn't have any problems" from smoking cigarettes.

Bev is now 38 years old and has smoked at least a pack of cigarettes a day since she was 12. Her periods also began about age 12, and over the next 10 years, she had a wide range of troubling symptoms she called "weird." She said at her initial visit,

Warning
Cigarette smoking causes earlier menopause, and this includes exposure to second-hand smoke.

Frightening
Many compounds in cigarette smoke are highly carcinogenic.

Bad Endings
Take a look at this young woman, who started smoking at age 12.

"No one could tell me what was happening to me. I had this dizziness, swimming in my head, I felt like my brain was in a fog, my body would shake at times, and I felt more and more anxious/depressed/foggy, and just never felt quite right. I felt like something chemical was happening in my body but none of the doctors could ever explain what was going on. Then in my early 20s, I was getting worse and could barely function. I would wake up with numb arms every night, feeling disconnected in my motor movements, and would have split second moments of memory glitches and not know where I was. I thought I was losing my mind. Then all of a sudden, my period came three times in one month, and I had intense panic attacks. I also had this weird muscle tension where I would realize my muscles would be tense and I would have to consciously try to relax them. My libido totally disappeared and has never returned."

"I had watched my body, and I realized that these weird things were happening at certain times of my cycle."

"In desperation, I went to a psychiatrist and an ObGyn. The psychiatrist put me on an antidepressant and said I was dysthymic. The GYN just though I was under stress. I also saw that my cycles were changing. I put 2+2 together, and figured that something must be affecting my hormones."

"I demanded that he humor me and do the hormone tests. When he called me with the results, I almost cried, I was so relieved and validated. I had high prolactin and really low estrogen, so he sent me to an endocrinologist who started me on Parlodel (bromocriptine). I felt a lot better, especially considering the state I was coming from, but I never felt 100%. I still felt there was more to it than just taking Parlodel, but I decided to settle for what relief I had at that point."

"I demanded that my GYN do hormone tests, but he just said I was too young and it wasn't necessary."

"I tried for over two years to become pregnant and never could, so I finally went on Clomid and got pregnant. I stopped smoking during my pregnancy until after my son was born, and I figured there wasn't a problem if I went back to smoking. But then I had a post-partum depression and went on Paxil, which helped, but I felt really tired all day and my sex drive was totally gone. About six months after the baby was born, I went back on Parlodel, which only made me feel worse. I felt like I had a hangover—fatigue, brain-fog, just no sense of clarity in my thinking. It really has such a dramatic effect on me."

"Then I had a miscarriage that they said was a blighted ovum and I had to have a D&C. I just didn't feel well all this time, so I finally decided I wanted to have this consult with you. I feel like

Dr. Vliet's Guide: Smoking hurts!
How Smoking Makes Pain Worse

- Diminished serotonin production

- Constriction of small arteries that serve muscles and nerves, which leads to diminished blood flow and diminished supply of vital nutrients to body tissues, nutrients needed for building, repairing and healing microtrauma from daily use.

- Reduced oxygen-carrying capacity of the red blood cells since smoking replaces oxygen with carbon monoxide. The loss of oxygen supply not only leads to fatigue, but also to a build-up of metabolic waste products in muscle tissues, causing more muscle pain.

- Decreased blood flow and nutrients to cells, along with a reduction in vitamin C from smoking, causes an increase in oxidative (free-radical) damage to nerve and muscle cells, and release of inflammatory prostaglandins and other body chemicals that intensify pain.

- Diminished stomach acidity and decreased absorption of many vitamins, especially the B group, needed for the brain and body to make pain-relieving neurotransmitters.

- Nicotine also increases pain perception by several mechanisms and as a stimulant, leads to increased anxiety and irritability, both of which are already present from the "stimulant" effect of pain itself.

- Nicotine withdrawal during sleep causes frequent awakenings, and loss of stage 4 deep sleep that is crucial for muscle repair, Growth Hormone secretion and keeping the brain healthy.

© 2003–2007 Elizabeth Lee Vliet, M.D.

there is something else going on hormonally that causes my severe fatigue, brain fog, and makes it hard to concentrate. It isn't all month long, but seems to come for a few days in a row and then lifts some, then later comes back. I just don't have a good sense of well-being. It always feels like there is something chemical going on and my body isn't quite adjusted. I find that my body is tensing all over, even if I am not stressed. My muscles hurt, my joints ache, and I feel like an old woman before my time."

When Bev and I reviewed her lab tests, I could see why she was still having so many problems. Clearly the cigarette smoking had damaged her ovaries over all these years, and she was having the problems that occur in smokers due to loss of estradiol.

"For the next two years, I was on a hormonal-roller coaster with anxiety, mood swings, a quaking feeling, intermittent brain fog, etc."

She had a really low day 1 estradiol of only 30 pg/ml (optimal is about 80–90 pg/ml), and her day 20 (luteal phase) estradiol level was only 105 pg/ml, which is only about *half* the healthy level at this time of the cycle.

Her low levels went right along with what research studies show for hormone levels in smokers. Her low estradiol also decreased sex hormone binding globulin (SHBG) and pushed more testosterone into the *free* fraction.

Too much testosterone in the free fraction can cause such problems as irritability, insomnia, anxiety, agitation, tense muscles because the testosterone is more available to over stimulate the receptors. This is why she would feel worse during her periods, when the estradiol was the lowest.

Fact

If estradiol is too low, it makes the symptoms of excess available testosterone even worse.

You may recall that she said her libido had vanished. So how can she have excess free testosterone and a loss of libido? This happens when estradiol levels are too low to properly "prime" the testosterone receptors in the brain so that the testosterone can work optimally for women, unlike the way it works in men.

Her low libido was aggravated by the high progesterone relative to her low estradiol in the second half of her cycle. Progesterone blocks testosterone from acting at its receptor sites. Progesterone break-down products (metabolites) act as central nervous system depressants much like Valium, Ativan, Xanax or Klonopin. All drugs or hormones that bind at these brain sites can cause low libido.

Shocking

Bev's bone density test (DEXA) showed early bone loss (*osteopenia*) at the *hip*.

In addition, higher levels of progesterone relative to the estradiol in the luteal phase of her cycle added to her brain-fog, as if she took Valium or Klonopin.

There is no question Bev had perimenopausal levels of estradiol, even though she was still having periods. Most of her brain symptoms—fuzzy thinking, "brain fog," memory loss and problems concentrating—occurred because her estradiol was too low. I explained to her that the cigarette smoking was a direct cause of her low estradiol, and had also probably contributed to her high prolactin. High prolactin *adds to* the smoking-induced suppression of her ovaries and decrease in hormone production.

Bev had already had saliva hormone tests done before I saw her. The report of that test said she had *"estrogen dominance and low progesterone."* This is exactly the same description I have seen on every single saliva test report I have ever reviewed! These reports have little relevance to what is actually happening in your body.

When I tested the more reliable blood hormone levels, she had *decreased estradiol* throughout her cycle, and a *normal rise in progesterone* in the luteal phase of her cycle.

The *blood tests fit exactly with what we would expect* based on her symptoms, and on the known consequences of cigarette smoking together, including bone loss.

Low levels of estradiol and cigarette smoking also cause changes in the pH of the stomach and intestine, affecting the body's ability to absorb nutrients, such as calcium, magnesium, iron, B vitamins, and others. Loss of these important vitamins and minerals made her "brain fog" and memory problems even worse.

All of Bev's problems were directly related to her smoking cigarettes for 25 years. Smoking had profoundly damaged her ovaries and brain pathways, including the pituitary, by several different ways, showing how damaging smoking can be for young women's fertility.

1. **Nicotine** disrupts chemical messengers that regulate the pituitary and prolactin release

2. **Nicotine** and the other chemicals in cigarette smoke kill off follicles, causing early ovarian decline and lower estradiol levels;

3. **Smoking** increases activity of liver enzymes that metabolize hormones, which means hormones are broken down or inactivated faster.

4. **Nicotine** interferes with normal production of mood and sleep-regulating chemical messengers;

5. **Smoking** contributes to *impaired absorption* of vitamins and minerals from the gut at the same time it *increases* the body's need for these same vitamins and minerals.

In 1986, lung cancer became the leading cause of cancer death in women. Most women still think breast cancer is the leading cause of death. The reality is starkly different.

Caution
Early bone loss is also common in women who smoke, primarily due to the lower level of estradiol.

Statistic
Every year since 1986, lung cancer deaths in women exceed the deaths due to breast cancer.

Shocker
Lung cancer and heart disease, both increased by smoking, together kill more than *10 times* as many women as breast cancer.

Cigarette smoking itself increases your risk of breast cancer. This risk is more pronounced for young, premenopausal women than for post-menopausal women. Tobacco smoke in the body contains many direct carcinogens, adversely effects immune system function, as well as the metabolism of estrogens and other important hormones. Breast cancer risk from smoking is a much *bigger increase in risk than the risk of taking hormones!*

With smoking, it is a "dose-dependent" relationship: the *more you smoke, the higher the risk.*

If you are still smoking cigarettes, give it up now. Take steps to prevent any more damage to your ovaries that can cause infertility and lead to even more serious problems later.

Alcohol

Alcohol is a socially acceptable, legal drug, widely available everywhere. Drinking among young people has risen dramatically in recent years, and more ominously, *binge* drinking is on the rise in adolescent and college age girls. Alcohol is widely touted as a sexual enhancer. It's legal, so it must be safe, right?

This legal drug takes an insidious toll on our health, especially for women. Compared to men, women don't have as much of the enzyme that breaks down alcohol, so alcohol is far more damaging, even if the amount consumed is similar to what a man drinks.

Let's look at all the ways alcohol is an endocrine disruptor that affects your hormones, sexual responsiveness, fertility, and your total health.

Folk wisdom has always said that alcohol increased sexual desire but took away the ability to perform! It decreases men's testosterone, causing impotence. It also acts as a depressant drug on the brain and nerves, so nerve endings in the clitoris and penis are less sensitive to sexual stimulation, leading to difficulties having an orgasm. The brain's sexual circuits are also dulled, another negative effect on arousal and orgasm.

How does alcohol affect the menstrual cycle and fertility? Studies from many countries have shown that regular use of alcohol disrupts the normal menstrual cycle, causes problems with ovulation and make it harder to get pregnant.

Fact
Premenopausal women who have ever smoked daily have approximately a two-fold increased risk of breast cancer compared to women who never smoked.

Warning
Women who are currently heavy smokers have *four times* the risk of breast cancer compared to the risk for non-smokers.

Sex? Not...
Women who are "just" social drinkers report more disruption of their sexual responsiveness.

Gender Matters: Alcohol Effects on Fertility, Menstrual Cycles, and Hormone Production

- Alcohol impairs the brain's GnRH "pulse generator" that triggers proper release of FSH and LH. This in turn causes low estradiol and reduced ovarian function in women

- Cycle length shows greater variability in women drinkers than in non-drinkers—some cycles are long, some are short, and there are more skipped cycles.

- Estradiol and testosterone levels decline earlier in women who drink alcohol regularly, which lead to a rise in FSH at younger ages. All of these changes lead to decreased fertility.

- Women drinkers have more cycles in which they do not ovulate, another way that fertility is impaired.

- Women who drink alcohol regularly have heavier menstrual flow and more painful menstruation (dysmenorrhea). In one study, this effect was seen in women who had just one 6-drink "binge" a week; these effects are also seen in women who average 3+ drinks a day.

- Alcohol use leads to markedly higher rates of premenstrual distress and severe PMS, regardless of age, income, educational level or occupation

- Women have greater sensitivity to brain damage and neurotoxicity from alcohol than men do.

- Alcohol causes a *decrease* in sexual desire, arousal, and orgasm in 70–75% of women drinkers.

- Alcohol causes early bone loss by decreasing absorption of calcium, increasing calcium loss in urine, and decreasing the action of bone-building osteoblasts, in addition to decreasing estradiol.

- Regular alcohol use causes an increase in early spontaneous abortions, and miscarriages, stillbirths and premature babies.

- Alcohol causes birth defects by acting as a teratogen: Fetal Alcohol Syndrome consists of growth retardation, small head circumference, mild to moderate mental retardation plus a variety of skeletal, joint, genital, heart, kidney, and skin effects.

© 2001–2007 Elizabeth Lee Vliet, M.D.

Alcohol also lowers production of estradiol and testosterone, leading to earlier onset of menopause. The table on the next page shows you how alcohol affects women more severely than men.

Hormone changes get little attention in most alcohol treatment programs, but it is an enormous factor that perpetuates alcohol abuse in a large percentage of women.

Caution
Your menstrual cycle hormone changes may actually increase your alcohol cravings.

One 28-year-old woman started binge drinking at age 12, soon after her periods began. She had several hospital admissions for alcohol abuse complications, and was struggling to maintain her sobriety. She described the premenstrual cravings quite graphically:

"I do fine staying off alcohol from the end of my period until I ovulate, and then all hell breaks loose. I feel like I have an uncontrollable demon inside me that won't let me alone and demands that I go get a drink!

"I have an awful time resisting these cravings when they start after ovulation and become especially intense the week before my period starts.

Warning
Daily alcohol use is an *independent* risk factor for breast cancer.

"That's the time I had my relapses and had to go back to the hospital. I feel like it is something chemical, like a switch is flipped in my brain, and I have to have that alcohol. It's a horrible feeling."

What chemical change with her cycle could explain this? The rise in progesterone in the second half of the cycle causes problems regulating blood sugars. Especially if the estradiol is lower than optimal as progesterone rises, your body has even more difficulty responding normally to glucose. You have more glucose fluctuations and drops in blood glucose that we call *reactive hypoglycemia*.

The drop in blood sugar is a powerful trigger for alcohol cravings. Alcohol behaves in the digestive process like sugars and it will quickly raise blood glucose. All the symptoms from falling or low blood sugar—anxiety, restlessness, low energy, etc.—are relieved quickly by alcohol, and you feel better for a short while. Then as alcohol levels drop, blood sugar falls, the symptoms return, and you crave alcohol again.

The drop in estradiol and progesterone just before your bleeding begins also causes a fall in brain endorphins and serotonin. These are your "feel-good" brain chemicals, and when they fall quickly, it causes more anxiety, insomnia, blue moods, irritability, and low energy. *Many women then "treat" these problems with a glass of wine, beer or liquor, and the cycle continues.*

Alcohol also affects metabolism of the hormones you take in birth control pills or for menopause and decreases their effectiveness, adding another factor to the potential for alcohol cravings.

Getting out of the vicious cycle means taking steps to stop alcohol *and* to stabilize the hormone fluctuations at the same time.

Alcohol increases the risk of breast cancer. This increased risk due to alcohol is *not* due to other variables, such as total calories, fat, fiber, vitamins or whether you take hormones. The age at which you begin drinking is important; the earlier you start drinking, the greater your risk, regardless of how much you drink later in life.

The first study to link alcohol consumption to breast cancer risk was published in 1977. Since then, we have many studies from a variety of countries showing similar results: even moderate alcohol consumption, *three or more drinks per week,* increases breast cancer risk from 20 to 70 percent. The more you drink, the more upper body fat you gain, and this further adds to breast cancer risk, as well as risk of diabetes and heart disease.

The mechanism for alcohol effect on cancer risk is not yet fully known. There is speculation that it may alter hormonal balance by increasing estrone and the androgens in fat tissue.

Alcohol causes a rise in the blood level of estrone by several pathways: alcohol stimulates the liver to make more estrone, and it also stimulates fat tissues to convert more of androgen (androstenedione) to estrone.

As you read earlier, estrone is the form of estrogen associated with a higher risk of breast and endometrial cancer. You can minimize the "estrone factor" in risk for both cancers by reducing or eliminating alcohol use, and by losing excess body fat.

In women taking hormones, alcohol raised the blood levels of estrone significantly. Among current hormone users in the Nurses Health Study and the Iowa Women's Health Study, the risk of breast cancer was increased *only* among those women who *also* drank alcohol. In both of these studies, the excess risk of breast cancer was *not* seen in all estrogen users, just those who also drank alcohol. Yet all you hear in the news is that "estrogen" increases breast cancer risk!

Scary
Risk of breast cancer is greatest if regular drinking begins during the vulnerable time of breast development in your teens.

Fact
Risk of breast cancer is increased even more if you drink more than 9 drinks per week.

A study from Italy published in 2000 found that alcohol use accounted for about 12% of the risk for breast cancer, making alcohol a highly significant, and avoidable, risk factor.

In addition to effects on hormone metabolism, alcohol also interferes with normal immune function and stimulates excessively high levels of insulin, another newly identified independent risk factor for breast cancer.

Fact
In women taking *oral* estrogen, estrone and estradiol levels increased more than *threefold* after drinking alcohol.

You may have heard that alcohol lowers the risk of heart disease. It turns out that this effect was primarily seen in men, not women. For men, the risk of heart disease decreased significantly even in the higher ranges of alcohol intake. In women, there was a slight decrease in heart disease risk only with the lowest levels of alcohol use each week. Women's bodies simply show more of the damaging effects from alcohol than men's.

Given all the negative effects on your ovaries, fertility, mood, sleep, memory and body weight, I encourage you to minimize alcohol use.

Marijuana

Fact
Women had a marked increase in deaths from heart disease at higher levels of alcohol use per week.

Few people today haven't heard of marijuana. THC, or tetrahydrocannabinol, is the primary brain-active chemical in marijuana that makes you high. The amount of THC varies greatly depending on the type of marijuana and where it is grown. All forms of marijuana affect brain pathways directly. It causes impaired memory, attention, and concentration, as well as difficulty thinking, diminished problem-solving, loss of coordination, and distorted perception.

For women athletes, marijuana interferes with timing, causing slower movements and impaired coordination, so you don't perform your best. It also impairs judgment, perception, ability to judge distances, and the ability to react quickly. These same marijuana effects also interfere with your ability to drive a car, causing similar incoordination and slowed reactions as alcohol does on standard "drunk driver" tests.

What many young people, and even doctors overlook, is that marijuana disrupts brain centers that regulate hormone production in both males and females. Luteinizing hormone (LH) is suppressed by marijuana so that it doesn't rise at mid-cycle to trigger ovulation. This is one way it can impair your fertility if used regularly.

Extracts of marijuana plants contain chemicals that compete with estradiol for binding at the estrogen receptor, *cannabidiol* and *apigenin* (a flavinoid phytoestrogen in marijuana). Marijuana *also can elevate prolactin*, a pituitary hormone that in turn suppresses the normal menstrual cycle and ovarian hormone production. So marijuana can decrease ovarian estradiol production, as well as compete with what estradiol you do produce for binding at the estrogen receptor.

If you are having trouble getting pregnant, keep in mind that marijuana leads to abnormal sperm development and significantly decreased testosterone in men. The hormone effects of marijuana can even cause men to develop enlarged breasts, called gynecomastia, and to have difficulty having an erection.

Marijuana also causes more frequent early miscarriages. Marijuana causes abnormalities in the baby, such as abnormal brain function, small head size, shorter height, and lower birth weight, even if the baby is carried full-term.

If all this weren't enough, a study published in June of 2001 found that the risk of a heart attack jumps nearly five-fold during the first hour after smoking marijuana, posing a particular threat to anyone with other risk factors for heart disease.

Researchers at Beth Israel Deaconess Medical Center in Boston found that heart rate can *double* after smoking a single marijuana cigarette. Marijuana may initiate a heart attack by causing a piece of plaque inside a coronary artery to rupture and form a clot, which then blocks the flow of blood to the heart muscle.

Marijuana also decreases blood flow to the heart by increasing blood pressure. This means that active chemicals in marijuana increase the heart's demand for oxygen, while at the same time decreasing the supply of oxygen in the blood.

Women are even more vulnerable to marijuana's other adverse effect, such as on the lungs. Marijuana contains similar cancer-causing compounds to those found in cigarette smoke, although the ones in marijuana are even more damaging to the lung than tobacco smoke.

Chemicals in marijuana are also irritating to the lung and can lead to immediate problems with chronic coughs, wheezing and even asthma in susceptible people. Women who regularly smoke marijuana, like cigarette smokers, have more frequent respiratory infections and pneumonias both from the suppression of

Caution
Women who smoke marijuana regularly have disturbances in ovulation that make it hard to become pregnant.

Warning
Endocrine effects of marijuana can damage sexual function and fertility in *both* men *and* women.

Warning
The risk of suffering a heart attack was 4.8 times greater in the first hour after smoking marijuana when compared to periods of not smoking the drug.

their ovarian hormones and from the direct toxic effects of the drug itself. THC and other chemicals in marijuana also disrupt normal immune function.

Fact

Smoking 5 joints a week is getting as many cancer-causing chemicals as smoking a whole pack of cigarettes a day.

Although some people say that they use marijuana because it "calms" them, it can also increase heart rate and actually cause anxiety. It can also lead to palpitations and anxiety as it is wears off. Either way, you may find that you are *more* anxious if you are using marijuana regularly. Since it also reduces the hormones of the ovary, such as estradiol and progesterone, you may also experience more anxiety as a result of lower levels of these hormones. This "recreational" drug is more damaging than you may have realized.

CNS stimulants: Cocaine and others

Cocaine and other brain stimulants such as ecstasy have the potential to disrupt the hormone-regulating pathways of the hypothalamus and pituitary that govern ovarian cycles.

Cocaine also changes how fallopian tubes function, interfering with your ability to get pregnant. We don't yet know exactly how this tubal abnormality occurs in cocaine users, but it is important if you have trouble conceiving.

Danger!

Women who abuse these drugs often have changes in their menstrual cycles, particularly if there is significant weight loss due to the appetite-suppressing effects of regular use.

Brain effects of these drugs can be profound. Dutch scientists reported in 2001 that women are more likely than men to suffer brain cell damage from regular use of the party drug *ecstasy*. The damage appears to selectively hit nerve endings that release serotonin, but may also damage brain cells that over see nerve signal transmission. Using sophisticated PET scans of brain function, recent studies in the U.S. have shown that only one "hit" of cocaine causes permanent changes in the brain that set you up for addiction and the vicious cycle of highs followed by severe crashes into profound, sometimes suicidal, depression.

Cocaine also causes constriction of the arteries serving the heart and can increase the risk of heart attack up to 25-fold during the first hour after use. This is one of the causes of "sudden death" that occurs in cocaine users.

Besides contributing to infertility and ovarian hormone problems, "Coke" can permanently scramble your brain, send your blood pressure soaring or kill your heart.

It's a deadly drug... more so if you already have any hormone problems.

Summary

I see women every day having problems with menstrually-triggered mood swings, headaches, body aches, low energy, loss of sex drive, changes in their menstrual cycle, trouble getting pregnant, or a number of other bothersome symptoms related to hormone changes.

Many of my patients haven't even considered that something that seems socially accepted like smoking, alcohol or "recreational" drug use could be directly linked to problems with their *ovaries* and hormones.

These are not simple pleasures or harmless ways to relax.

Just say NO to these chemicals that mess up your hormones!

Caution
At certain low estrogen stages of the menstrual cycle, the risk of coronary artery spasm and low blood flow to the heart is even greater with cocaine use.

Dr. Vliet's Guide

Life Style Habit	Actions	Ovary Effect
Cigarette Smoking	↓serotonin production ↓blood flow ↑norepinephrine (nicotine is a stimulant)	Toxic to follicles, increases liver breakdown of E2, causes premature menopause
Caffeine	Diuretic-depletes minerals Stimulant effects on brain Disrupts normal sleep (↓Stage IV) Alters serotonin-norepinephrine balance	May disrupt normal menstrual cycles and hormone production if used to excess
Alcohol	Depresses CNS Adrenalin rebound (when wears off) Interferes with ovarian function Damages muscle fibers ↓ absorption of B vitamins ↓ Stage IV sleep Damage to nerve endings	Even moderate use increases estrone levels, disrupts normal menstrual cycle, associated with infertility, decreases testosterone Increases risk of breast cancer even with moderate use.
Marijuana	Alters serotonin-norepinephrine balance Suppresses LH Elevates prolactin Competes with estrogen at receptors	Disrupts ovarian cycles, decreases hormone levels, kills follicles, impairs fertility, lowers hormone levels

© 2001–2007 Elizabeth Lee Vliet, M.D.

Chapter 7

Ovaries Shut Down:
The Toxic Role of Stress Overload
and Sleep Deprivation

Long Days, Short Nights, Overloaded Lives!

Many of my patients tell me they think they have Chronic Fatigue Syndrome, but when I ask them to describe a typical day, I'm not so sure a *medical* syndrome is the source of their fatigue!

Let's look at a typical weekday schedule for one of my patients, Harriet, a 36-year-old married school administrator and mother of three. Harriet sought a consult for "fatigue, insomnia, low energy, headaches, loss of libido and difficulty concentrating." This is a snapshot of her usual routine:

Harriet's Day

5:00 AM — Alarm goes off. She gets up, takes a shower, and then starts the family going

5:15–6:30 AM — rousts her husband, three sons, finishes fixing school lunches, prepares quick breakfast (cereal and milk), quick "tidy up" housework, gets dressed for work while watching the AM news, makes sure the kids have homework, books and lunches.

6:30 AM — husband leaves, taking one son to wrestling practice, and then goes to his office for 7:15–7:30 AM arrival.

6:45 AM — Harriet takes the other two children to school, then drives another 45 minutes to her office at a large urban junior high school

8:00 AM — Her workday "officially" starts and includes dealing with discipline problems, supervising teachers, preparing meeting agendas for teachers and PTA, reviewing school policy and curriculum issues with central office administrators, monitoring bus lines, meetings with local law enforce-

So Typical

Harriet's "workday" begins 3 hours before her "job"... and ends 5 hours *after* her job. No wonder she's exhausted!

Fuel?

Harriet has little sleep and she is nowhere close to a balanced, steady intake of "fuel" for her brain and body.

ment officials about drug and alcohol problems among students, meetings with parents, trouble shooting other administrative problems. Since teachers and principals patrol the cafeteria during lunch, she rarely has time to eat lunch, and usually grabs a soft drink 2–3 times though the day so the sugar and caffeine keep her going

5:30 PM — Leaves work to pick up two of the children at sports practices. Runs errands, picks up a few groceries.

6:45–7:00 PM — arrives home, fixes dinner, oversees the kids' homework (or takes kids to soccer or baseball practice or church youth meetings three nights a week; while waiting for the kids at practices, she pays bills, reads and sorts mail.

7:30 PM — Husband arrives home, dinner

8:00–10:30 PM — Helps kids with homework, does housework, washes several loads of clothes, and reviews her own work memos.

10:30 PM — gets the kids to bed, helps lay out clothes and books for the morning, prepares kids' lunches for the next day

11:45 PM — Goes to bed herself, but it often takes her a half hour or more to "unwind" and fall asleep, exhausted after another grueling day.

These are weekdays. Saturdays she's cleaning house, doing laundry, planning dinners, buying groceries, paying bills, balancing the checkbook, driving kids to various games, and running errands.

Her husband often works at his office on Saturday or takes the kids to events if he is available. On Sundays, they sleep "late," usually getting up about 8:30 or 9 AM to get ready for Sunday School and church. Sunday afternoons, Dad and the boys typically watch whatever sports events on television. Mom calls family, tries to get a few "odds and ends" done, and begins getting ready for the week ahead. Sunday dinner is the one meal of the week the entire family is usually together.

Not only is Harriet getting very little sleep, *but take a look at what she eats each day.* She has a small bowl of cereal and skim milk for breakfast—carbohydrates with little protein or fat to sustain energy and blood sugar over the morning, let alone the rest of the day. This breakfast will sustain blood glucose for about two hours.

She doesn't eat lunch; instead, she has a high sugar soft drink with a jolt of caffeine for an energy boost. The sugar boost lasts about 30–45 minutes before the "crash" of low blood sugar. She has another soft drink, and the cycle repeats. She doesn't eat again until dinner.

By then, her body has determined that it's in a famine and has increased its stress hormone cortisol, holding on to every last calorie to store as fat. No wonder she is eating less and gaining weight.

Harriet has a caring, stable marriage, loves her kids and enjoys her job. She does not perceive her life as overly stressful, just "busy." *She had no clue she was reaching perimenopausal levels of her ovarian hormones,* and no one she had seen for her health problems considered that issue. Her primary care doctor and gynecologist simply told her slow down, take some stress management classes, and "relax more."

In spite of her healthy outlook on life, Harriet's overloaded schedule, poor nutrition, and fragmented sleep were *physiological stressors* that had suppressed her ovaries. Her cycles were now longer with shorter, lighter bleeding days. Her progesterone was still in the lower end of ovulatory range, and her testosterone was only 10 ng/dl (100 pg/ml). No wonder she was tired, had headaches, trouble concentrating, no libido and couldn't sleep.

The three primary solutions were straight forward: I gave her a steady-dose birth control pill to restore her cycles and provide hormone stability. I gave her a pill with better estrogen to progesterone ratio, Orthocyclen.

We designed a balanced plan of quick, healthy, simple meals and snacks to sustain energy at work and give her body nutrients. I recommended appropriate doses of vitamins and encouraged her to take some time for herself and get some exercise!

June was 41 when I treated her. Her POD symptoms—fatigue, insomnia, headaches, difficulty concentrating, and lack of interest in sex—had an entirely different cause from Harriet's. She recently lost her parents, both deaths completely

Low hormones
She was only 36, but she was in Premature Ovarian Decline (POD). Her day 1 estradiol was only 20 pg/ml, and her day 20 estradiol was only 61 pg/ml (about one fourth an optimal E2 level.

Low fuel
Harriet didn't eat enough *food* fuel, and she certainly didn't have enough *hormone* fuel to sustain her schedule, or enough *sleep* to recharge her body.

However—
Although June ate well and exercised several times a week, these overwhelming life stresses affected her health and her ovaries.

unexpected and 3 months apart. She owned and operated a demanding restaurant business and worked long hours there.

After her father died, she took over and ran her father's automobile dealership—clearly a stressful, male-dominated business. She was a single mom with two children, and cared for a younger sister with a serious chronic illness. She had also just broken an engagement. Her losses of significant people were catastrophic, particularly so close together.

Her ovarian hormone levels were similar to Harriet's, except her stress hormone, cortisol, was significantly higher. She benefited from hormone management, and I also recommended a therapist for help with her grief, as well as prioritizing her goals for family and businesses.

These women are typical of the ones I see in my office every day. They lead more complex lives with multiple demands—at work, at home, and with extended family. Jobs that were once "men's work" have been added to traditional female roles.

Fact
You can't be alive and have *no* stress, because the body itself is undergoing the stimulation (stress) of constant change every moment of every day.

Society pushes us to operate at a higher level. We want and need to function at higher levels of physical and emotional energy as well as cognitive performance. We expect much of ourselves, and feel devastated when we can't achieve all that we want. These combined stresses take their toll.

Stress and What it Does to Your Health:

Stress is a constant, inevitable, even *necessary* part of life itself. We live with stress, all of the time. Stress, in its broadest sense, simply means a stimulus that causes change and adaptation to maintain *homeostasis*, or balance, of our body systems.

The stimuli that alter homeostasis are called *stressors*. They come from changes inside the body, like rising or falling blood sugar, or from outside the body, like a hot day that makes you sweat.

The stimulus, or stressor, may be an event in your life, or a thought or image that comes into your mind. We are constantly bombarded with millions of such stimuli every day. The brain monitors and modulates all incoming stimuli, and constantly guides the responses of body systems.

So if stress is constant, and our body always deals with it, how does it cause problems with our health? You read about stress and its body-wrecking effects: cancer, heart attacks, high blood pressure, infertility, allergies—and other problems.

Is there a balance between the stress that allows the body to *survive and thrive*, and the stress that slowly *destroys* us?

Why do some people thrive on the stress levels others find overwhelming?

Why do some people cope with catastrophic stress and others cave in over trivial events?

After decades of stress research, we now have a better understanding of the role that individual vulnerability plays in who becomes ill. Viruses, bacteria, and carcinogens alone do not cause illness in every exposed individual.

Most diseases we "moderns" develop are greatly influenced by the physical and psychological environment of our bodies. We now know that many factors play a role in determining who gets sick, how sick they get and how quickly they recover.

Our attitudes, the foods we eat, the vitamins we take, our hormone balance, our energy, our feelings of control and choice, our degree of social support, and our faith–all matter.

Think about it. Have you unwittingly made your body a compromised host, a fertile "soil" for viral, bacterial and carcinogenic invaders by the way you live, like Harriet?

Or have you developed lifestyle habits and thought patterns that serve as an "inoculation" against disease, such as the way June paid attention to her diet and exercise?

What Exactly is Stress?

Your body is faced with daily external situational and environmental stressors or internal body changes (*physiological stressors*). The body itself is the "final common pathway" through which all of these changes act and operate to product necessary responses.

The body has a range of responses, regardless of the particular stressor trigger. Our brain constantly perceives and processes information from the world and from moment-to-moment changes inside the body.

Our brain is a *physiological* organ, as well as the *psychological* organ of "mind" expressing personality and guiding behavior. Thoughts, moods, and behaviors governed by the brain are caused by both *physical* and *psychological* causes.

Still

Our lives may not be as *physically* demanding as the workloads of our foremothers, but our roles are certainly more stress-filled and mentally demanding.

Balancing Act

The balance between risk factors and our "resistance," or hardiness, helps determine whether we stay healthy or develop acute or chronic illness.

Choices

There is a lot we can do that will improve our ability to resist the ravages of stress.

Vital!

This critical two-way street is often overlooked in health care today, especially when related to women and hormone imbalances.

Many times, patients are diagnosed with a psychological or psychiatric disorder because of changes in mood or behavior. Doctors are taught that such symptoms have psychological causes, whether internal thoughts and feelings or external situations.

Keep in mind; the brain is a *physical* organ, so it is just as susceptible to *biochemical* changes that can trigger the same mood or behavior symptoms.

It is a fact of basic biology that falling or low estradiol causes brain changes in chemical messengers (physical changes) that cause anxiety episodes, depressed moods, or difficulty sleeping (psychological symptoms).

Psychological stressors lead to profound *physical* changes in every cell in the body: ovaries, blood, arteries, intestinal tract, thyroid, immune cells, pain-regulating neurotransmitters, nerve endings, blood sugar levels, brain chemistry.

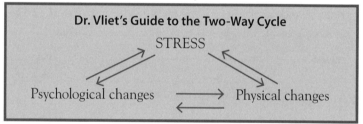

The Fight-or-Flight Response

The body's "stress response" is sometimes called the "fight-or-flight" pathway. When change hits, it activates the brain alarm center in the *locus ceruleus*, setting off a burst of norepinephrine and other chemical messengers that notify the rest of the body within milliseconds to respond.

The body reacts to the "fight-or-flight" signals in hundreds of ways: the adrenal glands rev up production of cortisol, another hormone that oversees stress response. Heart rate goes up to pump more blood. Eyes dilate, so we can see well. Blood vessels dilate to deliver more blood to the critical organs—especially the brain and heart and big muscle groups—and blood vessels constrict to decrease blood flow to less critical areas—intestines, hands, feet, scalp.

The liver makes more glucose and releases it into the bloodstream to maintain our energy. Muscles tense for action. Platelets are put on alert to help stop bleeding. All over the body, cells and organs are put on ready alert, all in a split-second.

What about the way we live today? Rushing around, going long hours without food, staying up late, getting up early, feeling angry, short-tempered, frustrated, overloaded.

These are all signals that continually activate the "fight-or-flight" emergency responses. Instead of a short-lived emergency like running from a wild animal as our Stone Age ancestors did, we now keep our bodies in a perpetual state of hyper alert.

It's like asking your body to run a 26-mile marathon every day, with no rest and recovery in-between, and not much food for fuel along the way. No smart marathoner does that! Yet, that's what is happening when you live a daily schedule like Harriet's.

What does this do our health over the long haul? Prolonged stress of any kind disrupts the body's balance, or homeostasis and causes symptoms related to the constant over activity of the "fight-or-flight" stress response pathways—headaches, muscle spasms, fatigue, fuzzy thinking, high blood pressure, irritable bowel, colitis, angina, eczema, frequent infections, irregular periods, acne, weight gain, allergies, hives, herpes outbreaks, anxious/panicky feelings, insomnia, depressed mood, angry/irritable moods, heart disease, cancers.

You shouldn't be surprised that prolonged stress can lead to suppression of the ovaries. It is part of Mother Nature's protective effects to prevent pregnancy if we are too physiologically "stressed" for our own health, and we are not able to sustain a healthy pregnancy. This is true in all species.

Mice lose fertility when kept in crowded cages with inadequate food and water and not enough room for their normal "territory." Our biology operates in similar ways to prevent further drain on the body's resources when it is already "running on empty."

You need ways to reduce the damaging effects of toxic stress, which in turn helps all your body systems work better.

Heads up! Anxious or depressed moods may have *physical* or hormonal causes, as well as *psychological* causes.

Calm? When the "emergency" is over, the body slowly settles back to normal pace and functions. Everything calms down…or does it?

Stress, Estrogen and Coping

Constant stress also suppresses ovarian cycles and decreases estradiol, testosterone, progesterone, and DHEA production. A stress-induced decrease in estradiol then contributes to an imbalance in norepinephrine, serotonin, dopamine, acetylcholine, and other brain-body messengers that regulate pain pathways, sleep, muscle repair, appetite, metabolism, memory, mood, energy, sex drive, and other functions.

Fact
Prolonged stress can also suppress your ovaries and cause loss of your hormones.

Women describe being able to coping successfully at other times of their lives, when their hormones were more optimal. Decreased estradiol also negatively affects the brain chemical messengers, causing a direct impact on women's ability to function optimally when their hormones are out of kilter.

45-year-old *Janie* said it well: "*I raised six kids as a single mom, worked full-time, took college classes at night, and I coped just fine with all that stress when I was younger. Now I hit perimenopause and I can't seem to deal with even the smallest stresses without falling apart!*"

Women's observations about coping better during times of optimal estradiol fits with what science now shows about the protective effects of this powerful hormone. For example, estradiol acts as an antioxidant, much like vitamins E and C, to scavenge "free-radicals" made constantly during metabolic processes.

Wrong medicine
A doctor's "pat-on-the-back" and direction to "relax more" or "take an anti-depressant" simply won't cut it.

Free radical production increases under stress, contributing to more cell damage. Antioxidants inactivate these free radicals and prevent their damage.

Estradiol also helps dilate arteries, including those that serve the heart. When you are under stress, adequate estradiol improves blood flow. All your organs work better with more oxygen, especially your brain!

The combined effects of estradiol helps improve our physiological reaction to stress and also regulate vascular metabolic, cognitive, and immune functions critical for us to cope with stress.

Once again, the role of stress is a two-way street: stress of all kinds suppresses the ovaries and decreases production of estradiol. This leads to insomnia, which decreases growth hormone release at night, and also increases fatigue and makes you feel foggy-brained. The stress of all these negative physical changes in turn leads to further decline in estradiol, which causes insomnia, which increases fatigue, and so on.

Stress also has adverse effects throughout mechanisms, too. Persistent stress and elevated cortisol shifts active forms of thyroid hormone into less active, or bound forms, to conserve energy. There is *less* of the available T3 so important for metabolism in muscle, the brain, and other organs. Lower free T3 results in more sluggish metabolism, more weight gain, more fatigue, and then more trouble coping with stress, another stress!

Chronic stress also causes excessive adrenal cortisol and other stress hormones. High cholestrol makes you fatter.

Release of excitatory amino acids (EAAs) occurs from the action of adrenal stress hormones on sodium, potassium, and calcium ion transport into and out of cells. Cortisol over activity alone leads to excessive build-up of the EAAs in the brain and nerves. Excess EAAs lead to over-stimulation of calcium-dependent enzymes in the nerve cells and generate more cell-damaging free-radicals.

The result is nerve cells die, leading to impaired conduction, abnormal pain regulation, and impaired memory, attention, and concentration. As stress persists, cortisol effects continue to build up over time, further damaging nerve cells in the brain's memory centers. This whole sequence is thought to be one way that memory, thinking, concentration and focus all diminish when we are under prolonged stress, such as illness or chronic pain. *Women often euphemistically call it "brain fog." Fibromyalgia sufferers call this "fibro-fog."*

Besides toxic effects on brain cells, excess cortisol impairs normal metabolism of collagen, which is the basis of healthy connective tissue, or fascia. You then have more muscle and joint injuries and pain. Wound healing becomes impaired.

Over-production of cortisol also disrupts the sleep cycle, which in turn means more fatigue, less growth hormone release, and less muscle repair at night. These negative changes further compound the sleep problems and muscle-damaging effects already occurring from the declining estradiol.

High cortisol levels and prolonged stress also increase the body's need for antioxidants, vitamins, minerals, and all the macronutrients. But lower than optimal estradiol means these aren't as well absorbed from the stomach and intestinal tract. Plus, when we are stressed and don't feel well, we don't take the time to eat nutritionally balanced meals—we may eat too much junk food, or overeat or under-eat. Poor nutrition then becomes another stress on our body.

Endless
It can feel like you are stuck in a quicksand pit—the harder you work to get out, the deeper you sink.

Brain-fog
If you are drinking a lot of soft drinks for quick energy, it makes the build-up of EAAs even worse.

See...
How it is all intertwined.

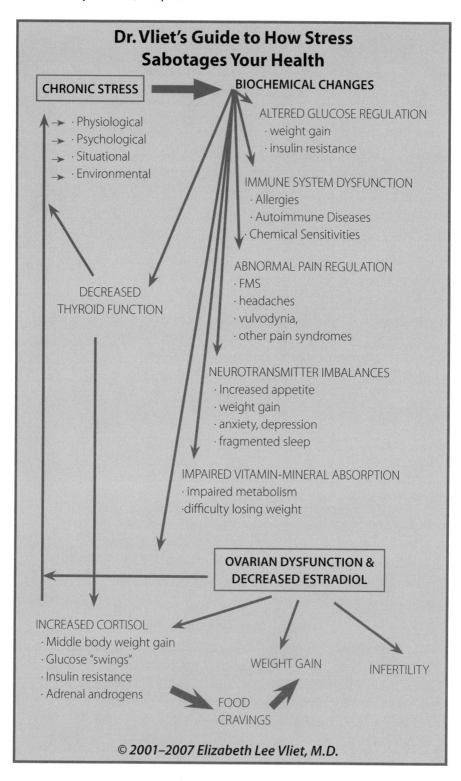

Dr. Vliet's Guide to How Stress Sabotages Your Health

CHRONIC STRESS ➡ **BIOCHEMICAL CHANGES**

· Physiological
· Psychological
· Situational
· Environmental

ALTERED GLUCOSE REGULATION
· weight gain
· insulin resistance

IMMUNE SYSTEM DYSFUNCTION
· Allergies
· Autoimmune Diseases
· Chemical Sensitivities

ABNORMAL PAIN REGULATION
· FMS
· headaches
· vulvodynia,
· other pain syndromes

DECREASED
THYROID FUNCTION

NEUROTRANSMITTER IMBALANCES
· Increased appetite
· weight gain
· anxiety, depression
· fragmented sleep

IMPAIRED VITAMIN-MINERAL ABSORPTION
· impaired metabolism
·difficulty losing weight

**OVARIAN DYSFUNCTION &
DECREASED ESTRADIOL**

INCREASED CORTISOL
· Middle body weight gain
· Glucose "swings"
· Insulin resistance
· Adrenal androgens

WEIGHT GAIN   INFERTILITY

FOOD
CRAVINGS

© 2001–2007 Elizabeth Lee Vliet, M.D.

Prenatal Stress: Does it Set Up Problems for Life?

We have discussed the effects of stress, mostly after puberty. But what about its impact on a developing baby? This is another adverse consequence of our high-stress lives. The damaging effects of prenatal stress have been found in studies of both humans and animals.

Stress effects in offspring include attentional deficits, learning disorders, hyperanxiety, disturbed social behavior, and impaired coping skills.

Many are similar to those of a biological depression, which suggests that stress on mothers during pregnancy can increase the possibility for children to develop depression later in life. The specific mechanisms are not fully known.

Stress-inducted brain changes include disturbance in the regulation of the hypothalamic-pituitary-adrenal pathways, decreased feedback inhibition of corticotropin-releasing hormone (CRH), higher overall levels of CRH in parts of the brain, elevated cortisol production in response to stress, fewer cortisol receptors in the brain's memory center, reduced effectiveness of the inhibitory activity of the brain's GABA (benzodiazepine) and endorphin (opioid) chemical messenger systems. If there is less effective function of the GABA and endorphin systems, there is more anxiety, pain and sleep problems.

Children of mothers overly stressed during pregnancy can experience delayed puberty because of alterations in the normal patterns of FSH and LH that oversee the ovaries and regulate menstrual cycles. Stress increases release of a brain hormone, corticotropin-releasing factor (CRF), which in turn inhibits release of the hormone, GnRH, that governs our menstrual cycles. If GnRH isn't released properly, the ovarian cycles don't occur normally, resulting in low hormone production, which in turn affects multiple body pathways.

The cumulative effects of persistent high cortisol levels and chronic stress adversely affect practically every pathway in the human body, especially women's ovarian hormone balance. If you want more information, read *Why Zebras Don't Get Ulcers*, by Robert M. Sapolsky, an excellent, humorous review of the damaging effects of excess corticosteroids over time.

Prenatal warning
High levels of the mother's stress hormones during pregnancy appear to cause long-lasting changes in the brain of the developing baby.

Stress
It is complicated, and has profound implications for all aspects of women's health.

Dr. Vliet's Guide to Adverse Health Effects of Excess Cortisol

- Middle and upper body fat gain, enlarged large breasts
- Hair loss
- Thinning skin with splotchy discolorations
- More fragile blood vessels, leading to easy bruising
- Elevated blood glucose, glucose intolerance and insulin resistance, leading to increased risk of diabetes
- Increased total cholesterol, LDL and triglyceride levels, lower HDL leading to increased risk of early heart attacks in younger women
- Disrupted formation of healthy collagen, the basis of healthy ligaments and tendons, leading to injuries, joint and back pain
- Fragmented sleep, leading to diminished Growth hormone, decreased muscle repair at night, and daytime fatigue. If your estradiol is also low, it adds to these negative effects of high cortisol.
- Disrupted thyroid function, leading to *less* of the available T3 that is so important for cellular metabolism throughout the body.
- Suppressed immune function, leading to more infections and illnesses
- Increased need for antioxidants, vitamins, minerals as well as proper balance of macronutrients, yet if you are stressed and don't feel well, you may not pay attention to the nutritional balance most needed
- negative effects on pain pathways, including increased brain excitability, via release of excitatory amino acids (EAAs), glutamate, and aspartate. This effect contributes to more pain and the constant feeling of anxiousness many women describe

©Elizabeth Lee Vliet, MD 2001–2007

Sleep Deprivation: Toxic to Your Ovaries and Your Health

"To sleep, perchance to dream: ay, there's the rub."

William Shakespeare—Hamlet, Act III

What? Premature menopause never entered my head.

Tossing and turning, waking up wide-eyed, looking at the clock, going back to sleep, waking up, looking at the clock. I have experienced episodes of disturbed sleep and thought I'd go nuts. I had always been a good sleeper until I hit age 37–38. I couldn't figure what was happening. My doctors thought it was the stress of a medical practice (made sense, given how busy I was), and I acquiesced to that idea.

Later, it dawned on me that I had been under a lot of stress at other times in my medical career and my life and did not have the same problems. What was going on? It turned out, probably from all the running I was doing at the time, my estradiol levels were actually quite low even though I had not yet hit 40. The loss of estradiol caused the frequent waking up.

A good night's sleep is more crucial to our health and wellbeing than most women realize. The quality of sleep is a major determinant of whether we are healthy, have an enjoyable life, and function optimally on a daily basis. Women are 50% more likely than men to suffer chronic insomnia. About 75% of women in this country get less than eight hours of sleep a night. Close to *1 in 5* women get less than six hours of sleep each night during the workweek.

Persistent sleep disruption and loss of sleep over time leads to drowsiness and fatigue, feeling "foggy" brained, memory loss, difficulties with concentration and focus, impaired judgment, depression, agitated-anxious moods, more suppression of optimal ovarian hormone production, muscle pain syndromes, disruption of the immune system, and even loss of libido.

A recent study even found that reaction times slow down when we are sleep deprived: *up to 50% slower after 17–19 hours awake than they are if you are legally drunk.* This study of people in their 30s and 40s looked at several measures: Mental and physical reaction times, accuracy, coordination, and attention span. The more hours without sleep, the worse they performed. And I haven't even listed *all of the negative effects* of sleep loss.

Based on the above, you see how lack of sleep costs society billions of dollars in lost productivity, and leads to over 100,000 car and truck accidents a year. And, if sleep deprivation is prolonged, it can lead to acute psychosis with full-blown hallucinations and delusions.

Sleep deprivation is regularly used in POW camps as a form of torture, and can lead to sudden death syndromes. If laboratory rats are robbed of sleep, they die within a few weeks. Sleep deprivation is too critical to ignore.

Sleep 101

We take sleep for granted although it seems rather mysterious. We breathe, yet it is as if we are unconscious. We dream of action and movement, but our muscles are completely paralyzed. What is sleep, really? What are the normal stages we go through each

Amazing!
"Within two weeks of starting on the estradiol patch, I was back to my normal sound sleep again."

Too many pills!
Women are also prescribed far more sleeping pills than men, but common hormonal causes of insomnia are rarely ever checked.

night? What does sleep actually do? Let's review some basics, since it is so critical to our well-being.

Non-REM

Non-REM sleep (NREM) are the four stages in which dreaming does not occur.

Sleep architecture is the medical term used to describe the normal pattern of sleep stages (shown in the Table below). Each is characterized by different electrical activity or "brain wave" patterns, measured on electroencephalogram (EEG) tracings, eye movement measures (EOM), and muscle activity (EMG).

Physiological responses such as dreams, penile erections, or clitoral engorgement only occur during REM sleep.

Problems with sleep (apnea, narcolepsy, and others) are evaluated in sleep laboratories to determine the specific type of disorder, which helps determine proper treatment.

You experience 70 to 100 minute cycles of all stages each night. You have more non-REM sleep in the first half of the night, and more REM (dreaming) sleep in the second half. NREM Stages 3 and 4, called "deep sleep" are the stages where the physical body's "wear and tear" are repaired and restored. Most Stage 3 and 4 deep sleep occurs in the first half of the night. Toward morning, REM sleep stages get longer and alternate with Stage 2 sleep.

REM

REM sleep is the stage in which dreaming occurs.

REM accounts for about 20% of our total sleep time, and on average, you enter REM sleep about every 90 minutes throughout the night. Just as Non-REM deep sleep restores the body, REM or dreaming sleep, is thought to restore the brain-mind and helps maintain normal learning and memory during the day.

Deep sleep is needed to restore the body, and repair daily wear and tear. GH oversees muscle growth and repair as one of its many functions. If these sleep stages are disrupted, such as by declining estradiol, then you lose the benefits of optimal GH to build new muscle tissue and repair the minor tears in muscle fibers. Loss of optimal GH means you are likely to gain weight, because new muscle isn't made.

Healing

Most of our daily amount of Growth Hormone (GH) is secreted in stages 3 and 4 each night.

Leptin is another hormone decreased by sleep deprivation. When leptin is present in normal amounts and cells properly respond to it, this hormone tells us when we are full after eating. If sleep loss persists, leptin decreases and you crave carbohydrates, even though you may actually have had enough total calories for the day. This is another reason we gain fat.

It is *not* true we need less sleep as we get older, but sleep *quality* declines for both men and women, for a number of reasons, even

Dr. Vliet's Guide to Some Common
Causes of Insomnia

- hormonal changes (ovary, thyroid, adrenal, pituitary, etc.)
- pregnancy—physical and hormonal changes
- drug and alcohol abuse (acute effects and withdrawal)
- tobacco (nicotine) use, nicotine patches
- excess caffeine (sodas, coffee, tea, chocolate)
- **stimulants** in "metabolic" or "energy" boosters: (examples include herbs with *ephedra,* also called ma huang, phenylpropanolamine (PPA)
- use of OTC weight loss products (many contain Gotu kola and other herbal stimulants)
- medical disorders, such as asthma, allergies, other types of breathing disorders, congestive heart failure, diabetes, fibromyalgia, sleep apnea, narcolepsy, restless legs syndrome, myoclonus, and many others
- medications, such as decongestants in allergy and cold medicines, theophylline (asthma), some antidepressants, testosterone or DHEA (if taken at night), corticosteroids (ex. Prednisone), beta-blockers, and many others
- jet lag, or shift work that disrupts normal sleep-wake cycles
- working late after the evening meal
- sensitivity to environmental chemicals, perfumes, cleaning products
- clinical depression, generalized anxiety disorders
- life stress, persistent worries, bereavement, post-traumatic stress disorders
- poor sleep habits (making your bed a home office doesn't help you relax!)

©Elizabeth Lee Vliet MD, 1995, revised 2001–2007

in healthy individuals. Poor quality sleep can be caused by many factors, such as hormone declines with age, obesity, alcohol use, cigarette smoking, use of decongestants, drinking coffee late in the evening, plus a number of medical disorders.

Unhealthy

Most of us really need eight hours of sleep each night, yet the overwhelming majority of Americans average between six and seven hours.

Sleeping pills interrupt normal sleep stages and alter the normal balance and progression of sleep stages. It is actually harder to get good quality sleep. Many people who take longer acting sleeping pills, such as Klonopin or Restoril or Dalmane, wake up feeling groggy and tired in the morning. Shorter acting ones, such as Halcion or Ambien, may wake you up too early because they wear off at 3–4 AM.

Eventually, sleeping pills make it harder for the body and brain to function normally and further impair energy, mood, and memory. These are some of the reasons I do not like women to use sleeping pills without first looking for the *underlying causes* of sleep problems, *including* hormone changes. *Sleep apnea,* for example, is one that *can be dangerous in combination with sleeping pills and causes many other health problems.*

Your Hormones and Sleep

Estradiol produced in the ovary is one of the primary hormones regulating the brain's sleep center. When estradiol declines—whether from menopause or other causes—we experience difficulty falling asleep and disruption of our normal stages of sleep, especially Stage 4, our deep, restorative sleep.

Bad for your sleep

People often turn to sleeping pills to treat insomnia, but this causes problems if you use them for more than a couple of weeks.

This is a common scenario I see in my patients. It doesn't matter what age you are; if you have a hormone imbalance and too little estradiol, it can lead to insomnia, whether it occurs from PCOS making too much testosterone and DHEA and not enough estradiol, or a post-partum hormone crash, or having a hysterectomy with removal of the ovaries and not enough estradiol replacement, or hitting perimenopause.

Low estradiol makes it hard to fall asleep several ways, such as by decreased serotonin activity and changes in the balance of other chemical messengers in the brain. You lay there, your mind obsessively stuck in worries from the day, unable to drift off to asleep. Women must have adequate estradiol for normal deep, restful sleep.

During the first few days of bleeding each month, many women report restless sleep. Some blame headaches or cramps, but falling estradiol and progesterone are more likely triggers for difficulty falling asleep, restless sleep, and early morning wakening. Both of these effects cause increased release of norepinephrine that acts like little jolts of electric current stimulating brain and body, keeping you awake or waking you up throughout the night.

As estradiol levels drop before a menstrual period, after ovulation, after a baby is born, from too much dieting or exercise, or at menopause, the fall also triggers the "alarm" centers in the brain. These centers then discharge a burst of an adrenaline-type chemical messenger, which "alerts" you and you wake up. The burst of adrenaline also hits the brain's heat-regulating center, short-circuits those pathways, and triggers a "hot flash or flush," followed by sweating that also wakes you up. These awakening episodes may be just a few, or may be many times a night. They leave you tired, groggy, and often grumpy.

Progesterone also has effects on sleep, but acts on different pathways from those regulated by estradiol. Taking progesterone doesn't *eliminate* the need for estradiol to restore sleep, as some books claim. A number of progesterone metabolites act at the same brain receptors as barbiturates and benzodiazepines. These progesterone breakdown products can have potent sedative effects.

How you take progesterone makes a significant difference in the sedative effects it produces. The liver "first-pass" metabolism makes most of these sedative breakdown compounds from progesterone, which means you have a much greater sedative effect if you take progesterone *orally*.

A *non-oral form*—vaginal gel, rectal suppository, sublingual troche or an injection—is directly absorbed into the bloodstream and bypasses the first step in the liver, so it has less sedative effects. Since progesterone can make you sleepy, there are occasional times when it is a useful addition to hormone therapy. For progesterone to be effective in helping you sleep, however, *estradiol has to also be restored to optimal levels.*

Taking progesterone every night for sleep must be balanced against its unwanted, potentially negative metabolic effects such as weight gain. If progesterone is used just to improve sleep for a woman who has had a hysterectomy, it can be effective in a lower dose (such as 25–50 mg) than what is needed to prevent excess buildup of the uterine lining.

Insomnia

If insomnia persists after your hormone levels are optimal and other simple causes corrected, I think it is important to have a sleep study.

No Zzz...

Falling estradiol disrupts the sleep regulatory cycle, and falling progesterone takes the lid off the GABA inhibitory pathways—much like stopping Valium suddenly.

Dr. Vliet's Guide to Normal Sleep Architecture

	TYPES OF BRAIN WAVE PATTERNS (EEG)	EYE MOVEMENTS	MUSCLE ACTION, VITAL SIGNS
AWAKE	mainly alpha waves, some beta	depends on task	Normal tone, able to have directed, voluntary movement
NREM Stage 1	mixed theta, beta waves; alpha <50%	slow, rolling	Relaxed, less tone; slower heart and breathing rates, lower blood pressure (BP)
NREM Stage 2	theta, bursts of sleep spindles, etc.	slow, rolling	Relaxed, less tone, slow heart and breathing rate, lower BP
NREM Stage 3 "Deep Sleep"	delta waves ("slow wave sleep") 20–50%	Slow	Relaxed, limp; Slow heart and breathing rate, low BP, release of Growth hormone
NREM Stage 4 (deep sleep)	delta waves now more than 50% on EEG	Slow	Relaxed, limp; slow heart and breathing rate, low BP; blood flow directed toward muscles, less to brain; GH released
REM (dreaming)	similar to waking	symmetrical, rapid, jerky	none (muscles are in effect "paralyzed"); penile erections, clitoral engorgement occur

© 2001–2007 Elizabeth Lee Vliet, M.D.

When Sleep Isn't Normal: Sleep Disorders and Your Health

Disordered sleep can take severe forms, such as *restless legs syndrome* (RLS) or *sleep apnea syndrome* (SAS). While RLS is not potentially life-threatening in the way that sleep apnea is, it does cause frequent awakenings. And because RLS interferes with deep stage 4 sleep that restores the mind and body, it is a cause of daytime fatigue, mood problems, and even weight gain.

If the sleep disturbance is severe, prolonged and includes significant apnea (stop breathing) spells that cause oxygen loss, the consequences can be more severe. Sleep apnea is a significant contributing risk factor for high blood pressure, cardiovascular disease, heart attacks, early morning sudden death, major depression, and sexual dysfunction. Such serious consequences occur from the dangerous drops in oxygen (02 saturation) in the blood when you stop breathing.

Oxygen saturation drops when you stop breathing. Low oxygen is made worse by the drop in estradiol, which causes a burst of catecholamines that trigger pounding heartbeats, palpitations, and unstable heart rate and blood pressure. This fall in estradiol and burst of catecholamines is the same trigger for hot flashes and night sweats. The result is that lower oxygen content in the blood creates less effective blood delivery to the heart due to both high blood pressure and too rapid a heart beat …all of which increase the possibility of a sudden heart attack.

RLS

RLS can occur in women with thyroid abnormalities or low iron stores (ferritin) or low estradiol.

Current therapeutic options for sleep apnea are limited to weight loss, surgery and/or continuous positive airway pressure (CPAP). It would be helpful to know whether hormone changes (as in PCOS, post-partum, perimenopause or menopause) play a role in the development of sleep apnea, and whether the use of hormone therapies to restore optimal balance, can alleviate sleep disorder symptoms. Recent studies from several countries show positive benefits of estrogen on sleep apnea. Both estradiol alone and estradiol with medroxyprogesterone acetate (MPA) regimens *decreased* sleep apnea significantly.

Warning

Sleep apnea plus the drop in estradiol with peri-menopause, menopause, or POD causes women to have a greater vulnerability to sudden death or heart attack than men.

Doctors previously thought fragmented sleep and the multiple awakenings women commonly experience in post-partum, peri-menopause or menopause were due solely to nighttime hot flashes. This sleep apnea study, however, showed that 40 percent of the waking episodes in the study were *not* associated with hot flashes. This explains why so many younger women with hormone problems report waking up frequently at night, without classic hot flashes.

Since sleep apnea is a more serious sleep problem, such positive findings about hormone therapy effects on sleep are promising for women with milder forms of insomnia. If your bed partner says your legs move all night, or you snore, or that you seem to stop breathing and then "jerk" back into a loud breathing, talk with a physician about sleep studies and insist on getting your estradiol level checked.

There are many mechanisms by which estradiol, alone or with progesterone/progestins, interacts with neurotransmitters and regulates brain centers involved in sleep pathways. Women have

Dr. Vliet's Guide to Sleep-improving Strategies

1. Go to bed when you are pleasantly tired. Try not to wait until you are so exhausted you can hardly move.

2. Establish a simple routine at a consistent bedtime. Likewise, have a regular wakeup time so your body keeps its normal rhythm.

3. Do not go to bed hungry, or too full from a heavy meal.

4. If pain interferes with sleep, ask your physician about proper medication.

5. If you need a nap, take one earlier in the day, preferably before 3PM. If you nap in the evening, you may wake up restless halfway through the night and then feel tired the next day.

6. Gentle exercise (like a short walk) helps you relax and feel genuinely tired. Don't overdo it, and do make it regular. Don't do an *aerobic* exercise routine just before retiring. It revs you up too much and makes it harder to fall asleep. On the other hand, *lack* of physical activity during the day makes sleep more difficult.

7. A glass of warm milk, along with a relaxing warm bath, really does help you fall asleep.

8. Avoid stimulants late in the evening (coffee, cola, tea, or chocolate) since they can keep you awake.

9. Once in bed, *comfort* is important. Make sure the bedroom isn't too hot; people sleep better in cool rooms. Make sure you have a comfortable pillow and mattress.

10. Fresh air and quiet create a more conducive environment for sleep.

11. If outside traffic sounds are a problem, try playing a recording of "white noise," such as ocean surf, to mask intrusive sounds.

12. Don't take your work to bed with you. I know this is easier said than done, but bedtime is not the time to rehash the concerns of the day.

13. Keep a pad and pencil by the side of the bed. If something does come to mind, write it down. You can then dismiss it and focus on relaxing thoughts or pleasing images that help you "drift off."

14. Darkness in the bedroom is more important than most people realize, since it helps the brain naturally produce melatonin, which maintains normal sleep. If your bedroom has a lot of light coming in the window, then wear a sleep mask. It's cheaper and safer than melatonin supplements or sleeping pills.

©Elizabeth Lee Vliet, MD 2001–2007

been telling doctors all along that our ovarian hormones *do* play a significant role in normal sleep, and when our hormones are out of kilter, we don't sleep well.

It doesn't matter how old or young we are, because this is a *hormone* effect, not an *age* effect. I have adolescent patients with low estradiol who have exactly the same fragmented sleep as my menopausal patients with low estradiol. My patients consistently say their sleep is better when estradiol is improved.

Physicians should not dismiss sleep problems in women as "just stress," and prescribe sleeping pills, if they haven't checked hormone levels. If women actually have sleep apnea, sleeping pills can cause more episodes of not breathing, making a bad situation more dangerous.

Findings
Researchers concluded that hormone therapy has a potential role in reducing sleep apnea.

Anger and Our Hormones: Toxic Effects of Negativity

I have noticed that many women are really angry about all they have been through. They are angry at doctors who have dismissed these hormone connections. I have *felt* the anger from many patients during consults. These women have both expressed and suppressed anger for many reasons: anger at losing significant relationships when sexual interest dies from lack of hormone catalysts; anger at having headaches; anger at feeling betrayed by the body and not having the energy to do what they want; anger at not feeling listened to or validated when they sought help; anger about not getting answers to feel better, and anger at losing quality of life. As one woman said, *"I think these hormone problems robbed me of my life and career!"*

Sleepless nights
Waking episodes and hot flashes are each separate and *independent* ways the brain responds to falling or low estradiol.

People cannot be separated into emotions *or* body. We are both. If the mind is tortured with angry, negative feelings, the body responds with an outpouring of cortisol a stress response that blocks healthy function of both ovaries and thyroid.

You have likely experienced the way anger causes physical symptoms: neck muscles tighten up and spasm, or you get a headache or diarrhea. Maybe you have hives, or your herpes breaks out again. There are a hundred ways anger is felt physically. Muscles bound by the threads of anger tension are *going* to hurt. Do a check right now. Think of something that makes you really angry, concentrate on it, and notice what happens to your neck and shoulder muscles.

What happens to your gut? What happens to your heartbeat? You can't avoid the physiological responses anger produces.

Cover-up

We smile to cover up the anger, trying to pretend all is well.

Recently, a patient shared a story that graphically demonstrated this anger-hormone connection. This young woman, in her mid-thirties, had a problem with cyclic acne and mood changes, along with memory problems that grew worse at the time of her menstrual period—pretty typical "low estrogen" type symptoms.

At her appointment, it was obvious that she was in pain. When I asked her about it, she said "*I really don't know what happened—my neck just started getting tighter and tighter, I am having trouble turning my head and it really hurts. I can't think of any injury. I skipped my period this month, but that's the only thing I noticed that was different.*"

She casually observed, "*you know, my patch seems to be wearing off sooner lately—it seems related to all the stress at my house—my sister-in-law and her three children came to live with us until her husband is transferred back here, and it has really been a zoo at home with my three kids and her three kids. And we don't see eye-to-eye on the way we discipline the kids, so it makes it really hard. I find myself feeling angry with her a lot of the time now. I can't say anything because she is my husband's sister. I get angry that she doesn't seem to appreciate what we are doing for them, and I get angry that she lets her kids do things I don't let mine do. Then I feel bad about myself for being so angry.*"

Vital

Hormone imbalance tends not to be a very visible problem.

CLICK. I realized the connection between her neck muscle spasms and pain, her missed period, and the estradiol patches wearing off sooner. *Her stress hormones were working overtime.* She unconsciously tensed her neck as she literally, and figuratively, "clenched" her jaw to keep from saying something she would regret.

But she didn't appreciate the connection and said, "*Oh, I'm really not that angry, we'll get through it, it's really no big deal.*" I adjusted her estradiol patch dose, and suggested massage therapy sessions for her neck. A month later, the pain pattern had affected her sleep, making her more tired and tense, and less able to "go with the flow" at home. She said at one point "*I can't remember what it feels like to feel normal anymore.*"

One day I received a letter from her. With big exclamation points she wrote that her neck pain was completely gone, and her menstrual cycles were more regular.

"It's amazing. Just as suddenly as all this had come, it dissipated. My sister-in-law and I had finally reached a point where we weren't speaking to one another and she moved out. My symptoms got worse over the next few weeks, and I realized how much anger and resentment I was harboring toward her. One day, just before Christmas, I called her, we apologized to each other, and I ended the conversation with 'take care'. I meant it. That night at dinner, I noticed, with complete surprise, that the pain in my neck was completely gone. When I thought back over things, I could see how the simple act of being pleasant to my sister-in-law released the intense anger that was keeping my jaws clenched and my neck muscles so tight. I was amazed at the difference in my body. There are still a lot of hurt feelings in this situation, but I feel I had a big breakthrough in making a choice that helps me feel better, both physically and emotionally."

Cause
The undercurrent of anger affected her physical body, her menstrual cycle, and how she metabolized the estradiol in the patches.

Her story illustrates a further point. Part of her body tension and hormone disruption was a result of anger, and part was a result of her negative judgments that she was "bad" because she felt angry. In our culture, women are taught that it is "ugly" or "bad" to express anger. We grow up with the message "if you can't say something nice, don't say anything at all." This gets translated into "if you can't be nice, don't be at all." So we clam up, tense up, jam the anger down deep inside.

No matter how badly we feel, we are taught to look pretty and be nice. We wear make up. We dress nicely. Above all, we smile. If we look pretty and smile, people—including doctors—then say, "So, how can you be having any problems? You look healthy, you look like you feel fine." Unless, of course, you are noticeably pale, gaunt, and have lost your hair.

Closed
If your emotions are "out of control," the stress feeds back to the body and leads to a physical shut down.

For women, showing you don't feel well is often a two-edged sword. If you convey how bad you actually feel, you may be accused of trying to "manipulate" others, or you may be labeled a hypochondriac. It's a catch-22.

My staff is often surprised when women come in for their appointments looking so good, after they have talked to them on the phone. In the front office, our patients are wearing their "public face." It is only in the privacy of the consult room that the public façade is dropped and their face shows pain, often with tears. But this happens only if they feel safe, listened to, and cared about.

Summary

When you see many doctors and still don't feel any better, you may feel angry. The anger is built on disappointment and frustration that may be understandable, but it leads you to the next physician carrying the baggage of negative emotions that can alienate the physician and staff from the start. If you are labeled difficult, complaining, or demanding, you become more alienated, feel devalued and discounted, and get angrier. The downward spiral perpetuates itself.

Your conscious mind may pretend the anger doesn't exist. You make your body carry the anger so your conscious mind can pretend it doesn't exist because it isn't "acceptable" for a *woman* to feel so angry. You're afraid people won't love you if you show your anger or, you may drive away those who could help you. You can fool me, you can fool your other doctors, and you can fool your family. But you cannot fool your body. Your body knows.

Anger is often a mask for fear. Take a time out, look inward honestly, and ask yourself, "If I am feeling angry, what am I afraid of? Is there fear hiding under the anger?"

You know. Your soul knows. Your body knows. Ask, and then listen. With answers, you can focus on ways of releasing the pent up corrosive feelings.

Anger and fear can be resolved. You must first admit they are there. Then commit yourself to release the negativity. It's OK to ask for help from others. None of the other medical approaches work optimally unless you add this one too. You must have good quality, restful sleep, and some relief from stress. Boiling with anger inside, however, will prevent both.

"Anger hormones" disrupt the balance of all the others in your body. Create an environment where it is safe to express and release your anger; it is essential to getting well.

You don't have to do it alone—there are friends, family, therapists, and others who can help you. A healthy balance of all aspects of your life is necessary for healing and to keep all your hormones in balance and functioning well.

Waves of pain
Like an undertow current at the beach sweeping you away, anger can drag you down and drown you if you don't learn effective ways to feel it, flow with it, releases.

Cure
Anger—whatever the source or cause—must be resolved for healing to take place.

Chapter 8
Lifestyle Habits and Cultural Issues—Unexpected Stress for Our Ovaries

Many factors affect the regulation of the ovary rhythm and hormone levels that can cause changes in your menstrual cycles. Some result in decreases in frequency of periods, some cause extreme changes in bleeding and some may stop your cycles altogether.

Many times we are too busy to notice these changes, or we may actually feel relieved to be rid of the inconvenience. After all, not many of us *like* the bother of bleeding every month. A lot of young women, particularly athletes, have told me that they were pleased when their periods came less often or stopped.

Other patients tell me that even their doctors dismiss the concern, saying things like "Oh don't worry about it. You probably don't miss the nuisance anyway."

There are hidden consequences to not having periods. The "convenience" of no periods means an underlying hormone imbalance that can cause adverse effects on your body and your future fertility.

The rhythmical nature of our menstrual cycles is governed by the brain's gonadotrophin releasing hormone (GnRH) or "pulse generator" that integrates all the hormonal, metabolic, and neural signals for the normal workings of the ovaries and reproductive function.

Before puberty, the brain has mechanisms to keep the GnRH pulse generator in check and prevent menstruation from beginning too soon.

After puberty, there are a variety of lifestyle factors, such as frequent use of cigarettes, alcohol, marijuana, cocaine, ecstasy and other drugs, chronic dieting, as well as the many chemicals, illnesses and environmental influences that can interfere with the brain's ability to properly regulate the menstrual cycle.

Excess stress (both physical kinds and psychological sources), being significantly underweight (such as anorexia nervosa), obesity, other metabolic disorders, and emotional losses—all of these can disrupt or even stop your normal menstrual cycle.

Lessons from the Track: A Young Woman's Wake Up Call

Exercise is good, right? We have all heard that it is one of the best "medicines" of all and we should exercise more. Certainly, a balanced program, designed for your needs and limitations, is an essential part of your health plan.

But what about the *amount* of exercise? We all know that *too little* exercise is detrimental, but can you exercise *too much*? Absolutely.

Exercise puts a physical demand, or stress, on our body. Too much can lead to injuries and shut down your ovaries, as this young athlete found out.

Tobra was 21. She started running track in high school and had a successful college career. Just before her college graduation, however, she had stress fractures in her spine, and was diagnosed with significant bone loss. Her trainer suggested she see me to discuss hormone options, and the possibility of adding other medication to preserve and rebuild bone.

Her menstrual periods began about age 11. She began running competitively at age 14, and by age 15, her periods stopped completely. At 19 she stopped running for a year because of injury. During this time her menstrual periods returned, although the flow was light.

When she resumed competitive running, she again lost her menses. By the time I saw her, she had not had any periods for the past three years.

In addition to the bone loss and lack of menstrual periods, she was having difficulty sleeping and would wake up feeling tired and slow. She was up multiple times at night to urinate, and had been embarrassed recently by urinary leakage, especially at the end of races.

She had trouble concentrating on her schoolwork, and said, "My short-term memory seems shot. I feel irritable a lot of the time, I cry over little things for no real reason, I don't have any interest in sex, and I have this awful fatigue much of the time now. I just don't feel like myself anymore."

Tobra didn't have any of the usual risk factors for bone loss, such as alcohol use, too many soft drinks, cigarette smoking, stimulant abuse, poor diet, or too little calcium. The extensive training schedule, running 5 to 10 miles a day every day was her only risk factor.

Even though running is a weight bearing activity, her intensive training suppressed her ovaries so she no longer menstruated. This also meant she didn't have adequate estradiol; her level was less than 20 pg/ml instead of well over 100 pg/ml as it should have been at that time in the cycle.

Her physical exam showed typical effects of low estrogen such as excess downy facial hair and decreased breast mass. Her DEXA test for bone mineral density (BMD) was far too low for her age, at both the spine and the hip.

Her doctor had tried to restore her periods with Ortho-Tri-Cy-clen birth control pills, but she had intolerable side effects and stopped. "*I was very emotional, sad, had mood swings, water retention and swelling, especially in my face and legs, along with weight gain and fatigue. I felt horrible and I could hardly run at all.*"

Since she did poorly on that particular balance of estrogen and progestin and the varying hormone doses, I suggested she try Ov-con 35, a steady dose pill with less progestin and more estrogen.

I also recommended Actonel, a medicine that prevents bone-breakdown and helps build new, healthy bone mass. She also needed to increase her food intake to provide better nutrition for her workouts and recovery, and she had to cut back her training to give her body more time to recover.

After a couple of months, she was sleeping better and had a higher energy level. At six-months, the markers of bone break-down had improved, and she was feeling well, with none of the mood problems she had with Ortho-Tri-Cyclen.

A year later, Tobra had stopped the birth control pill thinking she didn't need the hormones if she increased soy in her diet. She was drinking soy shakes, eating tofu instead of meat, and taking soy isoflavone capsules daily. *"I thought these were "healthy things to do,"* she said.

But when I repeated her BMD, she had quite a shock: she had lost another 5% of her bone mass.

Danger!
The dangers of soy... another 5% loss of bone and she was only 22.

I explained to her that soy alone would not restore lost bone, and could inhibit the positive effects of her own body estradiol. I recommended she restart Ovcon 35 and Actonel and stay on both for several years until her bone mineral density built up to a normal range.

She continued to do well on this regimen without any adverse side effects. Her bone density improves steadily each year. She now exercises for pleasure and fitness, keeping to a more realistic level that doesn't overstress her body.

Athletic Training and Your Ovaries

The medical term for exercise-induced ovarian suppression is *hypogonadotrophic hypogonadism*, or *hypothalamic amenorrhea*.

Effects
The combination of intensive athletic training and dieting can be devastating

This condition has been recognized for decades. But it has come to the forefront more recently more highly publicized women's events such as the Olympics and the emergence of competitors in "women's" events who are still pre-pubescent girls.

In Olympic circles, it is well-known that eating disorders and loss of regular menses are common among gymnasts, figure-skaters, divers, and swimmers, to name a few. Girls in these sports deal with demanding, incredibly rigorous, training schedules, spending hours every day in practice sessions and weight workouts.

They are also under tremendous pressure to have a "perfect body," at least for the skaters, divers, and gymnasts since judges also evaluate their "artistic presentation" (i.e. appearance).

Why?
Many athletes encounter declining performance, but don't have a clear picture of why.

Two major reasons make these issues of great concern:

First, many young non-athletic women are compulsively over-exercising trying to live up to the current images of beauty in our culture.

Second, with greater acceptance and encouragement of women athletes, we now have millions of school-age girls, teenagers, and college-age women participating in competitive athletics. Female athletes are pushing the envelope to optimize performance, to win. Competitive levels are now similar to men.

There is a lot more at stake today for elite women athletes: scholarships, multimillion dollar sport, and advertising contracts, endorsements, and cereal box covers await the best. The underlying message is that skill is not enough; *image* is everything.

Female athletes often feel pressured by agents and others to present the "complete package" of top performance and a "perfect" looking body. Training schedules keep them quite lean. Now, they often *diet* to keep weight down.

Go easy... Even relatively mild exercise can disrupt the normal menstrual cycle phases.

We must pay attention to the effect of athletic training on ovarian cycles and hormone levels. Research supports this relationship between exercise intensity and ovary effects. Both gymnasts and long distance runners have lost menstrual periods at a higher rate and for longer periods than control groups.

The findings also show that women who did not have regular periods had a much higher incidence of running-related fractures and lower bone density of the lumbar spine than did women who still had their periods.

The women runners who had ceased menstrual periods also had lower thyroid levels, so another important hormone was out of balance and wreaking havoc on body function.

Studies at Boston University by Williams and co-workers, published in 1999, found that short-term exercise can cause "egg" (corpus luteum) dysfunction even when exercise is limited to just one-half of the cycle, either follicular or luteal phase.

Luteal phase defect was found in 40% of women who exercised during the first half (follicular phase) of the cycle, and in 50% of women who exercised during the second half or premenstrual (luteal) phase.

This meant there were fewer ovulatory cycles, which could affect fertility. In the control group that didn't exercise, none of the women developed any corpus luteum dysfunction.

The researchers concluded the abrupt onset of training altered proper ovulatory function in the second (luteal) phase of the

---

What Happens With Dieting and Overtraining

- ovaries shut down
- menstrual cycles stop
- bone breakdown increases
- sleep goes haywire
- muscle declines
- energy fades

Slow down

Many fertility specialists recommend women cut back on exercise when they are trying to get pregnant.

cycle, regardless of *which* phase of the menstrual cycle phase the exercise occurred. This is why you should start slowly with a new exercise program and increase intensity gradually.

We are not certain of all the mechanisms by which exercise suppresses the ovaries, but we do know there are abnormal patterns of hormone secretion in women athletes.

Athletic training alters the GnRH pulse generator in the hypothalamus so that it fails to trigger the normal cyclic activity of hypothalamic-pituitary-ovarian pathways.

German research found that athletes with menstrual disorders also had significantly lower resting metabolic rates (RMR), even though daily caloric intake did not differ from athletes without menstrual disorders.

Estradiol plays an important role in our metabolism, so this study suggests that over-training and low estradiol decreased metabolic rate. That's the opposite of what we want: *we exercise to increase our metabolism not decrease it!*

Chronic Dieting, Anorexia, and Bulimia—Risks to Your Ovaries

Girls think they are too fat, so they start a diet. Dieting slows your metabolism, and makes it harder to maintain healthy weight as you age.

Unhappy

By the fourth grade, 80% of girls in the United States are already unhappy with their bodies.

Dieting damages normal ovarian and thyroid function, which has wide-ranging effects on your entire body and health.

The severest forms of dieting—anorexia and bulimia—are devastating to young women's fertility, and set them up for a lifetime struggle with weight.

Chronic dieting is also often the precursor to obesity, insulin resistance, and diabetes because metabolism was altered.

Why are so many young girls, adolescents, and young adults so obsessed with weight and body size? One explanation lies in the way we are brainwashed to believe we must be *thin* to be successful, happy and attract a man. The distinct message is that if we are not thin, we are not worthwhile.

Women in fashion magazines and advertisements are thinner than ever, despite years of concern about sending the wrong message about healthy *female* body size. These images begin in early childhood and continue our entire lives.

Think about it. What is the image of "*woman*" we are conditioned to believe is desirable? The ideal "woman" in ads is thin; young; muscular; usually white; beautifully groomed; with long legs; sexy feet; perfect white teeth; flawless skin; long thick hair.

Most of all, this woman is extremely thin. Size 2 or size 4 thin. She has no body fat; her bones protrude at the shoulder, clavicle, and hip.

We think that is how we are supposed to look. Then we berate ourselves if we don't.

Thinness, (which usually occurs from *under nutrition*), is one of the most frequent "suppressors" of normal menstrual cycles and healthy hormone production in young women.

But even women without full-blown anorexia push themselves to degrees of thinness that cause irregular cycles, low estradiol production, difficulty getting pregnant, and early bone loss.

A 1985 study of women aged 20–29 found that dieting for only 6 weeks (approximately 800–1000 kcal/day) caused plasma estradiol levels to decrease to *menopausal* concentrations during the final 2 weeks of dieting.

In two out of every three women, menstrual cycles were disrupted. It took 3 to 6 months for regular cycles to resume after dieting ended.

The authors concluded that *even mild dieting* interferes with ovarian hormone production, and causes disturbances of the menstrual cycle.

Women are affected by cultural images of being thin far more than men. Our identity is tied up culturally with our appearance rather than our career. **Ask women to chose thinness or health. Thin wins 99 times out of a hundred.** We feel that, at all costs, we must *look thinner and younger.*

Women restrict calories, restrict fat (and count every single dirty little fat gram), cut meat, cut dairy, and so on, until nutrition is so imbalanced, the body shuts down and metabolism slows to conserve fuel.

Self
We are not conscious of how such images profoundly influence us and shape our sense of self and self-worth.

Don't
Pushing ourselves to reach this "ideal" thin body profoundly perturbs all our body systems.

That's when you feel cold, tired, and irritable, have dry skin and lifeless hair. You worry you have *chronic fatigue* and spend thousands of dollars on medical consultations, tests, and supplements.

But still, you persist with the dieting, always focused on a *thinner* body, obsessed with wearing a size smaller. I commented to a patient that she was killing herself with dieting and food restriction. I was shocked when she said, *"Then at least I will die thin!"*

Unhealthy
Women with full-blown anorexia nervosa lose their menstrual periods completely.

Low ferritin is one dieting-induced physiologic stress that causes fatigue, and the likelihood of menstrual cycle disruption. Dietary intake of iron is often insufficient for girls, particularly those who cut red meat to lose weight or decrease dietary fat.

Losing iron in your menstrual blood, coupled with dietary deficits, also causes low ferritin. Low ferritin is a stresses the body because it impairs optimal delivery of oxygen to the body.

A study of competitive swimmers found low ferritin levels in 46.8% of the girls tested, compared to none of the boys. These women did not have full-blown anemia evident on their red blood cell counts, but they nevertheless had iron depletion with serum ferritin (iron stores) levels less than 12 micrograms/L.

Iron
The average American girl today gets only 40–45% of the recommended daily iron.

The researchers did not find ferritin levels lower over the course of the swimming season, so they did not conclude the training caused the low ferritin. The cause was low dietary intake along with loss of iron during menstruation.

Menstruating girls and women should supplement with iron because of monthly blood loss. Men don't have this monthly source of iron loss and usually get plenty of iron from red meat and other dietary sources.

Dieting ultimately makes you sick, in addition to disrupting your ovaries and their critical hormones. A truly healthy *female* body cannot co-exist with such extreme degrees of thinness.

The ovaries simply won't tolerate it. Much like a petulant child pouting in the corner, they shut down and refuse to make the hormones we need.

Dieting-induced ovarian suppression and loss of estradiol and testosterone means you push yourself into premature menopause, even though you may only be in your 20s.

We have earlier ovarian decline than our mothers did and are entering perimenopause at younger and younger ages. I am convinced this constant dieting is a factor, and also contributes to infertility. Dieting pushes the body to skip or stop menstruation, sending estradiol production lower than normal, and ovulation occurs less and less often.

Female hormones are designed to help store fat so that we can sustain pregnancies and nourish a growing baby. You won't get pregnant without a minimum percent of body fat because it is the signal to our regulatory systems that there is enough food for mother and baby.

Thyroid hormones are affected because the active, free hormone converts to the inactive bound portion as a protective response to low food intake in order to conserve energy.

Sadly, I can't fight Hollywood and the media machines that perpetuate these images, but hope this gives you perspective on the choice between health and thinness.

If you are tired and run down, cold, losing hair and sex drive, and your periods are barely there or don't come at all, you need a thorough nutrition evaluation and complete hormone tests, including both ovarian and thyroid hormones, not just a TSH check.

Restless legs syndrome
Low ferritin also leads to "restless legs" syndrome that disrupts sleep, another physical stress.

Another Diet Pitfall: The Low-Fat Diet and Your Ovaries

Being female
Pushing our bodies to such thinness thwarts Mother Nature's plan to keep us fertile.

Extremely low fat diets may not be all the hype would have us believe, especially for women. It was studies done primarily on men that researchers Dean Ornish and Nathan Pritikin found a reduced risk of cardiovascular disease with diets having less than about 15% fat. Women have *different* biological needs.

Optimal production of ovarian and adrenal steroid hormones that support fertility and pregnancy require a minimum level of fat in the diet so that the liver can make cholesterol, which then becomes the building block for estradiol, progesterone, testosterone, DHEA, cortisol, and aldosterone.

When women do not eat enough fat in the diet, the body cannot make hormones and the metabolism slows down, along with other effects such as mood changes, sleep problems, loss of libido, joint and muscle aches, dry skin and hair, brittle nails, and other problems.

Without adequate fat, several crucial vitamins can not be absorbed. These fat-soluble vitamins are A, D, E and K, which help the body with many functions, including the synthesis of important enzymes, proteins and prevention of cell-damaging free-radical build-up.

Warning
Extremely low-fat diets decrease your hormones!

Then, since many sources of fat are also sources of protein, a very low-fat diet is often low in protein, especially high-quality animal protein.

Too little protein causes *increased* production of sex-hormone binding globulin (SHBG), which in turn means a higher percentage of ovarian hormones that are present are now attached to this carrier protein in the bloodstream. "Bound" hormones are not then available in the free, active form for cells to function properly. Even less of your hormones are free to do their critical metabolic jobs throughout the brain and body.

Getting enough?
How much fat is enough? For women, 20–30% of calories as fat is a healthy range for optimal hormone production.

As a result, you become tired, listless, lethargic and "dull" on a diet like this, symptoms easy to confuse with hypothyroidism, yet due to an entirely different cause.

A 27-year-old patient found these problems when she reduced fat to 8–10% of her total calories. It almost cost her the ability to become pregnant. She saw me for the following problems: *joint pain, extreme fatigue, hair loss, daily headaches, dry skin and premature wrinkling, and waistline weight gain* in spite of the rigorous diet. She only had 3 or 4 periods a year, with the flow scant and shorter. Her gynecologist said not to worry since there couldn't be hormone problems at her age. She had not been able to get pregnant even though she and her husband had not used contraception for two years.

During her evaluation, she admitted being on an extremely low fat diet. Our analysis showed inadequate protein and an excess intake of simple carbohydrates and sweets.

Danger
On her bone density test, she already had significant bone loss (osteopenia), even though she was only 27.

My detailed hormone analysis identified markedly low estradiol, progesterone, testosterone, and DHEA. She also had a very low free T3 even though her TSH of 1.45 was optimal. Low free T3 is a compensatory, protective reaction to inadequate nutrition.

I recommended changes in her diet, increasing fat and protein into desirable ranges. Eight weeks later, she said *"Adding more fat and protein really seemed strange at first, after all the years of feeling brainwashed by the no fat gurus. But I had more energy and my sweet cravings disappeared...like someone turned off a switch! Pretty soon, my hair even started to get fuller and thicker again. I felt like I had my body back."*

Her new eating plan provided balance that gradually restored her ovarian and adrenal hormones, and her free T3 returned to the desirable level as well.

Until the diet changes could take effect, I also suggested that she use a low dose of bioidentical 17-beta estradiol, testosterone, and cyclic natural progesterone to help restore hormone balance. After six months her hormone levels had returned to healthy levels, and her cycles were now regular. She was able to go off the supplemental hormones.

A year later, she called to report she had a *healthy baby girl.*

Warning
When SHBG is high, there is less *free*, active estradiol and testosterone.

Occupational Hazards— Forewarned is Forearmed

There are many occupational groups with increased risk of certain diseases and/or injuries, because of exposure to industrial hazards and/or chemicals.

Flight attendants, a group that has been predominately female, get overlooked. I spend a fair amount of time in airplanes, and I talk with a lot of the flight attendants, particularly after they find out what I do. I see in their faces, based on years observing women with hormonal problems, changes in skin and hair.

I hear about their problems—insomnia, headaches, fatigue, no libido, allergies, memory problems, PMS getting worse, gaining weight for no reason, and on the list goes.

My observations and conversations with a limited "sample" of flight attendants does not make a scientific study, but I see patterns that are similar to what I see in women who come to our offices for hormone evaluations. These connections need to be explored.

Why are flight attendants any different from other groups of women in their age group? There are some unique aspects to this career that may contribute to women having earlier than usual "perimenopausal" type hormone changes.

We have already discussed the many adverse effects from poor nutrition, cigarette smoking, and sleep deprivation. Practically every flight attendant I have ever talked with has commented about their poor eating habits while traveling. When they do get to their destination and grab a meal, it's often airport fast food—high in saturated fat, sugar, salt, and preservatives. This isn't the way to a healthy body or healthy ovaries.

Early menopause
Women living at high altitudes, above 7,000 feet, commonly have earlier menopause than women at lower elevations.

Since most planes are pressurized to an approximate elevation of 8,000 to 10,000 feet, so flight attendants are spending a lot of time in an environment equivalent of living on a mountaintop.

Amazing what sound nutrition can do to get your "hormone power" back!

Air is drier at these elevations, contributing to dehydration, and exposure to ionizing radiation is more intense. Ionizing radiation causes many different types of damage to the body, depending upon the exposure.

Each of these elements can *independently* cause early menopause, or at least a decline in ovarian hormones, especially estradiol.

If you are flight attendant with a number of years in this career, and have begun experiencing changes in your menstrual cycles or having other symptoms I describe, I encourage you to pursue having a comprehensive hormone evaluation and bone density testing, as described in Section IV. Your health is worth it!

Dr. Vliet's Guide to Flight Attendants Risks

The role of flight attendant *combines* a number of risk factors that contribute to early ovarian decline and low hormones:

- hours at high *altitude*
- exposure to *ionizing radiation*
- loss of normal *sleep*
- frequent changes in *sleep schedules*
- frequent *time zone changes* that affect circadian rhythms
- *dehydration*
- *erratic nutrition*
- marked increase stress of travel under today's security risks
- exposure to *secondhand cigarette smoke* (for those who have been in this career longer, since smoking on planes was only banned on all planes in the U.S. in recent years)

© 2001–2007 Elizabeth Lee Vliet, M.D.

Negative Self-talk, Self-image

I am talking about the impact of our "inner tapes," those thoughts and feelings that go around and around our minds, some good, some critical, some self-doubting, and some chastising. Some are there from childhood scars; others are there from present day disappointments or wounds from careless comments of people around us.

An example of negative "inner talk" many of us share is summed up well in this ad from the 1990s, written for Nike by *women* writers:

"Fear of Failure
Fear of Success
Fear of Losing Your Health
Fear of Losing Your Mind
Fear of Being Taken Too Seriously
Fear of Not Being Taken Seriously Enough
Fear That You Worry Too Much
Fear That You Don't Worry Enough
Your Mother's Fear You'll Never Marry
Your Father's Fear That You Will

....it's not so surprising that there are a lot of conflicts and a lot of fears."

Negatives

"Negative tapes" in our mind are the stresses to the body... and affect hormone balance.

This ad poignantly describe the double bind in which women often find themselves. All of us have these doubts and worries due in large measure to the culture in which we live. The psychological pressure creates more physical stress in our bodies, which in turn affects our hormone balance and leads to physical and psychological symptoms.

We are also bombarded with psychological messages that say *someone else* will take care of us, that "someone else" is often a husband, a doctor, an attorney, or a businessperson. The weight of the entire culture supports this message. As a result, we may not feel confident in our own decisions.

It is not surprising that health care has become another *paternalistic* system, one in which women are "told" what is best by authority figures. In this male-dominated system, women are labeled as worriers, hypochondriacs, neurotic, anxious, and hysterical and overutilizers of medical care when we go in as patients, trying to explain unusual or puzzling symptoms that fall outside the physician's specialty box.

Outside authority?

Women are given the unconscious impression that there will be an outside authority to tell us what to do.

In addition, women are the usual caregivers for everyone else, far more than men. Many women tell me they feel overloaded with the responsibilities of caring for everyone around them and hardly have a moment to call their own. They feel "selfish" for taking time out to take care of themselves. Some of my patients tell me that they feel guilty taking time to read, saying *"I found myself constantly justifying the value of the information for the amount of time I spent on myself reading this!"*

Time

Most of my patients constantly struggle finding time and space for themselves in their lives.

Burden

We struggle with the burden of our perceived inadequacies alone.

Eventually

Over time, the cumulative effect plays out in our body and disrupts our ovaries' ability to make critical hormones.

I thought about this overload of care-giving responsibilities as I read the tragic headlines about Andrea Yates, the young mother with post-partum psychosis who killed her five children. Even with her own catastrophic post-partum illness, she had also been caring for an invalid father with Alzheimer's, and her five very young children. She was even home-schooling them, in spite of the obvious toll on her own health.

We see the disastrous, horrifying consequences that can occur when a woman reaches her breaking point. To me, the tragedy is how she, and the children in her care, were failed by all those around her—the family who didn't "see" that she was drowning in illness and overload. In my opinion, she was failed by the medical professionals who didn't evaluate the hormone connection in her postpartum depression, and the doctors who didn't "see" her psychosis and stopped critical medication prematurely.

Ultimately, she was failed by a legal system woefully unprepared to comprehend the enormity of a psychotic mental illness and "see" that it is more than simply knowing right from wrong.

Fortunately, her tragic story had a somewhat better outcome when she was recently retried and found *not guilty by reason of insanity.* The new verdict doesn't bring her children back, but it does allow her to be in a hospital, not prison, and receive treatment.

Summary

The collective impact of all these stressors, both psychological and physiological, produce profound changes in the body, whether they are lifestyle choices or societal stereotypes and cultural biases.

The health of our ovaries as well as the rest of our body is affected. The consequences vary from woman to woman, but overall, there are similar patterns to the symptoms women experience, regardless of age.

Recognize these factors and their very real consequences on your health. Make appropriate lifestyle changes to improve your health. And, if you have any of the symptoms or body changes described, see someone knowledgeable and have your hormones checked properly.

Don't compromise your needs.

You are worth some care taking too!

Chapter 9

Ovaries At Risk:
Unusual Effects of Viruses and Medical Illnesses

Mysterious, puzzling, and bizarre are words that often run through my mind as I listen to the experiences of my patients as they describe *when* their hormone symptoms began. Many unusual triggers have led to sudden and premature menopause in patients I have evaluated, as in this list.

Perhaps our ovaries are more at risk, and sensitive, than doctors appreciate. My patients and I are on a journey, rather like a detective, to understand the causes and triggers of their problems and find solutions to help regain their health.

While sometimes we may never know for certain what triggered the premature ovarian decline, we are usually able to identify clues in women's experiences, and then correlate with the science that explains and validates women's own observations.

Women often ask me which type of specialist they should see for these problems—is an internist or endocrinologist or a gynecologist better? My short answer: whichever specialist listens, will do complete testing, and offers options to help you improve your health. Many of these problems cause symptoms that cross the "specialty" boxes of our current health care system. The point is to get the problem *correctly* identified and *properly* treated. So go with the person who is best qualified to help.

Toxins from Ticks, Spiders and Viruses

Lyme Disease, transmitted by the deer tick, has gotten a great deal of attention in recent years. Just one tick bite can cause peculiar problems. You may be familiar with these symptoms—bull's eye rash, diffuse joint pain, muscle aches, and persistent fatigue. But

Got these?
Tick bite?
Black widow spider bite?
Viral illness?
Chlamydia infection?
Hemorrhage following delivery?

Caution
Don't get caught up in doctors' "turf" issues over who is "supposed" to check your hormones.

I doubt you have read much about *tick bites* triggering *premature ovarian decline*, or *premature menopause*.

Wisdom
I have learned that with the human body, very few things are "impossible."

In fact, the doctors I have discussed this with have usually said "Impossible." There usually isn't much conversation or discussion. Most doctors simply dismiss the idea with the comment, "It can't be" and move on.

I have a number of patients for whom I could find no other trigger in their medical or lifestyle or family history to account for the sudden onset of menopause-like symptoms except the tick bite, or a spider bite, or severe viral illness such as "mono" (infectious mononucleosis).

These types of illnesses can trigger an inflammation of the ovary that we call *oophoritis*. Since we don't have good tests to measure oophoritis, however, it often goes undiagnosed.

The symptoms are similar to low estradiol in PMS, menopause, or other causes, so the connection with the bacteria, virus, or "bug" is usually missed.

Sometimes this isn't critical, because the treatments may be the same, regardless of cause. But with Lyme disease or Chlamydia, it is important to ferret out the cause because you may need antibiotic therapy to prevent long-term complications.

Oophoritis
Inflammation of the ovary that can be viral, bacterial, toxic, or autoimmune.

So if you have a bug bite or viral illness and then notice changes in your menstrual cycle or you start having hot flashes, night sweats or other menopause-like symptoms, make sure that you insist on a thorough hormone evaluation.

In patients I have seen, these unusual triggers have caused such significant loss of ovarian hormones that women developed osteoporosis in their thirties. You, and your doctors, need to take these issues seriously. Examples of my patients show what can happen when these types of oophoritis are missed.

Linda had a sudden, full-blown menopause at 30, in spite of excellent health with no risk factors for early menopause. I first saw her about ten years after her symptoms began because she was "*tired of being so tired all the time and just not feeling well.*"

She said hot flashes, night sweats, restless sleep, joint and muscle pain, fatigue, and *abrupt loss of her period* began shortly after she had been bitten by a black widow spider, which made her quite ill. She was certain the toxins in the spider venom triggered her menopause, but "*My doctors just blew me off and pooh-pooed that idea. They said I was too young for this to be menopause!"*

She was treated for many years with antidepressants for a low-grade, depressed mood, loss of energy, and problems sleeping. There was not a great deal of improvement. She also tried many different herbs and vitamin supplements, but nothing seemed to restore her former sense of well-being.

The character and pattern of her symptoms, the obvious sign of losing her periods, and the bone loss, convinced me that she had been thrown into menopause by the toxins in that spider bite. There simply were no other risk factors and no history of early menopause in her family.

Now that we have found a hormone combination that works well for her, she has regained much of her former vitality and is also rebuilding bone to replace what she lost. Today, she feels angry, and sad too, that her insights were discounted and she spent so many years not feeling well.

I've had quite a number of patients, mainly from the east coast where deer ticks are widespread, who had clearly documented Lyme disease followed soon after by the usual symptoms of ovarian failure, including loss of periods.

Coleen was in her 20s when diagnosed with Lyme disease. This was followed by severe, intractable PMS with marked mood swings, joint aches, muscle pain, chronic fatigue. She also gained 30 pounds she couldn't lose, no matter how diligently she followed a diet and exercise program.

Her periods didn't stop completely, but her menstrual cycles and bleeding pattern changed dramatically: her cycles were closer to 35 days with heavy bleeding and severe cramps. Even though she too had no other risk factors for early ovarian decline, her hormone profile told the story.

Thyroid and adrenal tests were excellent, but she had lost bone density and had a Day 20 estradiol of 98 pg/ml even though her progesterone was excellent at 18.5 ng/dl, showing she still ovulated. The high progesterone in the face of *low* estradiol caused her mood problems and changes in bleeding pattern.

After we found a steady dose birth control pill (Ortho-Cyclen) that worked well, her symptoms improved markedly, and she no longer had the monthly "crazies" with her mood swings.

Spider Bite
She said, *"My symptoms of menopause all started after that black widow spider bite. But my doctors dismissed it!"*

Too early?
By the time I checked both her hormone levels and her bone density, she had developed osteoporosis even though only 40 years old.

Both of these women, as well as most of the ones I have seen with similar stories, had seen multiple doctors and spent thousands of dollars on sophisticated medical tests. Of course, no one checked the basic ovarian hormone levels that might have confirmed what the women suspected all along.

Chlamydia and Other Sexually transmitted Diseases

Chlamydia is one of the most common sexually transmitted bacterial infections in the United States, but it is notoriously difficult to diagnose.

In the early stages, it often causes such subtle, vague, and indolent symptoms that women don't know they have been infected and mistake symptoms for "stress."

One woman began in her late twenties having problems with painful bladder problems and recurring vaginal infections that were increasingly difficult to treat. Then, in her early thirties, she started having with menopause-like symptoms.

After 25 years of suffering bladder pain, chronic vaginal infections, debilitating fatigue, loss of sex drive and unexplained infertility, an infertility specialist in New York finally diagnosed her with Chlamydia, and said this had been the cause of her problems all along.

I saw her for a consult a few months after she had begun treatment for the Chlamydia. She said:

> "I went to the top doctors in New York. They never checked for it and I certainly didn't know I might have been exposed to it. I started trying to get pregnant in my 30s but I never was able to. I finally went to a fertility specialist who was the first doctor that checked me for Chlamydia. He put my husband and me on antibiotics and finally it resolved. It affected me terribly for so long. I had very painful periods, really bad PMS with terrible hormone swings, and I was told I needed estrogen and was put on Premarin years ago, even though I had it all over my medical charts that I had severe allergic reactions when ever I got around horses! I was so angry that I suffered all that time now knowing what was wrong with me, and not knowing why I never could get pregnant."

Once she had been successfully treated for Chlamydia, her ovaries began to cycle again, the bladder problems gradually

---

Warning

Sexual transmission of viruses and bacteria may lead to similar oophoritis syndromes and loss of healthy hormone production.

Tragic

"After the Chlamydia was treated, my ovaries started working again and I could feel my ovulation— but here I am now at 48 and it is really too late for me to try and have a child."

resolved, the recurring vaginal infections stopped, and her PMS improved. She had already scheduled the consultation with me, and decided to see what additional suggestions I had for her hormone management, even though she could see that the antibiotic treatment for Chlamydia had a dramatically improved her cycle function and symptoms.

Fact
The unrecognized Chlamydia caused her ovarian dysfunction and inability to become pregnant.

At our meeting, I found that her estradiol was still low at 30 pg/ml, and her testosterone was also low at 17 ng/dl. This fit with her residual symptoms of insomnia, hot flashes, difficulty with short-term memory and loss of interest in sex. I recommended increasing the dose of her estradiol patch and adding a low dose of natural testosterone. Since she had such an excellent response from her antibiotic treatment for the Chlamydia, I did not make any further changes to her therapy.

Chlamydia organisms must live inside cells of the body to survive. We call this type of organism an *obligate* intracellular parasite. It is difficult to diagnose because it hides in white blood cells (macrophages and monocytes) that travel throughout the body in the blood.

Nasty travelers
Camouflaged in our own cells, Chlamydia organisms can be carried via the bloodstream to other parts of the body, like the ovaries and joints.

Chlamydia has long been known to cause *pelvic inflammatory disease* (PID) as well as infertility. Chlamydia infections, however, can cause additional problems that may surprise you.

Both Chlamydia and the sexually transmitted bacteria that cause gonorrhea, can also lead to *inflammatory arthritis* and are one of the most common causes of arthritis in young women.

There is another type of joint inflammation, however, that is far more common in women, at a ratio of about *eight* women sufferers to every one male: TMJ, or *tempromandibular joint pain-dysfunction syndrome*. TMJ causes significant pain, debilitating quality of life, lost productivity, and costs sufferers thousands of dollars for evaluation and treatment.

There is now evidence that a hidden Chlamydia infection can play a role in the enormous female preponderance of TMJ, and also contribute to decline in ovarian hormones.

Fact
Chlamydia can trigger oophoritis and affect hormone balance.

Drs. Henry, Hudson and Gerard examined the synovial fluid of TMJ sufferers for the presence of Chlamydia, thinking that it could be an example of an inflammatory arthritis from infection with this organism. This study, published in 1999, is the first to show that, in fact, Chlamydia organisms are present in large numbers in the synovial tissue lining the jaw joint of patients with TMJ.

Women hit harder
All of the patients with both Chlamydia and TMJ were women, with an average age of 34–37 years.

But not men?
None of the males in their study tested positive for the Chlamydia organism in the synovial tissue.

Numbers
By the age of 50, 10% of women have diagnosable thyroid disorder. By age 60, it jumps to 17%. This means millions of women.

After finding that so many women with TMJ also had the Chlamydia organism present in the jaw joint, these dentists concluded that TMJ dysfunction and pain can be an unrecognized inflammatory, infectious arthritis. If TMJ is caused in some women by Chlamydia, then early treatment with the right antibiotics may help prevent this debilitating syndrome.

If Chlamydia can be disseminated through the bloodstream to infect the jaw joint, it can also travel to infiltrate the ovary. Since Chlamydial infections often go undetected, particularly in women, there is a strong possibility that this organism may be a trigger for an infectious *oophoritis* that can lead to early loss of the ovarian hormones, as well as cause an *arthritis*.

Early disruption in healthy function of your ovaries can lead to the whole gamut of symptoms I have described.

Don't let this happen to you. Practice safe sex, and ask your doctor to test for the sexually-transmitted infections at your annual pelvic exam.

Thyroid Disorders and Your Ovaries

The statistics are eye-opening: Thyroid disease affects more than 10 million women, and is *eight to twenty* times more common in women than men.

According to the Thyroid Foundation of America, more than half of the people with thyroid disorders are undiagnosed. Why talk about thyroid in a book about ovaries? *Because the thyroid gland is a critical regulator of ovarian function and fertility.*

The thyroid gland and ovaries are in constant direct hormone communication with each other, as well as with the brain through the hypothalamus and pituitary, the two glands that oversee ovarian function.

Younger women today have a high incidence of subtle thyroid dysfunction that we call *subclinical*, and it can affect the ovaries as well as leave you feeling sluggish and moody. PMS symptoms intensify and you may have difficulty getting pregnant.

I have evaluated hundreds of women over the years with undiagnosed thyroid disorders that caused ovarian problems. In younger women, thyroid disorders are more damaging to reproductive function than in men. As you get older, and *hypo*thyroidism goes untreated, it can lead to high cholesterol by impairing the body's ability to remove "bad" LDL and VLDL cholesterol particles from the circulation.

The specific effects depend on which type of thyroid problem you have—*hypo*thyroidism (low thyroid) or *hyper*thyroidism (excess thyroid), and what age it occurs.

Thyroid imbalances also cause a wide range of both physical and emotional symptoms, from anxiety, agitation, depression and mania to rapid-cycling "bipolar"-type syndromes. Many of the same symptoms can be caused by loss of the ovarian estradiol. That is why it   is even more critical to check all of these hormones carefully when symptoms appear.

If overactive thyroid (*hyper*thyroidism) goes untreated, serious health problems include atrial fibrillation, congestive heart failure, osteoporosis, muscle wasting and weakness, anxiety, agitated depressive syndromes, persistent insomnia, and cognitive difficulties similar to attention deficit disorder.

These multiple effects are not surprising when you consider that thyroid hormones help translate our DNA code guiding cells to make and use nutrients, vitamins, hormones and other various building blocks used by the body and brain.

Let's look at the thyroid hormones and how they are regulated, since they are intimately involved with the normal function of our ovaries and fertility.

Danger
Untreated hypo-thyroidism also leads to high blood pressure, early heart attacks, stroke, marked weight gain, clinical depression, and dementia.

A Guide to Your Thyroid Hormones

The thyroid system is controlled by the brain's master control center in the hypothalamus. The hypothalamus produces TRH, or *thyrotropin releasing hormone*, that stimulates the pituitary to produce and release TSH, *thyroid stimulating hormone*.

TSH circulates in the blood and directs the thyroid gland to make T4 (*thyroxine*). T4 made in the thyroid gland is converted in the gland and in body tissues to the more active form, T3 (*triiodothyronine*)—if all the pathways are working properly.

The thyroid gland has several important enzymes, such as thyroid peroxidase (TPO), that are essential to convert T4 to T3. If the body doesn't make enough T3 from T4, this can lead to symptoms of thyroid disorder even with supposedly "normal" standard thyroid function blood tests.

Great Imitator
Thyroid disease causes just about every physical, mood or cognitive symptom ever described!

T4 and T3 circulate in the bloodstream to serve the entire body and also report to the pituitary and hypothalamus about the thyroid gland's production—not enough or too much or just right. This feedback determines how much TRH and TSH to make which in turn directs T4 and T3 production.

Very little T3 and T4 occur in the free, active form in the blood; over 99% of the T3 and T4 is attached or "bound" to three carrier proteins: *thyroid binding globulin* (TBG), *transthyretin* (TTR), and *albumin*.

For example, only about 0.2% of T3 is in the free, unattached form. This means that anything in your diet or medications that changes the balance of the carrier proteins can have a huge impact on how your thyroid hormones work.

The whole process of thyroid regulation is similar to the thermostat in your house that registers hot or cold relative to where you set the temperature. If it's too hot or cold, signals go back to the heating or cooling system and direct it to turn off or on. If the thyroid gland is *not making enough T4 and T3*, then the pituitary puts out *more* of the stimulating hormone, TSH.

This means an *underactive* thyroid gland shows up with a *high* TSH, usually greater than 5. Many patients think that a low TSH means *hypothyroidism. It is the opposite.*

A *low* TSH means the pituitary senses *too much* thyroid hormone in the bloodstream and shuts *off* the stimulating hormone.

If TSH is too low (less than 0.5), this indicates an over-active thyroid gland.

Thyroid hormones are essential for normal body metabolism, brain development and normal reproductive function in most species, especially humans. T3 and T4 regulate our ovarian cycles along with many aspects of brain and nerve function, from growth of neurons, to the movement of nerve cells to the proper areas for their function. They oversee the formation of normal nerve cell junctions (*synapses*), and formation of the protective fatty sheath (myelin) around nerve cell extensions (*axons*) that connect one cell to another.

Human brain development occurs at specific windows throughout our time in the womb. Proper levels of thyroid hormones are critical during these times. If we don't have thyroid hormones and iodine in the right amount, at the right time, and in the right

Beginnings
Thyroid hormones are also crucial for fetal brain development during pregnancy.

Opposite
Just remember, it's the reverse of what you expect: low TSH = *hyper*thyroid, high TSH = *hypo*thyroid.

Cross-talk
There are thyroid hormone receptors on the ovary, and ovarian hormone receptors on the thyroid

balance, permanent brain damage occurs leading to neurological and learning disorders. This type of brain damage, and the symptoms that occur later, depends on *when* in pregnancy, and *how severe*, the disruption was.

Worldwide, low thyroid hormone during brain development is one of the leading causes of learning disorders, attention deficit disorders and other subtle types of neurological/cognitive dysfunction. Learning disorders and mental retardation are common in areas of the world where iodine is deficient in the diet.

Although iodine is added to salt in the United States, chemicals in our environment can interfere with adequate dietary iodine so that it cannot be used normally by the thyroid gland to make thyroid hormones.

This is another way that exposure to synthetic chemicals during pregnancy can have damaging effects: by interfering with normal thyroid hormone action when the baby's brain is developing in the womb, these chemicals profoundly affect the brain's ability to function normally the rest of your child's life.

How do *your* thyroid hormones affect your baby? Some cross the placenta, primarily as thyroxine (T4). If you are pregnant and exposed to chemicals such as pesticides that can interfere with your ability to make enough T4, less T4 is available for your baby's developing brain.

I described above that T3 is the most active form of our thyroid hormone, especially in the brain. Most of the T3 for our brain is actually made there from T4 and by the action of a particular enzyme, *thyroid peroxidase* (TPO).

This type of enzyme deficiency could explain why, even though serum T4 and T3 levels are normal, an infant or young child can have hypothyroidism causing learning and neurological deficits.

Another study, published in April 2001, of 182 Swedish fishermen's wives, found that the women who ate more fish had higher blood and body fat levels of persistent organochlorines and PCBs and also had lower levels of their thyroid hormones than did women who ate very little fish.

This suggests that the chemical contamination of foods can affect thyroid hormone levels in adult women. These findings are especially important for women during pregnancy because of potential long term damage to the baby.

Issue #1

Pesticides may also damage TPO, making it unable to help make enough T3.

Issue #2

High soy intake also blocks the action of TPO.

The Role of Iodine and Iodine Deficiency

Iodine is a critical element needed by the thyroid gland to make its thyroid hormones in the process called *iodination*.

You can see how the balance of iodine available to the thyroid gland is important for optimal thyroid hormone synthesis. Excess iodine intake over time may lead to hyperthyroidism, more so in older people.

Too much iodine intake over time may disrupt thyroid hormone actions and also cause hypothyroidism and goiter, as we see with the high incidence of goiter in some areas of Japan where seaweed is eaten regularly. Normally, however, our thyroid gland regulates its iodine metabolism several ways to maintain balance.

Iodine 101
There are three iodine molecules added to make T3, and four to make T4.

Many areas of the world have soils deficient in iodine, and that includes major areas of the Midwestern United States, the so-called "goiter belt." Adding iodine to salt in this country helped decrease the incidence of goiter, but it is rising again in recent years, in part because so many people (women especially) have cut down on salt.

A recent study from Switzerland showed a similar pattern. High goiter rates in iodine-deficient areas were virtually eliminated with the introduction of iodized salt. Then in 1991–1992, researchers saw a rise in goiter rates again, for several reasons: reduced intake of salt, increased use of foods prepared with non-iodized salt, and more diverse diets. The Swiss health officials recommended people use iodized salt again. I think we should follow this recommendation as well.

Careful
Iodine deficiency can produce hypo-thyroidism and increasing likelihood of goiter.

There is another reason for iodine deficiency to reappear: many chemicals in the environmental POPs "endocrine disruptor" group can interfere with our ability to use the iodine in our diet. This is caused by a number of mechanisms.

POPs interfere with the function of the enzymes needed to manufacture T4 and T3, and interfere with thyroid hormone action at receptor sites in the hypothalamus and at other body receptors.

There may be many other ways that our sensitive thyroid pathway can be disrupted by POPs in our environment. For example, PCBs, nitrates, organochlorine insecticides, thiocyanate exposure, and possibly many other compounds may cause impaired iodine utilization. This is how symptoms of hypothyroidism develop slowly over time.

If the iodine content of your diet is low, your thyroid gland will initially adapt by increasing iodine concentration from the bloodstream, by enhancing iodination to make T4 and T3, by decreasing iodine storage in the gland, and by better recycling of iodine from breakdown of thyroid hormones.

TSH will also stimulate the thyroid gland tissue to grow (hyperplasia), which adds more hormone producing tissue.

Risky
Long term, both iodine deficiency and goiter are risk factors for one type of thyroid cancer.

There is a wide range of people's response to iodine deficiency, depending on your genetic makeup, your diet, medications you take, and environmental chemical exposure. Some people develop an enlarged gland (goiter), others have only a mild increase in TSH, and still others have marked symptoms of hypothyroidism even when measures of T3 and T4 are normal.

But over the long haul, low iodine intake dramatically *decreases* levels of both thyroid hormones, T3 and T4, in several areas of the brain by 30–50%. This leads to subtle brain symptoms of hypothyroidism such as depressed mood, memory loss, scattered thinking, a feeling of "fuzzy brain."

As hypothyroidism progresses, there is disruption in the brain pathways that regulate the ovaries and other endocrine systems, leading to decrease in these other hormones. Later, the hypothyroidism may become overt and obvious as it affects more body systems.

Another reason for young women to be aware of iodine deficiency is that there is an increased risk of cancer in later life. See the chart in Chapter 5 for the pathways to explain this.

Timeline
You may have adequate iodine in your diet, but be unable to use it due to exposure to such chemicals.

Hypothyroidism

Hypothyroidism is more common than hyperthyroidism, and is more likely to go unrecognized because the symptoms are subtle. Its manifestations can be so varied that they are easily confused with other problems.

Gynecologists may miss thyroid dysfunction because it so closely mimics other more common gynecological disorders that also cause breast discharge (galactorrhea), excess facial and body hair (hirsutism), loss of menses (amenorrhea), infrequent menses (oligomenorrhea), and even infertility. (See Chapter 14 for hypothyroidism and fertility)

Hypothyroidism can cause different sysmptoms at different times in our lives. Let's look at some of these patterns, based on when they occur.

Hypothyroidism before Puberty:

Girls who become hypothyroid before they reach puberty will *typically be shorter* than if thyroid function had remained normal.

Causes

Iodine deficiency, chemical goiter-inducers (goitrogens), and thyroid toxins promote tumor growth in the thyroid gland and have also been linked to breast cancer.

They may also have either *delayed* puberty, or a different syndrome called *precocious puberty*, which leads to premature menstrual bleeding, breast enlargement, a milky discharge (galactorrhea) from the breasts due to a parallel rise in the brain hormone, prolactin and normal pubic hair growth does not happen.

So if a girl has breast development and vaginal bleeding but no pubic hair, it is an important clue to check the thyroid carefully.

Loss of memory and concentration from hypothyroidism can also severely affect school performance.

If premature puberty is caused by low thyroid function, these changes generally reverse when treated with thyroid hormones. It is important to identify and treat hypothyroidism quickly before puberty so that girls reach their normal height and have healthy ovarian and cognitive function.

A 10-year-old girl I saw recently illustrates how important this can be. *Sandie* was an active soccer player who got plenty of daily exercise, ate a healthy diet and didn't have more than an occasional soft drink. But she kept gaining weight, felt sluggish, had trouble concentrating at school, and her grades were slipping. She felt so tired when she came home from school she took a nap.

Not normal

Thyroid connections to infertility can be missed if thyroid antibodies are not checked, even if TSH is "normal."

Her mother was worried about these changes. Because so many people in the family have thyroid problems, she thought this might be happening to Sandie. They had consulted a pediatric endocrinologist at a local Children's Hospital, and had been told that Sandie's thyroid and ovarian hormones were "just fine."

At her consult, I discussed with Sandie and her mother all the changes they had noticed, particularly the decline in school performance. Earlier doctors had not asked about this, and her mother had not realized it might be important to mention.

Her first evaluation had not checked thyroid antibodies, free T3, free T4, or the glucose and insulin responses after eating. I reviewed our findings of rising TSH of 3.8, low free T3, low free T4, and markedly elevated thyroid antibodies.

Normally, I might not start thyroid hormones when the TSH isn't over 5, but I was very concerned about Sandie's change in cognitive performance at school, and the amount of weight gain she had even with all her exercise. She also had findings of insulin resistance that went along with this weight gain, and made her at more risk of diabetes later.

My clinical opinion was that she had an early thyroiditis which was negatively affecting brain function, metabolism and weight, even though the TSH was still in the high "normal" range.

Her mother was very eager for Sandie to try thyroid medication, and I decided this was reasonable, as long her TSH wasn't pushed too low. I started Sandie on just 12.5 mcg of T4 the first two weeks to see how she did on a very low dose, then increased to 25 mcg daily.

After four weeks, her mother reported, *"It was like a miracle! She has more energy to play soccer, she doesn't take naps in the afternoon, she has lost 7 pounds, and best of all, she's alert and able to concentrate again at school. She is so happy about how much better she feels on this little bit of thyroid. I can't believe the difference in my daughter!"*

This is a time when carefully evaluating the patient and her needs, rather than just focusing rigidly on lab tests alone, tipped the balance toward use of thyroid hormone. This young girl will likely have much better health in the years ahead because her mother was persistent in seeking answers that made sense to her from her observations of her daughter.

Hypothyroidism occurring in adolescence:

Adolescent girls normally have some degree of menstrual irregularity until their cycles develop their particular rhythm. But significant menstrual irregularity is common if hypothyroidism occurs in adolescence because low thyroid hormones cause lack of ovulation. There may also be heavy bleeding, not a normal pattern for adolescents.

Hypothyroidism may cause a rise in prolactin from the increase in brain TRH that stimulates TSH and prolactin release, or from thyroid effects on dopamine pathways that regulate prolactin.

Hypothyroidism also leads to a decreased breakdown of the *androstenedione* (an androgen made in the ovary) as well as *estrone*, an estrogen produced in body fat from androstenedione.

Hypothyroidism also converts more estradiol (E2) to estriol (E3) causing abnormal feedback to the pituitary, so it releases more FSH and LH that disrupt ovulation and increase ovary production of androgens (androstenedione, DHEA and testosterone).

Mom knew
Her mother wasn't satisfied with this answer, as she watched her daughter change from a vibrant, energetic, athletic girl into a tired, chubby, lethargic person.

So satisfying
I found it very meaningful to see this delightful 10-year-old get her energy and enthusiasm back—not to mention her "A" grades.

Higher levels of androstenedione cause more acne, and excess body hair. Higher levels of both hormones add to the gain in fat around the waist. The increase in fat around the middle (called central or truncal fat) doesn't respond well to the usual weight loss efforts and causes more likelihood of insulin resistance.

Then, the more you diet, the slower your thyroid hormones and the higher the increase in cortisol, your stress hormone. You get fatter and fatter!

Increased production plus decreased breakdown of androstenedione means girls have serious weight gain, acne and excess body hair. These same symptoms occur with other disorders, such as PCOS.

PCOS and hypothyroidism are different, so you need a careful evaluation of the thyroid and ovary hormones to determine the problem.

Hypothyroidism occurring in adult women or during pregnancy

Besides robbing your energy, mental clarity and mood, hypothyroidism can have a profound impact on the health and function of your ovaries.

Because thyroid hormones play such a big role in the brain, mood changes may be one of the earliest clues that something is amiss with the thyroid gland. The thyroid link with depression has been known for a long time, yet not often taken into account when evaluating women.

For example, one study published almost 20 years ago, showed that 20% of a series of psychiatric inpatients with depression had elevated thyroid antibodies (*antimicrosomal* antibody, *antithyroglobulin* antibody). This rate was much higher than the 5–10% observed in people without depression.

These patients had subtle thyroid dysfunction contributing to the depression. But they all had "normal" standard thyroid tests, which is why the hormone connection was missed. Except for the depression, they had no apparent symptoms of a thyroid disorder.

This illustrates again why I think it is so important to check thyroid antibodies in women with symptoms like depression or fatigue, even if their TSH is normal.

Careful

If prolactin is too high, it can cause breast enlargement, milky discharge, weight gain, depression, headaches and cycles with no ovulation.

Warning signs

Sometimes depression is the first clue to a subtle thyroid disorder

Next step

As the thyroiditis and hypothyroidism progress, disruption of the menstrual cycle is often the next thing that occurs.

Dr. Vliet's Comparison Guide

Normal Puberty	Precocious Puberty of Hypothyroidism
৯ Pubic hair growth	delayed pubic hair growth
৯ Normal bone growth	delayed bone development
৯ Breast enlargement	breast enlargement
৯ Vagina + estrogen effects	vagina + estrogen effects
৯ Vaginal bleeding	vaginal bleeding
৯ TSH normal	*TSH elevated
৯ FSH, LH normal	FSH, LH may be consistently elevated
৯ Normal prolactin	*prolactin elevated, often proportional to rise in TSH
৯ Normal SHBG	*SHBG decreased, with elevated free E1, E2 and elevated free androgens (hirsutism, acne, truncal weight gain)
৯ Normal menses	amenorrhea or menorrhagia
৯ No breast discharge	may have galactorrhea

*These three laboratory findings are not seen in normal puberty. If these are abnormal, it can help point to an underlying hypothyroid condition.

© 2001–2007 Elizabeth Lee Vliet, M.D.

If you have normal, regular menstrual cycles, and then become hypothyroid, it typically causes longer or shorter cycles. Bleeding patterns also commonly change, becoming much heavier, often with severe menstrual pain and cramping.

Hypothyroidism also leads to loss of normal ovulation, which makes it difficult to get pregnant. Even milder forms of thyroid decline, especially early stages of autoimmune disorders like Hashimoto's or Graves disease, may also cause a defect in the luteal (ovulatory) phase progesterone and estradiol production, also contributing to infertility.

Untreated hypothyroidism during pregnancy also causes higher incidence of pregnancy-related high blood pressure, which in turn increases the risk of toxemia (also called *pre-eclampsia*) before delivery.

Various studies also indicate untreated hypothyroidism *doubles* the risk of early spontaneous abortions, stillbirths, and premature births, while it triples the risk of congenital abnormalities in the

Warning Women who become pregnant with unrecognized hypo-thyroidism have an increase in miscarriages in the first three months.

Answer

You can reduce these risks if the thyroid problem is corrected.

baby. Even with thyroid hormone supplementation, however, women who had hypothyroidism still have a higher risk than normal of having a baby with a congenital malformation.

If you were treated in the past for hypothyroidism and then become pregnant, you should have your Ob doctor or an endocrinologist monitor your thyroid medicine carefully. You will often need higher doses to keep the optimal range as the ovarian hormones change during pregnancy.

Dr. Vliet's Summary: Effects of Thyroid Hormones on Your Ovaries and Ovarian Hormones

Hypothyroidism:

◊ Abnormal thyroid activity has direct effect on hypothalamus-pituitary-ovarian axis (pathway); may also cause elevated prolactin which also interferes with normal ovarian cycles:

⬇

 Irregular cycles, lack of ovulation, decreased hormone production

◊ Decreased SHBG (more estrogen and androgens in free form)

⬇

[handwritten annotation: also associated w/ hypo- which also w/ PCOS? NO]

 Chronic excess estrogen ➜ heavy bleeding

 Excess androgens ⟶ excess face and body hair, acne, middle body weight gain

◊ Decreased metabolic clearance of androstenedione and estrone, WITI I increased peripheral conversion (aromatization) of androstenedione to estrone:

⬇

 Chronic excess estrone E1 ➜ heavy bleeding

 Excess androgens ⟶ excess face and body hair, acne, middle body weight gain

◊ Increased rate of metabolism of estradiol (via 16-alpha hydroxylation) to make more estriol

⬇

 abnormal feedback to pituitary, abnormal gonadotrophin release chronic anovulation

⬇

◊ ovary produces more androgens plus more free androgens from decreased SHBG

⬇ ⟶ infertility

more hirsutism

© *2001–2007 Elizabeth Lee Vliet, M.D.*

The high levels of ovarian hormones increase the binding proteins that carry thyroid hormones T4 and T3 in the bloodstream during pregnancy, it leads to a decrease in the free, active thyroid hormones present.

If you are on thyroid medication when you become pregnant, it is wise not to stop your medicine abruptly. If you just stop thyroid hormones, and don't taper down slowly, your own thyroid gland can't immediately start to make all it needs. This means you can be hypothyroid until the gland fully takes over again. This could cause problems for the pregnancy as I described above.

Only small amounts of the mother's T4 and T3 cross the placenta, so it isn't likely that your replacement dose of thyroid hormone will harm the baby unless you are taking so much that you are hyperthyroid (TSH lower than 0.5). Just be sure that your doctors checks this regularly during pregnancy.

Hyperthyroidism

Problems from excess thyroid hormone activity are also quite varied, and hit most organ systems in our body. Symptoms range from mood effects and heart palpitations to bone loss, hair loss, muscle weakness, and yes, even weight gain and fatigue, which many do not associate with excess thyroid hormones.

Hyperthyroidism in the early stages may also be overlooked and misdiagnosed as an anxiety or panic disorder, or even "bipolar" illness because of the mood changes it can produce.

The specific effects will depend on how severe the excess, when it happens and how long it has been present, just I described for hypothyroidism.

Hyperthyroidism before puberty

If a prepubescent girl becomes hyperthyroid, she may have delayed sexual development and begin menstrual periods later than usual. This appears to be caused by lower body fat in hyperthyroid individuals, since we know that a certain threshold, or set-point, of body fat is needed before menstruation begins.

Physical development in other areas is generally normal, although a girl who is hyperthyroid may be thinner and taller than her peers. Excess thyroid increases bone growth, making bones of the legs and arms longer, but bones are often less dense because excess thyroid causes too much bone breakdown.

Check-ups
TSH should be checked at least once every trimester so that the dose remains correct as the hormones change.

Vital info
If your thyroid condition is particularly unstable, your doctor should check the TSH and other levels more often.

Difference
Hyperthyroidism may cause infertility, although it's effects on menstrual function and fertility are different from hypothyroidism.

Fine hair, but

The higher estradiol and estrone, along with a lower *free* testosterone, helps to explain why your skin is softer, with fine downy hair, when you have excess thyroid.

Watch out!

If hyper-thyroidism goes undiagnosed, it causes low bone density and a higher risk of osteoporosis.

Warning!

Graves Disease is the most common cause of hyper-thyroidism during pregnancy.

Excess thyroid activity also causes scattered thinking, hyper-activity, and difficulty with focus that can be mistaken for an attention-deficit hyperactivity disorder.

If you have hyperthyroidism and you are put on the stimulant Ritalin thinking the problem is ADHD, it can worsen the learning disorder, and cause serious heart rhythm problems. Demand a careful medical evaluation and ask to be checked for thyroid problems instead of starting medicines like Ritalin or Adderall based only on evaluations of learning and behavior.

Hyperthyroidism occurring in adolescents and adult women

Excess thyroid can make the cycle longer or shorter so the luteal phase doesn't develop properly. This elevates FSH and LH, which often causes loss of ovulation and diminished menstrual flow. The decreased menstrual flow results from too little endometrial lining is built up, which makes it harder for a fertilized egg to implant properly.

But sometimes, hyperthyroid women still ovulate normally, unlike those with hypothyroidism. So, if you miss menstrual periods, you could be pregnant and should have a pregnancy test.

Excess thyroid activity causes an *increase* in sex-hormone binding globulin (SHBG), an opposite effect from hypothyroidism. This means that *less testosterone* is in the free, available form even though the total amount of testosterone is often increased.

Hyperthyroidism also increases the conversion of androgens to estrogens and shifts estrogen metabolism preferentially to estradiol and estrone.

Since hyperthyroidism suppresses appetite, in addition to being a major metabolic "stressor," it often leads to nutritional deficiencies that aggravate the menstrual disturbances and contribute to infertility.

Excess thyroid activity also causes restless sleep, increases the rate of bone breakdown and can cause serious palpitations.

Hyperthyroidism in pregnancy

It is much less common for a woman to develop hyperthyroidism and toxic thyroid excess (*thyrotoxicosis*) during pregnancy, but it does happen in about two out of every 1000. It is an urgent medical condition because the thyroid-stimulating immunoglobulins in Graves' disease are able to cross the placenta and may cause thyrotoxicosis in the baby as well as the mother.

Hyperthyroid states are sometimes missed in the early stages because some of the symptoms, such as nervousness, feeling overly warm, excess sweating, elevated blood pressure, and rapid heart beat *mimic the early changes of a normal pregnancy.*

Thyroid blood tests, along with checking for signs of excess thyroid (tremor, eyes protruding, lid lag, hyperactive reflexes) help confirm hyperthyroidism. If you are pregnant and develop hyperthyroidism, I recommend that both an experienced endocrinologist and your OB physician monitor your progress.

Women with autoimmune thyroid disorders such as Graves' disease or Hashimoto's thyroiditis may notice that their thyroid symptoms are easier to control or may even diminish after they become pregnant.

This is because the high progesterone levels of pregnancy suppress the mother's immune system so that the mother's body does not destroy the "foreign tissue" of the developing baby. This is one reason women with Graves' disease become rapidly hyperthyroid again after delivery, when progesterone falls rapidly.

Huge problem Postpartum thyroid disorders occur in anywhere from 5% to 10% of women, a significant problem during our reproductive years.

Post-partum Thyroid Disorders: Hypothyroidism, Hyperthyroidism and Autoimmune Thyroiditis

Thyroid imbalance can lead to serious mood problems, including severe forms of post-partum depression and post-partum psychosis. Autoimmune post-partum thyroid problems often go undiagnosed because doctors today do not routinely test for thyroid antibodies, even though we have published reports in the medical literature about this problem going back many years.

If the thyroid problems are associated with elevated thyroid antibodies, it is called autoimmune post-partum thyroiditis, and it may manifest as either hyper (overactive) thyroid or hypo (underactive) thyroid.

Women with elevated thyroid antibodies prior to pregnancy are at much higher risk of developing severe post-partum thyroiditis after delivery that can lead to a serious post-partum psychosis. Autoimmune disorders of all types, but especially autoimmune thyroiditis, commonly return with a vengeance after delivery

Common symptoms to watch for: severe, unrelenting fatigue, markedly depressed mood, hair loss, dry skin, memory or concentration problems, difficulty losing weight, constipation.

when progesterone levels fall and the immune-suppressing effects of this hormone are now gone.

For example, a 1982 Japanese study found that over 5% of women had post-partum thyroid dysfunction, either hyper or hypothyroid conditions. This translates to millions of women.

Continuing problem

Over 50% of the women with post-partum thyroid problems had a lifelong thyroid problem within five years after delivery.

A 1984 study of Swedish women found that the rate of hypothyroidism with positive thyroid antibodies was even higher, at almost 10% of reproductive age women. They found that in women with hypothyroidism, microsomal antibodies were always present. The severity of the disease correlated closely to the level of antibodies measured during pregnancy and post-partum.

Studies since that time have confirmed these findings, but doctors are still not seeing the importance of measuring thyroid antibodies.

There are many symptoms of post-partum hypothyroidism and these same symptoms may also occur from decreased production of the ovarian hormones in the post-partum phase. You have to check all of the hormone levels.

It is possible to have both a thyroid problem and also have a post-partum depression or psychosis.

You may only need thyroid medication, or you may need both thyroid hormones and antidepressants, or all thyroid tests may be normal and you may only need antidepressant medicine.

Cause

If the cause of your symptoms is low thyroid, antidepressants alone won't "fix" it!

We cannot assume that all "low energy, depressed mood" states are "just" due to post-partum depressions. Since antidepressants are more expensive and have more side effects than thyroid medications, it is important to rule out the thyroid first.

Postpartum thyroid dysfunction is not limited to the immediate postpartum period. Effects may become permanent. Dr. Premawardhana from the University of Wales in the United Kingdom recently found that permanent hypothyroidism developed in about 33% of the young women with postpartum thyroid problems.

Another 20% developed hypothyroidism over the next 3–5 years, even though they had normal thyroid function in the first postpartum year.

This young woman's story shows how crucial it is to correct thyroid problems early, and to monitor your complete thyroid function carefully and regularly.

After the birth of her third child, *Juliana* had a serious bout with post-partum hormone problems that almost cost her life, and that of her baby. She had milder episodes of post-partum depression with her two earlier pregnancies, but neither she nor her family were prepared for what hit with this one.

Within a few weeks, Juliana was having suicidal thoughts and hearing voices telling her to smother her new baby. She and her husband, Doug, were obviously frightened and he insisted she talk with her obstetrician, who referred her to a psychiatrist. She was immediately put on antipsychotic medication along with an antidepressant, *but no hormone testing was done.*

She continued serious struggles with depression and intense thoughts of harming herself and her baby, despite three psychiatric hospitalizations and multiple medications—all since the birth of her last child.

Her husband and family were getting desperate. The psychiatrist was now recommending in-patient care again, this time for electroconvulsive (ECT) treatment.

Aware of the risks, her husband was frightened about this approach. He was convinced that there were hormone connections in all this. He didn't want Juliana to have ECT until this had been checked. He said *"She only gets depressed after her pregnancies, so it just makes common sense to me that we should be checking her hormones but no one will do that."*

Although they lived about a day's drive from my office, a friend suggested Doug arrange a consult, since Juliana clearly wasn't getting better and it was now six months after her baby was born. Her lab results came back a week before her appointment, and just prior to the other doctor's decision to start ECT, although I was unaware of the newest development. As usual I gave directions for the lab to send a copy of the report to me and to the patient at the same time.

Doug saw how many of the hormone studies were significantly out of range. He talked to her obstetrician, who agreed the results were abnormal, but didn't recognize the *brain* effects of such profound imbalances.

He said to Doug "This isn't a hormonal disorder, it's psychiatric. She needs the psychiatric medicines and the ECT, hormones won't help." Her psychiatrist also realized the hormones were

Caution
Thyroid disorders can be indistinguishable from "psychiatric" disorders and also cause suicidal depressions and/or psychosis,

Get started
To save time and make the initial visit more meaningful, there are certain lab tests I request ahead of time.

Rx

I was convinced that her psychosis was caused by the hyper-thyroidism. I thought she would not need the antipsychotic medicine if I could correct the thyroid excess.

Working together

It was complicated and challenging, but a gratifying experience of everyone working together in a therapeutic partnership.

There's more risk

Women with post-partum thyroiditis are at higher risk for later development of thyroid cancer

abnormal, but since the gynecologist did not want this treated, he felt Juliana needed to go ahead with ECT.

Doug called our office in a panic. "Is it really safe for her to have ECT with all these hormones out of whack?" It turned out that Juliana had a severe post-partum thyroiditis with markedly elevated thyroid antibodies, and her TSH was so low it was barely detectable. She was seriously *hyperthyroid*. ECT was not safe in this situation.

She also had significantly low estradiol and high prolactin, each of which can alone cause depression.

Hyperthyroidism coupled with low estradiol would further aggravate the potential for heart arrhythmias during ECT.

With her psychosis getting worse and the family's concern for the safety of both Juliana and her baby, we immediately made arrangements for her to be seen and start treatment for the endocrine imbalances.

The complexity of her situation required a combined approach to address the thyroid disorder, her low estradiol and high prolactin, and the side effects of her psychotropic medications.

She had what is called an extra-pyramidal syndrome (EPS) from the antipsychotic medicine Haldol. This caused her to have slowed movements, muscle stiffness, difficulty swallowing, a blank facial expression, and a restless crawling feeling, a sensation similar to being buried in an anthill!

Since she lived so far away, I was concerned that we needed time to observe her responses and make certain she was not in danger of hurting herself or her baby as we made these changes. Her family kept her children while we worked to start new medications and taper off some of the psychiatric ones, especially the antipsychotic medicine that was causing so many side effects.

I knew that if I started her on a birth control pill right away, it would *increase* the thyroid binding proteins and keep some of the excess T4 and T3 from being such a problem. I also gave her medicine to treat the extra-pyramidal side effects of the Haldol.

By the end of that first week, both her family and I could tell a major difference. Her anxiety, depressed mood and suicidal thoughts were lifting with the added estrogen, which also diminished the hyperthyroidism by shifting her excess thyroid hormone into a less active state.

A lower dose of Haldol, plus the addition of Ativan, helped relieve the agitation, slowed movements, muscle stiffness and the awful crawling sensation. She and her family could tell she had turned the corner.

It was a frightening time for everyone, and her treatment certainly required thought and a careful adjustment of medications to find the balance that saved her. I continued to work with her and her husband on the medication adjustments for another six months as her hormones changed.

She did not have another psychiatric hospitalization and did not need ECT. Within six months, she was able to go back to work. By the end of that year, she was off all psychotropic medicines. She remained stable on just the birth control pills.

Splits

No wonder our fragmented, medical care can't find someone to put the pieces together and relate it to the ovaries!

As I write this, it has been 10 years since I first saw her and started her hormone therapy. She has had no further episodes of the severe depression or the psychosis that required hospitalization, and no further need for antipsychotic medicines.

But there is an important update that illustrates another reason we must treat these post-partum hormone aggressively and they need to be monitored regularly. Recently, I found a nodule on Juliana's thyroid, and sent her for a biopsy. Even though only in her mid 30s, Juliana had thyroid cancer.

She had surgery to remove her thyroid gland, and is now on full replacement thyroid hormones. Occasionally after her thyroid was removed, she has needed antidepressants with her thyroid medicine to prevent depression.

Even though antidepressants and antipsychotics may help depression and abnormal thoughts, they don't treat endocrine problems that can have other effects and later health risks. Endocrine causes can be missed if the hormone evaluation was not part of the work-up for post-partum depression and/or post-partum psychosis.

I find myself wondering whether such a comprehensive evaluation could have helped prevent the tragedy with Andrea Yates and the deaths of her five children.

The chart below summarizes these important thyroid effects. If you think you may have a thyroid disorder, turn to Chapter 17 for a discussion of what to have tested, medications available, and how to work with your doctor to get started safely.

Dr. Vliet's Summary: Effects of Thyroid Hormones on

Your Ovaries and Ovarian Hormones

Hyperthyroidism:

◊ Abnormal thyroid activity has <u>direct effect on hypothalamus-pituitary-ovarian</u> axis (pathway); leads to higher baseline FSH, LH that interferes with normal ovarian cycles:

ﾝ Irregular cycles, lack of ovulation ⟶ Infertility

◊ Increased SHBG (less estrogen and androgens in free form)

ﾝ Lower free E1, E2 ⟶ reduced menstrual flow, other symptoms of low E2

ﾝ Low androgen activity → low sex drive, low bone mass, loss of bone strength

◊ Preferential metabolism of estrogen to estradiol and estrone, not estriol; and *increased* conversion of androgens to estradiol and estrone:

ﾝ Higher estradiol, estrone → soft skin, downy facial hair

◊ Abnormal feedback to pituitary, aberrant release of gonadotrophin may lead to anovulation ⟶ Infertility

© *2001–2007 Elizabeth Lee Vliet, M.D.*

Oophoritis and Adrenalitis: Autoimmune Disorders Affecting The Ovaries and Adrenal Glands

There is a wealth of published medical literature, particularly in the international journals, that addresses these overlooked autoimmune disorders that can lead to premature ovarian decline, infertility, chronic fatigue, fibromyalgia, and immune system disturbances.

Most of the research I find that supports the existence of an autoimmune "attack" on the ovaries (*oophoritis*) comes from work done overseas in the past several decades.

Without reliable measures of the antibodies, our understanding of these conditions is limited and it is difficult to prove their existence, particularly since it is hard enough to get many physicians to check levels of ovarian hormones using the reliable tests *we do have.*

You may have one of these disorders without a good way to test for them, other than checking levels of the hormones made by these glands, and levels of the pituitary hormones that oversee their function.

You can have the same symptoms from *any of these autoimmune endocrine syndromes*–adrenalitis, oophoritis, or thyroiditis. Not only that, the symptoms are so varied and vague that doctors don't typically associate them as ovarian or adrenal or thyroid in origin; they are more likely seen as part of a depressive syndrome.

Some of the common symptoms I see are sleep difficulties (restless sleep, trouble falling asleep, waking early, multiple awakenings at night—all of which are also listed in the diagnostic criteria for depression!), impaired memory and concentration, marked fatigue, bone loss, hair loss, muscle pain, joint aches, bladder problems, vasomotor instability, low blood pressure, loss of interest in sex, low libido, vaginal dryness, premature skin aging, increased allergies, and chemical sensitivities. The symptoms appear everywhere in the body.

When I evaluate a patient, sometimes it comes down to looking at the entire picture of symptoms, and then using years of clinical experience and intuition to make a judgment that the *gestalt* suggests autoimmune oophoritis, thyroiditis or adrenalitis. I may

Testing Difficulties There is no reliable antibody testing for ovarian or adrenal antibodies like we have for thyroid antibodies.

A problem Another issue making diagnosis difficult is that symptoms are *non-specific.*

Connected Women with an autoimmune disorder affecting one endocrine pathway may well have other glands affected as well.

not be able to prove it objectively, however, given the limitations of existing lab tests.

The ovarian hormone decline that occurs in the autoimmune oophoritis is similar to thyroid hormone decline that occurs in thyroiditis. Both of these autoimmune disorders produce symptoms that may be similar and overlap, due to a combination of factors that include loss of optimal hormone production and the autoimmune response itself.

Too low
Although there is still some menstrual function, ovarian hormone levels are lower than healthy levels.

These women typically have a family history of autoimmune disorders. They probably had a triggering event that affected the immune system such as exposure to environmental chemicals (pesticides and others), exposure to an infectious agent (viral, bacterial, or fungal illnesses), or exposure to a biological antigen, such as tick or spider bites.

The women I have seen with this type of ovarian decline are typically much younger than a normal menopausal age, may still have FSH in the "normal" range, and will still have some degree of menstruation though it isn't regular cycles and healthy flow.

An autoimmune attack on the ovaries can damage them, and alter production and availability of the ovarian hormones to cause complete premature ovarian *failure* (POF) with loss of menstrual periods and low levels of ovarian hormones.

POD
True premature ovarian failure is defined by a high FSH (greater than 20) in a woman younger than age 40.

Premature ovarian *decline* (POD) is earlier in the process, with loss of ovarian hormone production sufficient to cause profound symptoms and even infertility, but without complete loss of menses or an FSH over 20.

POD is a part of the continuum that many doctors do not realize is there. Consequently, if the FSH is still less than 20, they tell women "you aren't menopausal." They overlook that most of the time, it takes several years of declining hormone levels before the FSH will rise that high.

You can have "low estrogen" symptoms that disrupt life, even if your FSH is only 10 or 12! Many fertility specialists consider an FSH over 10 means you don't have enough remaining follicles for fertility treatment to succeed.

My message continues: the medical community shouldn't get so caught up in "the numbers" that we miss the person and her suffering. The best way to determine whether you suffer from one of these syndromes is a complete set of tests to check the various aspects of endocrine function, as described in Chapters 16 and 17.

Overactive or Underactive Adrenals: Impact on Your Ovaries

Two other adrenal disorders fall into the category of illnesses that can disrupt your ovaries and lead to abnormal ovarian hormone levels. If you are feeling "hormonally challenged," be aware of these conditions, and learn how to get properly tested and where to seek treatment.

Adrenal **corticosteroid** excess (**Cushing's Syndrome**): Steroids produced by the adrenal glands include glucocorticoids ("cortisol," the "stress" hormone) and mineralocorticoids.

When Cortisol is Too High: Cushing's Syndrome

Excess cortisol causes marked fat deposits around the middle of the body, breasts, upper back and arms, as well as a rounded puffy face that is called "moon facies."

Excess levels of cortisol, whether due to excess production by the adrenal glands, or a pituitary disorder, or from corticosteroid medications, such as for asthma or allergies or arthritis, may lead to Cushing's Syndrome. People commonly develop cortisol excess due to taking corticosteroid medications, such as Cortef, or Prednisone, and others.

One young woman I evaluated was given prednisone treatment for optic neuritis, a painful inflammation of the optic nerve that can lead to blindness if not treated aggressively with corticosteroids. The optic neuritis resolved quite well with this treatment, but over the next few months, she began developing more intense PMS, insomnia, hot flashes, irritability, fatigue, and menstrual headaches that she had not had.

A naturopathic doctor (N.D.) told her she had "adrenal exhaustion" and started her on a high dose DHEA, 50 mg daily. She became more irritable, had greater difficulty sleeping, started craving sweets, developed severe acne, and began losing "handfuls" of hair in her brush each day. In a panic, she arranged a consultation to have all of her hormone levels checked to get to the bottom of her problems.

I did a complete laboratory workup, and her ovarian hormone, likely caused by the corticosteroid treatment. Both her estradiol

Excess cortisol causes:

high blood pressure

high cholesterol

high triglycerides

high glucose

excess insulin

increased risk of diabetes

repeated infections

thin skin

thinning hair

easy bruising

muscle weakness

increased bone loss

weight gain

and testosterone were too low, and her DHEA was excessively high from the supplements she was given.

Thyroid and adrenal function tests were good. Her ovaries had been knocked down by the corticosteroids, and the effects made worse by the DHEA supplements.

Excess DHEA causes:
irritability
insomnia
acne
hair loss (scalp)
facial hair
weight gain
sweet cravings

I treated her successfully with an estradiol patch, which in turn led to her ovaries functioning better to make more testosterone. Since her ovaries were still making good levels of progesterone and she was having regular periods, she did not need supplemental progesterone.

In nine months, her ovarian function normalized completely and she stopped using the estradiol patch. She is one example of many women we see with ovarian imbalance or decline from corticosteroid medication.

I am not advocating that you avoid such treatment: there are clearly times it is critical. Just keep in mind that too much cortisol from your own adrenal glands, or from medicines, may interfere with your ovaries. Check hormone levels if you start having symptoms.

High cortisol is actually more commonly caused from life stress, loss of optimal estradiol, illnesses, infections, chronic pain, surgeries, loss of optimal thyroid function, biological depression, high progestin birth control pills, medications such as decongestants and steroids used to treat asthma and arthritis, to name some of the most common ones.

These problems are best treated by addressing the underlying cause, such as changing medications or improving "stress relief" strategies.

I typically find that if the cortisol is elevated because of thyroid disorders or loss of estradiol, once we have restored estradiol and/or thyroid balance the cortisol usually falls in line. If cortisol is high due to a suspected adrenal disease such as Cushing's syndrome, or to a pituitary disorder, your physician will likely suggest further testing.

Once a specific adrenal or pituitary cause is identified, treatment can be individualized and directed to the cause. See Chapter 17 for more detailed information on testing and treatment options.

When Cortisol is Too Low: Addison's or Adrenal Insufficiency (AI)

Cortisol and other hormones produced by the adrenal gland are critical for survival. If the adrenal gland is making too little of these hormones it leads to serious illness and major disruptions in multiple body pathways, including the ovaries.

If you have been under severe, unrelenting stress for long periods of time (many months to several years), your adrenal glands can lose their ability to respond properly with increased cortisol and you enter the phase of called "adrenal insufficiency." Fortunately, it is rather straightforward to test for adrenal insufficiency by first checking serum electrolytes and an 8 AM serum cortisol.

True Adrenal Insufficiency (AI) has low cortisol (an 8 AM cortisol less than 7 to 8), low sodium and high potassium.

AI may arise for unclear reasons not related to persistent, severe stresses, and then called *Addison's disease.* True Addison's disease is uncommon, but it is a very serious medical disorder and needs proper treatment by an endocrinologist experienced with its complexity and life-threatening medical complications.

Addison's disease typically causes loss of menstrual periods or very light flow. This occurs due to ovarian suppression from the loss of optimal adrenal hormones, or as a result of the same illness that triggered the adrenal insufficiency.

Women with very low adrenal hormones typically experience *extreme fatigue, poor appetite, marked weight loss, brownish pigmentation of the skin* (commonly elbows, knees, knuckles, and mucosa inside the mouth), *muscle and joints aches, loss of pubic and underarm hair, thinning scalp hair, and low blood pressure.*

AI is almost always associated with severe weight *loss,* not the *weight gain* of high cortisol. If you are overweight, it is very unlikely you have "adrenal exhaustion" and low cortisol.

Wasted!
She did not have adrenal exhaustion; she had "ovarian exhaustion!"

The term
"Adrenal exhaustion," is significantly over used based on unreliable saliva tests.

Caution

Be wary of people who tell you to take over the counter adrenal "boosters" for fatigue.

Summary

There are many medical disorders and illnesses that affect the ovaries along with other systems. I have shown you some examples in this chapter, although this is certainly not a complete list of every possible illness that affects your ovaries.

There is a great deal of overlap in the symptoms from imbalances of your thyroid, ovarian, adrenal, glucose-insulin pathways.

If you want a clear picture of *what* is out of balance and *how* to fix it, you must have a careful, complete, systematic hormone evaluation, rather than just relying on a list of symptoms to make a "diagnosis."

You should get the ovarian hormones checked if you have problems similar to those I have described. Doctors don't often want to do this, saying it isn't necessary, it is too expensive, or the levels vary.

None of these reasons hold up when you look at the science of how our body systems are affected if our ovaries do not make optimal levels of their hormones. These excuses are not valid, either, when women are suffering, and not getting answers to their problems.

Push to get the answers and treatment options you need.

It is *your* health at stake.

Chapter 10

Ovaries at Risk: Unrecognized Problems from Surgery, Medications and Herbs

I have evaluated several thousand women for symptoms they thought were related to hormone imbalance. The onset of these symptoms and menstrual cycle changes often followed a surgical procedure or illness.

One such procedure is a *bilateral tubal ligation*, often called just a "tubal" or BTL. Most of these women said they were not told that such problems were possible after such a "simple" procedure. When they sought explanations for symptoms, they were often told it couldn't possibly be related to having their tubes "tied." But it is true—there can be premature decrease in ovarian hormone levels after a tubal ligation.

Questions have been raised about "Post-tubal Ligation Syndrome" since the 1950s. In fact, I found articles in the British medical literature published over forty years ago that described this problem.

In 1951, Williams found that as many as 31% of women had abnormal uterine bleeding after a tubal ligation, and 16.5% ended up having a hysterectomy to control new bleeding problems.

This was *triple* the rate of hysterectomy in the women who had not had a BTL. A number of other studies in the 1970s found that hysterectomy rates were much higher (from 5 to 33%) in women who had a BTL than in women who had not.

Specialists felt the disruption in ovarian function from the BTL led to abnormal bleeding or other problems that eventually had to be controlled with hysterectomy.

Finally, a U.S. study, published in 2000, looked at menstrual cycle effects following BTL and supported exactly what I have

It's true
If you have experienced such changes after a tubal, you are not imaging it

Excuse me?
These changes indicate a decrease in hormone levels, but this study unfortunately did not check ovarian hormone levels in these women.

seen in my patients all these years. The researchers compared 9,514 women who underwent tubal ligation between 1978 and 1987 with 573 women whose partners underwent vasectomy in that same time frame so that the women did not need to have a BTL for contraception.

They found that women who had tubal ligations were *more likely* to report persistent *cycle irregularities, painful* menstrual periods (*dysmenorrhea*), and *decreases* in the *number* of bleeding days and in the *amount* of bleeding.

Without reliable hormone measures, they could not confirm the lower levels I see so commonly in my patients.

In spite of the problems reported by the patients in this study, the authors concluded that BTL was *"safe and effective"*…and the results provided "welcome reassurance" regarding tubal ligation since there were no changes in the menstrual cycle!

I can't see how they reached that conclusion, but this certainly shows why women today feel they are not informed about possible hormone problems after a BTL.

Why does this procedure cause hormone and bleeding problems? One theory is that the surgical process of cutting, cauterizing or tying off the Fallopian tubes also affects ovarian blood flow, leading to impaired function of the ovary and lower hormone production.

Fact
Decreased oxygen delivery shifts hormone production toward making less estradiol, while a normal amount of progesterone is still made.

Many gynecologists tell me "it isn't possible" to interrupt the ovarian blood flow with a tubal ligation and, even if that did occur, it wouldn't affect hormone production by the ovary.

Dr. John Cattanach, an Australian gynecologist, did an analysis of this hypothesis and published a plausible explanation of how a tubal ligation could lead to diminished estradiol production in the ovary afterwards.

Tubal ligations are done at the isthmus, the narrow part of the Fallopian tube. Dr. Cattanach explained that at the isthmus, the ovarian branch of the uterine artery is so close to the fallopian tube that this artery is "almost certainly occluded, or at least interrupted, by most of the usual forms of tubal ligation."

That leaves only part of the other end of this artery to become the main blood supply for the entire ovary, which means both less blood flow and increased pressure in the artery.

We know that whenever the arterial pressure is too high, as in hypertension, it can damage the small blood vessels called arterioles. This damage means impaired oxygen delivery to the cells of the ovaries, which in turn can decrease hormone production.

The chemical reactions in the ovaries that convert cholesterol to estradiol and progesterone require between 3.3 to 8 times more oxygen to make 1 mol of estradiol than to make 1 mol of progesterone.

When I measure hormone levels in the second half of the cycle in women with tubal ligations, I consistently find estradiol is *lower* than normal, while progesterone is in the upper end of normal range, altering the usual ratio of these two hormones.

This is exactly what Dr. Cattanach predicted, based on damage to ovarian blood flow. High progesterone when estradiol is lower than it should be is another cause of PMS and heavy menstrual bleeding, commonly described in many of the early studies of BTL, and as my patients also describe.

As more time elapses after a BTL, the gradual decline in blood flow causes lower than optimal estradiol levels for most of the cycle. Lower estradiol begins to cause menopause-type symptoms, even in women who are "too young" for menopause.

After a BTL, younger women may have irregular cycles, lighter menstrual flow, insomnia, mood changes, more PMS, or even hot flashes. I often hear these symptoms described by women who had a tubal ligation.

High progesterone levels stimulate more prostaglandin production by the uterus, and more prostaglandins mean more cramping, so I am not surprised to see more cramps and pain following a tubal if progesterone is high and estradiol is too low.

I am not saying that you should avoid a BTL if you want reliable, permanent contraception. Certainly it is a safe, effective approach. But if you have the procedure, be aware of possible to have changes in your ovarian function and hormone production afterwards.

If symptoms develop later, have your hormone levels rechecked and compare with your earlier test results. Then you can

Results

When I check luteal phase levels, I find low E2 and higher progesterone as Dr. Cattanach predicted.

Ow!

A high progesterone to estradiol ratio, can cause problems with painful, crampy menses.

choose to supplement your hormones rather than settle for a diagnosis of "stress" or depression.

Statistics show that antidepressants are over-prescribed for women. I think this is because physicians do not evaluate the endocrine issues. If you have good objective information to determine the correct cause of your problems, you can explore options for feeling better… and may not need antidepressants.

Smart
Test hormone levels when you are feeling really good *before* you have a tubal ligation.

Hysterectomy—Another Cause of Premature Hormone Loss

Another common surgery is the hysterectomy, or removal of the uterus. Many doctors recommend that for women under age 48, the ovaries should not be removed, so that women will have their hormone production until natural menopause.

At first glance that rationale makes intellectual sense, except when you consider that rarely do surgeons *check* hormone levels later to determine whether the ovaries still produce optimal hormone levels.

Doctors just assume the ovaries continue to work fine after a hysterectomy. Even more patronizing, doctors tell women with *one* ovary removed, "Don't worry, the other ovary will take over and make enough hormones. You'll be fine." Try telling *that* to a man who has lost one testicle.

Fact
30–60% of women have menopausal levels of estradiol and testosterone as early as 2–3 years following removal of the uterus.

Since the early 1970s, studies have shown that after hysterectomy premature hormone loss is far more common than we thought, even though the ovaries were left in place. I have included a number of these references in the Appendix should you have a hard time convincing doctors of this real concern. Most of these studies came from England, Germany, Italy and other European countries.

In the United States, this issue has not been taken as seriously. It is not clear to me why doctors here don't think follow up checks of ovarian hormone levels are necessary.

Dr. John Studd, an internationally known menopause researcher from London, is a strong advocate for follow up tests of women's hormone levels after hysterectomy when ovaries are left intact.

Dr. Studd attributes doctor's missing the hormone factor to two factors: the loss of menstruation as a marker of the phases of the ovarian hormone cycle, and to doctors' *assumptions* that "vague" symptoms such as insomnia, anxiety, low libido, and depressed mood occur because of psychological reactions to losing the uterus, to feelings of lost femininity, or fear of aging.

This focus on assumed psychological issues completely overlooks the physical hormone effects on brain chemistry.

There is objective confirmation of this endocrine connection in such symptoms: FSH is elevated in 25% or more of women who had removal of the uterus but still have ovaries. I certainly find these same objective confirmations in my own patients' lab results for hormone levels.

Hysterectomy is often accused of causing depression, inability to function sexually, and a host of other problems. But the newer, carefully designed prospective studies do not support that removal of the uterus causes major depression or other psychologically damaging consequences in the majority of women.

In fact, just the opposite has been found in a number of recent studies: incidence of depression (as a mood state, not the illness), is about *half* the incidence found prior to surgery, with women showing *improved* psychological and physical well-being—including sexual enjoyment—after hysterectomy.

Surgery is usually done today only when there are clear indications it is needed, such as severe endometriosis, excessive bleeding, painful periods, intractable PMS, severe fibroids that cause abdominal distension and pain with intercourse.

We certainly see many patients who have low hormone levels and don't feel "back to normal" following a hysterectomy, but even these women are grateful the surgery took care of the bleeding or pain.

Why the discrepancy between the general perception of hysterectomy versus the positive outcomes from studies like these?

I think the explanation lies in several facts:

1. Even after surgical menopause induced by removing the uterus and the ovaries, only about 25–30% of women start hormone therapy. Only half take it for longer than 5 years.

   This means a huge number of women with no ovaries are going without any replacement of the very hormones needed for a myriad of body and brain systems.

Still? The majority of gynecologists and primary care physicians miss the diagnosis of premature hormonal decline after removal of only the uterus.

Missing I don't believe it is the loss of the uterus; I think it is the loss of their crucial metabolic hormones that leads to so many problems.

Not!

Women who still have ovaries are assumed to be making enough hormones, but this is rarely ever checked objectively.

Sad Fact

Most women still do not get "optimal" replacement of their ovarian hormones after a hysterectomy.

This has got to change!

No hormone levels are checked after a hysterectomy. There is typically no individual-ization of type, route or dose of estrogen or testosterone.

2. The data shows that most women, in fact, do *not* make adequate levels of ovarian hormones even though the ovaries are still there. Studies have even shown (Lehmann–Willenbrock/Reidel, 1988; Watson/Studd, 1995) objective evidence of inadequate estrogen levels even if ovaries remained: there were adverse cholesterol changes and loss of bone, respectively.

3. Even if women *do* start hormone therapy after a hysterectomy, the usual approach is to simply give estrogen, usually Premarin. Testosterone is rarely replaced. It doesn't have to be this way.

I work hard to help my patients achieve optimal hormone replacement, and most are amazed at the degree of well-being that returns. I consistently find it isn't the removal of the uterus that causes so many problems; it is the lack of adequate hormone therapy afterwards.

4. Whether with ovarian removal, or early ovarian decline, women lose most of their testosterone production as well as their estradiol. Testosterone enhances energy level, libido, sense of well-being and mood, bone and muscle formation and also (along with estradiol) improves the vaginal tissue to relieve dryness that causes pain during sex.

Even though medical studies going back to the 1950s show the benefits, and safety, of testosterone replacement, the vast majority who have had a hysterectomy *still* are not offered testosterone therapy.

5. Depression following hysterectomy is assumed to be a psychological reaction to losing the uterus. Dr. Studd's view is that "the more plausible cause of depression is the varying degree of ovarian hormone deficiency, which is often overlooked and untreated following hysterectomy."

I certainly agree; my clinical experience clearly shows that depressed moods, low energy, sleep loss, anxiety, and loss of libido are alleviated with good hormone management.

A long-term prospective study published in 1992 found no depression at 4 months after hysterectomy, but it did develop after 24 months. This supports that depression is not likely to result from an emotional reaction to hysterectomy but can occur as the ovarian hormones decline over time.

What does this mean for you? If you are only 30 years old and have a hysterectomy, and even if you keep both ovaries, you can still develop menopausal hormone levels in your thirties, on average, within three years of the surgery.

In fact, even if the ovaries work well for many years, studies show that you will become menopausal about 4 to 5 years earlier than average.

But if no one is checking your hormone levels, the hormone cause of symptoms is missed. Fatigue, headaches, depression, insomnia, loss of sex drive, and other symptoms are more likely to be labeled depression, chronic fatigue, anxiety or stress.

How do women become prematurely menopausal after a hysterectomy? The reasons are very similar to those described for the BTL. This time, the decrease in blood flow is more severe because the uterine artery has to be "tied off" (clamped) when the uterus is removed. Otherwise you would have uncontrollable bleeding.

When the uterine artery is tied off, it means a loss of over 50% of the blood flow to the ovary from the ovarian artery. The ovary still gets some blood flow from another, smaller artery in the wall of the pelvis, but this does not make up for what is lost from the uterine artery. You can imagine how difficult it is for the ovary to work optimally if blood supply, along with oxygen and nutrients, is *reduced over 50%*.

If you have spent years suffering, not feeling well, and going from doctor to doctor trying to find a way to relieve symptoms and to feel better, ask your doctor to check your hormone levels! It is not difficult or overly expensive to do. You deserve to have your hormone concerns taken seriously and properly tested.

Fact

A *gradual* decrease in estradiol and testosterone just may not produce *noticeable* symptoms for two or more years after a hysterectomy.

Remember

Even if you keep your ovaries, you won't be guaranteed fully functioning ovaries until natural menopause, on average at 51.

Common Medications: Unexpected Pitfalls and Problems for Your Ovaries

The 21st Century "Tonic": Serotonin Boosters and Mood-Managers

"Just give her a happy pill." Prozac (and its new packaging as Sarafem), Zoloft, Paxil, Celexa, Luvox, Cymbalta, and Effexor are the most frequently prescribed group of medications for women under 50 in the United States.

For women especially, these drugs are doled out rather like the turn-of-the century *Lydia Pinkham's Tonic*, a popular "women's remedy" for a host of ailments from anxiety, depressed mood, irritability, and premenstrual problems, to headaches, insomnia, low energy, muscle pain, excessive "worrying" and a variety of others.

Shocking
Over 30 million Americans have taken these "serotonin enhancers" (SSRIs) at one time or another.

Our 21st century mood-altering medicines have a reputation for being so safe and effective that they are commonly prescribed for both FDA-approved reasons like depression and obsessive-compulsive disorder, as well as many off label uses, such as chronic pain, bulimia, attention deficit-hyperactivity disorder, borderline personality disorder, hypochondria, fibromyalgia, migraine headaches, social shyness, and most recently PMS and PMDD. Most of these conditions are more prevalent in women.

Of all the prescriptions written nationally for SSRIs, less than 10% are written by psychiatrists. Primary care physicians, gynecologists, neurologists, and rheumatologists prescribe most. As a result of their use for so many conditions other than depression, and being prescribed by non-psychiatrists, there are some emerging concerns: doses are now often larger than originally studied, and medicines are commonly combined with many other prescriptions.

"Mother's Little Helper"
About 65%–70% of all SSRI prescriptions are written for women.

The typical woman I see, even if she is in her teens, is already on an average of 5 to 8 different prescriptions.

When SSRIs are *properly used*, they have significantly fewer side effects than older antidepressants like the tricyclics (TCA, such as amitriptyline or Elavil, Pamelor, doxepin and others.

But overall, I do not think they are really needed as often as they are prescribed for women.

Danger!
The more medicines you take, the greater your risk of serious side effects and drug interactions.

First of all, many younger women have symptoms such as those above for a variety of endocrine reasons, not "psychiatric" in origin. Two common problems—low estradiol and low thyroid—discussed in previous chapters, cause many of the same mood symptoms. Women may need different treatments instead of simply using psychiatric medications.

What about taking these medications over a number of years, as many women often do? These medicines may have effects on ovarian function that you, and possibly your doctor, haven't realized.

Erratic menstrual cycles caused by declining ovarian hormone levels or thyroid disorders may cause "mood swings" or ups and downs in moods similar even to "bipolar" illness. Women are then prescribed "mood-stabilizers" such as Depakote (valproic acid), Tegretol (carbamazepine), Neurontin (gabapentin), or lithium.

These medicines can disrupt neuroendocrine pathways that regulate the ovaries and alter thyroid hormone production. Lithium, for example, commonly causes hypothyroidism, by interfering with the manufacture of thyroid hormones, and also triggers potential autoimmune reactions in the gland itself.

So if your mood symptoms were actually caused by an undiagnosed thyroid problem, you can see how your problems could get worse if you are put on lithium, based only on looking at symptoms.

Both SSRIs and "mood stabilizer" anticonvulsants such as De-pakote, Tegretol, and others can increase release of the pituitary hormone prolactin via their action on another brain chemical called *dopamine*.

Prolactin is the hormone that regulates nursing after delivery. Another effect of prolactin is to suppress the return of ovarian cycles and ovarian hormone production, helping prevent another pregnancy while a mother is still nursing a new infant.

Most of the antidepressants today act on pathways in the brain that either directly or indirectly increases prolactin. Even though you are not nursing, if you take a medicine that causes high prolactin, it leads to menstrual irregularity, a decrease in the ovarian hormones, and possibly infertility.

SSRIs, or serotonin-reuptake inhibitors, boost serotonin by inhibiting reuptake by the nerve cell, a process that normally *inactivates* serotonin. SSRIs serve to boost and prolong serotonin action. Brain cells get flooded with available, active serotonin that increases transfer of messages between nerve cells. These medications also may work by stimulating the growth of new nerve cells and connections, called *neurogenesis*.

Increased serotonin activity at receptor sites in the brain and body is usually a desirable therapeutic action of these medicines. Too much serotonin activity, however, can cause unwanted side effects such as fatigue, headaches, loss of sex drive and orgasm.

Another downside of increased serotonin action is a *decrease* in activity of the chemical messenger *dopamine*, which inhibits prolactin release. If dopamine is too low, prolactin is no longer inhibited correctly in a non-pregnant woman, and levels rise.

Higher prolactin then decreases the normal FSH–LH regula-tion of the menstrual cycle, inhibits normal ovarian cycling and decreases hormone production.

Warning
Many psychiatric meds increase prolactin… which then can suppress your ovaries, and decrease your hormones.

Be Aware
SSRI effects can mask other health issues, including hormone causes of similar symptoms.

Of course
SSRIs have subtle side effects not easily recognized.

Fact

Women often take SSRIs for years and years... leading to increased risk of serotonin excess.

Prolactin Effects

High prolactin also leads to weight gain, breast enlargement, milky discharge from the breasts, headaches, fatigue, and depressed mood.

Caution

Shake off your complacency about these medicines and review the potential problems carefully before you turn to SSRIs as "magic bullets."

Estradiol, progesterone, and testosterone all decline, even if you are in your teens or twenties and far from menopause. When the SSRIs are prescribed year after year, you are more likely to have side effects from too much serotonin effect relative to dopamine.

Dopamine is a critical chemical messenger in the brain's sexual circuits, so if you lose dopamine activity, sexual response is blocked. This is how SSRIs and other antidepressants cause loss of sex drive and decrease your ability to have an orgasm.

So if you are on a tricyclic antidepressant or a serotonin-booster medication for a while and have any of these symptoms, it is important for your doctor to do a blood test for prolactin.

If prolactin is too high, you should talk with your doctor about medication changes. For example, bromocriptine is a medicine designed to increase dopamine and reduce prolactin.

Other medications commonly prescribed for women also act on these same brain pathways and can cause increased prolactin:

1. **Anticonvulsants**, such as the mood-stabilizers I mentioned above. These are also commonly prescribed for seizures, migraine headaches, muscle and nerve pain syndromes.

   The anticonvulsant Depakote has another potential risk to your ovaries. Some studies have found it causes an increase in ovarian cysts and an increased risk of developing poly-cystic ovarian disorder (PCOS). This may happen due to elevated prolactin, or it may be through another unknown mechanism.

2. **Antipsychotics** chlorpromazine [Thorazine], haloperidol [Haldol], droperidol [Inapsine], thioridazine [Mellaril], thiothixene [Navane], risperidone [Risperdal], pimozide [Orap], quetiapine [Seroquel] and others.

3. **Antinausea medicines** such as Compazine and Reglan.

Many medications have more, and different, side effects in women than in men. Most testing was done on men because they don't have all the "noise" of hormone fluctuations that can confound the study. It is precisely these hormone changes, however, that can alter how women's bodies metabolize medicines!

As an example, let's take a look at some heart side effects that are more likely to occur in women.

Heart Side Effects of Common Medicines— A Hidden Danger for Women

Long QT Syndrome (LQTS), a disturbance in the electrical conduction system of the heart, is a new concern for women taking tricyclic antidepressants, SSRIs, antipsychotics, antihistamines, decongestants and a number of others.

The electrical impulse system of the heart keeps your heart pumping at a steady rate, so any disruption can lead to a potentially serious disturbance in heart rhythm, called *torsade de pointes*.

This abnormal heartbeat decreases blood flow to the brain and body, and may cause fainting spells (*syncope*).

Or, the abnormal heartbeat can degenerate into *ventricular fibrillation*, a very serious rhythm disturbance that can cause sudden death from cardiac arrest.

Why talk about this in a book about ovaries? Because many young women take multiple medications for mood, headaches, allergies and other problems, which creates potential problems for the heart, even though it doesn't appear directly related to the ovaries.

Women naturally have a longer QT interval in their heart beat cycle than do men, which means they are more susceptible to these medication side effects.

Hormonal imbalance added to multiple medications is an explosive mix that makes LQTS and torsade de pointes much more likely.

That's another reason I am so concerned about the over-prescribing of medications for women without baseline blood tests of the ovarian hormones.

The presence of an eating disorder (anorexia nervosa or bulimia that cause electrolyte imbalances), and dehydration are other risk factors that can lead to LQTS and *torsade de pointes*.

If you have episodes of irregular heartbeat, fainting, or significant tachycardia after starting a new medicine, talk with your doctor promptly. Our understanding of these medication effects on the heart changes rapidly.

As more women demand better information, new studies are including women as well as men to clarify how to use all medicines more safely. In the meantime, you can reduce your risk by learning about serious drug interactions and talk with all your physicians about everything you are taking.

Why not?
Many medications have been on the market for years without being subject to safety analyses by gender.

Effect
LQTS is much more common in women than men, and usually occurs at times in the menstrual cycle when estradiol is falling or low.

Caution
Heart arrhythmias can also happen due to fluctuating and falling levels of estradiol.

Dr. Vliet's Guide to Causes of LQTS

There are over 50 different prescription medications that can cause LQTS (and that doesn't include herbs that may also have this effect), including

- ✷ TCA antidepressants Elavil (amitriptyline), Sinequan (doxepin), Tofranil (imipramine), Norpramin (desipramine);
- ✷ SSRIs such as Zoloft (sertraline), Prozac and Sarafem (fluoxetine), Paxil (paroxetine);
- ✷ "atypical" antidepressants such as Effexor (venlafaxine),
- ✷ antiarrhythmics (such as quinidine, Norpace, Tambocor, Pronestyl, and several others),
- ✷ antipsychotics (see list above that cause high prolactin),
- ✷ antibiotics (Biaxin, Tequin, Levoquin, Zagam, Bactrium-Septra, erythromycin),
- ✷ anti-migraine medicines (Amerge, Imitrex, Zomig),
- ✷ the GI stimulant Propulsid,
- ✷ and some of the newer antipsychotics such as Risperdal.

You can locate more detailed and updated information by checking the website www. QTdrugs.org, or by contacting the Sudden Arrhythmia Death Syndromes Foundation at 800-786-7723.   *© 2003-2007 Elizabeth Lee Vliet, M.D.*

Other Common Medication Pitfalls for Women

Antibiotics

Caution
Women who over-use antibiotics are at risk for frequent or persistent yeast infections that create many problems.

Antibiotics are certainly necessary, and clearly life-saving. But antibiotics are also widely *over*-used today, often for minor problems that will get better on their own in a week or so, or would respond to simple remedies. Prolonged use of antibiotics also alters hormone metabolism in the liver by increasing the metabolic breakdown of estradiol, progesterone and testosterone.

You may not notice antibiotic-induced effects on your ovarian hormones because you are accustomed to daily variation throughout the menstrual cycle. But if you are using an estradiol patch or tablet, you may need a brief increase in the dose during antibiotic therapy to prevent return of hot flashes, or mood changes, or insomnia, because the antibiotic increases liver metabolism of estradiol.

Likewise, if you take oral contraceptives, adding an antibiotic may increase the rate of hormone breakdown in the liver, which *could mean your birth control pill is less effective for contraception.*

Beta-blockers

Beta-blockers are often used for migraine headaches, mitral valve prolapse, some types of anxiety, and to control blood pressure. These are safe medicines overall. But here are a few cautions.

Beta-blockers can inhibit the conversion of T4 to T3, leading to symptoms of hypothyroidism. This can lead to significant problems that in turn disrupt ovarian function.

Beta-blockers also impair glucose-insulin pathways, leading to problems with insulin resistance, and even diabetes. Women already have these problems at a higher frequency than do men, so you have a double whammy when medications have these side effects.

Warning

Beta blockers have some unique problems for women, especially if taken for a long time.

High progestin birth control pills

The progestins in birth control pills, particularly those pills with high progestin-low estrogen formulas, are common causes of fatigue, depression, headaches, low libido, muscle and joint pain, vaginal dryness or vulvar pain.

I have treated many young women for vulvodynia caused solely by several years of using a high progestin-low estrogen pill such as Loestrin, Mircette or Alesse.

Progestin-only contraceptives like Depo-Provera or Norplant are often worse, because they contain no estrogen and act to suppress your own estradiol production.

Suzette is a woman in her early 30s who was experiencing severe depressive symptoms, including mood swings, irritability, and sudden tearfulness for no apparent reason. She also reported feeling tired all the time, hot flashes, insomnia, joint and muscle aches. "*I feel like I've had a long bout with the flu,*" she said. Suzette had difficulties having an orgasm, and had lost her interest in sex, causing a serious strain on her new marriage.

Unwanted Effects

Weight gain, marked fatigue, difficulty concentrating, and decreased sex drive are common with beta-blockers

What triggered all this? She noticed the problems began within a few months after her gynecologist started her on Loestrin to keep her periods lighter and reduce menstrual cramps. "*I did pretty well at first,*" she said, "*and then I noticed that my depressed mood, irritability and low energy got worse and worse the longer I was on these pills.*"

I changed her oral contraceptive to Ovcon-35, with much less progestin and slightly more estrogen, which improved her symptoms. I told her to use a low dose of estradiol alone for the days between Ovcon pill packs to keep her estrogen from falling abruptly, which triggered her migraines. The estradiol didn't prevent a normal period, because bleeding occurs with the drop in progestin when she stopped Ovcon.

Cause These medicines can also intensify symptoms caused by hormone imbalances.

At her first follow-up appointment two months later, she said:

"I feel like someone flipped a switch on me. I don't have that deadened feeling, I don't feel depressed, I am not crying, my angry outbursts are gone, I sleep better, I have my energy, I don't have all those headaches, and I am getting my interest in sex back. It was remarkable to feel so much better in such a short period of time. It also surprised me that my joint pain was gone after you cut down the amount of progestin I was getting. I never knew that what's in a birth control pill could make such a difference!"

Her laboratory results showed other interesting findings related to the higher progestin content of Loestrin: her 8 AM cortisol was higher than normal, indicating a "stress response" activated by the low estrogen-high progestin pill. This returned to normal after being on Ovcon for six months.

Her free T3 and T4 thyroid hormones were lower than optimal, another potential side effect of birth control pills.

Although her TSH was still in a desirable range, her thyroid hormones weren't as effective as they should be when she was on Loestrin because a higher percentage was attached to the binding proteins in the bloodstream, making them less active.

BCP effects High progestin BCP such as Loestrin, Mircette, Alesse, or Seasonale, cause more weight gain, headaches, depressed mood and low sex drive.

Thyroid changes are common contributing factors to symptoms of depression, tiredness, and waistline weight gain when women are on the wrong birth control pills. This is another reason to integrate the evaluation of thyroid and ovarian hormone pathways.

Soy, Supplements, Herbs and OTC Hormones: Pitfalls for Your Ovaries

Women today are inundated with articles, ads, and multi-level sales schemes pitching a myriad of herbs, soy-containing products, "natural" progesterone–"wild yam" creams, over-the-counter forms of DHEA and melatonin—all touted as "magic bullets" for menopause, PMS and perimenopause. Many types of herbs and supplements have the potential to cause *harmful* effects, particularly if you already have a decline in your ovarian hormones, a thyroid disorder, allergies to plants and pollen, or any problem with liver metabolism. Remember, plants can produce potent poisons that humans have used for killing animals (and other people) for thousands of years.

Plant Estrogens (Phytoestrogens):

The phytoestrogens, found in several hundred different plants, are biologically weaker than the native human estrogens. *Your body cannot make the identical ovarian estradiol from the phytoestrogens in soy or yams.* All of the phytoestrogen chemical building blocks require chemical conversion in the laboratory because our body does not have the enzymes to make these changes.

Even worse, high concentrations of phytoestrogens, such as soy isoflavones, can overwhelm your declining estradiol at receptor sites and interfere with the action and production of the body's "natural" estradiol, even though phytoestrogens are less potent than estradiol.

Studies also show high soy intake in premenopausal women suppresses our ovary production of estradiol and progesterone by 20–50 percent. That's a significant loss, especially if you already have symptoms of hormone imbalance.

Research from several countries shows that phytoestrogens and isoflavones compete with our own estradiol and progesterone at the body's receptor sites. For example, genistein, a soy isoflavone, has different binding strengths depending on *which* estradiol receptor (ER) is considered: it has a six-fold greater affinity for the ER-beta than for ER-alpha. Genistein can act either as an estrogen *blocker* at low concentrations or an estrogen *enhancer* at high concentrations. At higher concentrations, the estrogen-enhancing effects of genistein have *stimulated* the growth of breast cancer cells.

If you have problems with your ovary hormones, eating a lot of soy can make matters worse, especially if you are trying to get pregnant, or having problems with infertility.

If you have already lost significant bone, soy-induced ovarian suppression can cause further bone loss. In China and Japan, where diets are high in phytoestrogens, women do not typically describe hot flashes, but they *do* continue to have bone loss after menopause, and osteoporosis is a serious problem in most Asian countries today.

Effects
BCP can affect cortisol and thyroid too—all need to be checked to determine causes of symptoms.

Not so!
Women have the mistaken belief, reinforced by clever marketing, that everything "natural" is automatically "safe" and without side effects.

Different
Phyto-estrogen effects at the human estrogen receptors are not the same as our own estradiol.

Research indicates that phytoestrogens alone do not provide enough estrogen effect to protect against bone loss and decline in cognitive function.

If you are frustrated with nightly insomnia, which can be triggered by declining estradiol, too much soy can make your sleep problems worse by reducing your ovary's estradiol production.

No substitute

Taking phyto-estrogen supplements does not provide or restore what your ovary made.

Low estradiol contributes to sleeplessness, anxiety and high blood pressure, which can in turn be made worse by some herbs. *Ginseng*, for example, is often recommended by herbalists as a "natural" source of estrogen and given to women to "balance their hormones." Yet ginseng can cause high blood pressure, insomnia, anxiety, or agitation in usual supplement doses. Furthermore, based on recent studies, ginseng has little or no measurable estrogenic effect. It doesn't even do what many of the ads claim.

I am aware of studies that show increased soy intake is associated with lower cholesterol, higher HDL (good) cholesterol, and lower blood pressure. But there is a drawback that you don't hear about. *Soy isoflavones block your thyroid gland from converting T4 to the more active T3.*

Studies as early as the 1970s show soy isoflavones have marked anti-thyroid effects and cause hypothyroid disorders in infants fed soy formulas. This is not *mentioned* in the current hype for adding soy foods to your diet—including all those protein drinks, protein powders, protein snack bars and isoflavone supplements.

Guilty!

Soy isn't as innocuous as the ads claim. Soy supplements can interfere with ovulation and your hormone levels.

Most American women don't know this, and flock to soy supplements based on all the clever marketing claims, not knowing that the products sold in the U.S. are those more likely to cause thyroid problems. Don't forget, having optimal thyroid function is critical to the health of your ovaries. If your thyroid hormones aren't working properly, you won't have normal ovarian hormone production either!

Some of these negative effects of soy can be reduced by eating only *fermented* soy products (such as tempeh, miso, and tamari), which are ones more commonly consumed in Asian cultures.

There are now excellent double blind, randomized, prospective placebo-controlled studies (the "gold standard" type of medical research studies) showing the isoflavone supplements have *no effect* greater than placebo on any of the menopausal symptoms measured, including objective measures of estrogen effect.

These studies were interesting because the hot flash frequency decreased in *all* participants, but there was *no difference* in flash/flush frequency between placebo and isoflavone groups.

Earlier studies that did not include placebo comparisons tended to over-estimate the value of phytoestrogen products such as soy on reducing hot flashes without realizing why. This is a big factor with symptoms like hot flashes, since there has consistently been an unusually high positive response to placebo in studies on how to control hot flashes.

Fact

The high intake of soy-based foods in Japan is one factor contributing to high rates of hypo-thyroidism and goiter there.

Funding for both of these studies was provided by the company that manufactured the particular isoflavone supplement (Promensil) and one of the study authors served as a consultant to the company. It is unlikely that there was a bias *against* Promensil.

You have probably also read recently about the Asian high-soy diet being associated with a lower risk of breast cancer. A sales pitch for soy supplements pills and protein powder drinks usually comes along with such articles or advertisements.

What's not often mentioned is that in Japan and other Asian countries, there are additional factors that also contribute to their lower risk of breast cancer. Asian women generally drink very little alcohol. Drinking even 2–3 alcoholic beverages (wine, beer or liquor) several days a week can increase breast cancer risk four times greater than in women who don't drink alcohol.

Asian women have a far lower fat intake, particularly animal fats that are a risk factor for breast cancer. They are far more physically active throughout their lives than are American women, and studies clearly show that regular exercise lowers risk of breast cancer.

Cause

Red clover (or soy) isoflavones can *cause* infertility, as seen in a variety of animals.

Be careful about using soy products in your childbearing years. I think important information like this is left out because companies want to make money selling you supplements, regardless of whether you need them, whether they work, or whether they do harm. Millions of women are using these products every day, so that's why I reiterate the potential negative effects.

Lessons from Women's Experiences

Rose is a 43-year-old woman who came for a consult describing "Severe vaginal burning, painful intercourse, lack of lubrication, and diminished orgasm." At her first appointment, she said,

"I have been through the mill—I have been to about a dozen different doctors including two different gynecologists and a urologist, who put a scope up my bladder. One Gyn checked an estrogen level and told me it was normal, but it was just done once on the day I went to the office and no one asked what cycle day I was on. After I read your book, I realized the cycle day was important to understand the test result. I went to a vulvodynia specialist and all they did was give me a prescription for citrate and glucosamine and said I could have surgery to remove the damaged tissue. I certainly didn't want surgery, so I tried the glucosamine and it has helped a little but I still had the burning. I felt like they were just treating the symptom not getting at the cause. Another doctor told me it was happening because I was in a stressful relationship. I didn't know what to think by then."

Effect
Asian women have many reasons for low breast cancer risk, not just soy intake.

I explained to Rose what her lab studies showed about potential causes of her vulvar pain. I also told her about the many endocrine and metabolic factors causing vaginal and bladder pain problems in women. I think it is damaging to just write them off to "relationship problems."

As we discussed her problems further, an interesting fact came to light. After reading that soy was really good for you, Rose began eating a lot of soy foods, taking soy isoflavone supplements, buying tofu and eating it instead of meat, and she even stopped drinking regular milk and switched to soymilk. This was about two years before she started having vulvodynia.

Cause
Rose had dramatically increased soy in her diet... about two years before her pain began.

"I heard soy was so good," she said, *"I changed everything to soy and I cut out fat in my diet and was eating only about 10% fat, if that much. I was so good at watching the fat, I was doing better than what they recommend at Pritikin!"*

So what affected her ovarian hormones and in turn, contributed to the vulvar pain? I explained above that high intake of soy phytoestrogens actually decrease your estradiol and progesterone production, anywhere from 20 to 50 percent. Since she was getting into her late 30s, her ovaries were slowly decreasing their hormone production anyway, and the soy-induced inhibition just added to this loss.

Your liver manufactures cholesterol from the fats in the food you eat, and from triglycerides. This occurs even if you don't eat foods that are themselves high in cholesterol. Rose was eating such an extremely low fat diet that her body simply didn't have enough fat to make the normal amount of ovarian hormones.

Rose's serum estradiol levels were abnormally low throughout her menstrual cycle, both before and after ovulation, but her DHEA and progesterone levels were still quite good and well into the normal range. Her thyroid and adrenal function were excellent.

The loss of adequate estradiol was the primary cause for her vulvar pain. She later sent a letter saying much better she felt, and commented that she was shocked that no one had checked her hormone levels before this.

She ended her letter with *"My health was regained by me listening to my own inner guidance and intuition of what was right for me, because I thought this was somehow a hormone problem."*

Sue Ellen is now 38. Five years ago, she began having night sweats, hot flashes, severe fatigue, insomnia, irritability, and mysterious crying spells a week before her period. When I saw her, she said,

> *"I am tired of being tired. I'd like to feel energetic again. I am tired of feeling so cold all the time, and feeling so irritable. I'd really like to have my sex drive back, both for me and for my husband. Sometimes I feel sick, totally weak, and lose my mental functions. I'm tired of having to restrict my foods so much because they say I have all these food allergies. I'd like to know if I really have them, because sometimes just having to watch what I eat all the time is another major stress in my life. I'd like to age gracefully and not look so dried out and wrinkled at my age!*
>
> *"Since all this began, I've seen several doctors and several alternative practitioners. The MDs all just told me the typical 'it's normal to be tired and not sleep well when you have three children', and I thought the alternative practitioners were going to be helpful but I quit seeing them after spending too much money and seeing no improvements. The last person I saw was a naturopath who put me on Progon B (progesterone) sublingual capsules. When I tried to talk with her about my total lack of libido and my skin problems, she just said it was caused by stress. I was so upset, I stopped seeing her after that."*

She had other upsetting changes: a "brownish" pigmentation around her mouth, and an "orangish" cast to her skin. Her face wrinkled more than usual, her scalp was dry, flaky and itchy and she said she felt "dry all over." She couldn't have an orgasm easily, and was especially bothered that her libido had "completely disappeared."

You do need some! Women need 20–30% fat intake for the body to have the necessary "building blocks" to make steroid hormones (estradiol, progesterone, testosterone, DHEA, cortisol).

Effect Soy in her diet "competed" at the estradiol receptors with what little estradiol her body was making.

Results

On the Progon B, Sue Ellen had serious skin breakouts, acne flare-ups, eczema of her ankles and elbows, boils on her buttocks, several episodes of pink eye, and frequent sinus infections.

Sue Ellen's evaluation showed a number of causes of her multiple symptoms: her estradiol level was extremely low at 36 pg/ml, her testosterone was too low at 23 ng/dl, her DHEA and progesterone were still in the healthy normal ranges, which meant an excess of both these hormones relative to her low estradiol and testosterone. Progon B gave her an excess of progesterone, and when this was *added* to her own body's progesterone and DHEA, it caused the acne, other skin eruptions and her worsening allergies. Remember, progesterone suppresses your immune system. Excess progesterone effects caused her low libido, irritability, and blood sugar fluctuations.

She also took so many vitamin and herbal supplements that she had side effects from these too. She was taking excessive doses of the B vitamins, vitamin E and omega 3 and 6 essential fatty acids.

Her other supplements included chaste berry (Vitex), nettle, dandelion, Siberian ginseng, licorice, horsetail, rosemary leaf, ginger root, yellowstock root, plus high-dose vitamin A.

All these phytoestrogens helped further lower her estradiol, leading to dry skin, sinus infections, vaginal dryness, low libido, insomnia, night sweats, fatigue, and irritability.

I frequently see women who are seriously over-doing it with excess vitamin doses and multiple, potentially conflicting, herbs and supplements.

Making Matters Worse

She was taking the progesterone under the tongue (sublingually), which makes the excess even greater than if this same amount had been taken orally and swallowed.

Additional Herb and Supplement Cautions

There are several additional cautions for women who have ovarian hormone imbalances:

&❧ **St. John's Wort** should **not** be taken with prescription hormones, as it decreases the effectiveness of the hormones by 50%. This is due to the way the herb increases liver metabolism of the hormones.

If you take St. John's Wort with a birth control pill, you risk losing the contraceptive effectiveness because of the drug-herb interaction. Unless you want a "St. John's" baby, forget taking this herb.

&❧ **DHEA**—I do not recommend that you take over the counter DHEA. Most over-the-counter products contain doses higher than women need and can lead to androgen side effects such as weight gain, sweet cravings, acne, facial hair, loss of scalp hair, irritability, restless sleep/insomnia, agitation, anxiety, and muscle spasms.

In addition, women with ovarian or thyroid hormone imbalances need to be sure that they are not already making *too much* DHEA, as in PCOS, before adding this hormone.

You need reliable blood tests, *not saliva tests*, of *all* your hormones before deciding whether DHEA is needed.

ᴥ *Melatonin.* Studies show that this popular sleep aid has some adverse effects for women. Daily use of melatonin causes high cortisol levels in women, but not in men. High cortisol causes more fat around your waist and upper body, interferes with immune function, and may also *impair fertility.*

Taking melatonin every night for sleep also commonly leads to headaches, tiredness and depression during the day.

Effect

High doses of vitamin A and beta-carotene commonly cause an orange discoloration of the skin, and can also cause hair loss.

Summary

Adverse medication effects, as well as drug-drug interactions, and herb-drug interactions are far more common than most people, physicians included, realize.

Be aware that all these seemingly innocuous medicines and herbs may affect your ovarian and thyroid hormone balance.

Remember, herbs may be wildly popular today, but many are metabolized by the same liver pathways that metabolize prescription medicines. Taking them together can significantly change the rate of breakdown of one or the other.

In Section IV, there is a list of commonly available herbs and their potential adverse effects. Several reputable sources for additional information are listed in Appendix 2.

The Comprehensive Database of Natural Medicines is an excellent authoritative guide, based on solid worldwide research. It is published by a team of pharmacists who also publish *The Prescriber's Letter* for health professionals.

Let your doctor know about any herbal supplements you take, just as you would any other medications, so that if you develop problems, he or she all the information to properly evaluate your symptoms.

In addition, keep in mind that physicians have many patients to see each day. They may not always remember, or think to ask

Caution

Be careful about interactions and watch the *combined,* total daily doses in multiple products.

Sleep?

If you are having trouble sleeping, don't just pop melatonin pills. You need a thorough medical evaluation of the cause.

you, what supplements or herbs you take. Doctors need gentle reminders now and then.

At every appointment, always tell your physicians *all* the supplements, herbs or over-the-counter products you take. Bring to your appointment a list of what is in each one. This is for *your* safety.

Keep in mind, if you have had a surgery involving the uterus or ovaries, *insist* on having your hormones properly checked when you start having symptoms.

Good studies show that these common surgeries *do* cause earlier loss of optimal ovarian hormones in a significant percentage of women.

OH?
Doctors have assumed, incorrectly, that hormone levels don't matter. I hope I have shown you they *do*.

Chapter 11

Ovaries Out of Balance: PMS, Endometriosis, Bladder and Vulva Pain

I have been struck by patterns in the way women describe the *same* symptoms as the *same* time in their menstrual cycle.

This became more striking when working with "PMS" in 1983, a time when menstrually related problems were not taken very seriously in most medical settings. I was a full-time medical school faculty member seeing patients and developing a curriculum in what we now call "mind-body medicine." Once other physicians learned of my interest, they referred many young women for evaluation.

Most were in their teens and twenties. There was a common thread in descriptions of their experiences whether they had ever heard of PMS or not.

One 16-year-old described the week before her period as having "horrible" mood swings.

Obvious! There were so many common patterns, there *had* to be a hormonal link!

> *"I feel like I am losing control, I crave chocolate, and I drink (alcohol) more. I am depressed, bloated, and sleepy and I feel so tired. I also get constipated, my breasts swell, and hurt, and I ache a lot. I don't usually have headaches, but I get them along with all this other stuff. It goes away when my period starts, but I feel like I am going to explode until then."*

It was similar with a *29-year-old* young woman,

> *"About a week before my period, I start getting really cranky and edgy, I snap at people and don't mean to and then I feel bad about myself," she said. "I don't sleep well, I feel like my appetite is out of control and I can't seem to get enough to eat. It seems like all I want to eat is junk food and ice cream or at least something sweet. I get these times of feeling dizzy and light-headed in the*

afternoons or late morning, and then I feel anxious and hyper. I feel so bloated and sluggish and don't feel like doing anything much at all. Once my period comes, I feel fine again."

Interesting

Even at different ages, the descriptions were often the same, at the same "time of the month."

And even a 14-year-old had similar problems.

"My mother wanted me to see you about this because she thinks my hormones are out of whack," she said shyly. "It feels crazy talking about this, but I get scared because the week before my period is such a nightmare. I am so mean nobody wants to be around me.

"My friends say I'm a real bitch. I fly off the handle at everybody, I'm out of control, I cry for no reason, I'm screaming at everybody, and I feel like I have to scratch myself until this tension goes away. Sometimes I feel like I want to pull my hair out, it's so awful. I don't like telling anybody how I feel because they'll think I'm crazy.

"I'm fat and puffy and achy and I feel totally miserable. I sneak all this chocolate because I can't seem to leave it alone, and then my face breaks out and I don't want to be around anybody. I can't sleep at night and I can't stay awake at school.

"I feel like my body is some alien thing and I hate it. But it's weird, because when my period comes, it all goes away like it wasn't ever there. Makes me feel like I was in a bad dream for a couple weeks. Then I wonder if I imagined it all. But it keeps coming back the same time every month."

A 35-year-old described her experience this way:

PMS facts

Close to two hundred symptoms have been associated with PMS.

"It is overall achy feeling, like I have the flu. I feel depressed, irritable, and mad at the world. I am much more anxious, and I often cry for no reason and then feel silly. I get these ache and cramps in the lower part of my abdomen and have this backache that really gets me down. I have a lot of water retention, and I get constipated and that makes me feel even more bloated and miserable. But I am so hungry I eat too much, and it drives me nuts because I crave chocolate so much. I have this dull headache a lot of the time, and I don't sleep well. When my period comes, it all clears up and I feel normal again."

Today, after thousands of PMS consults, the patterns are similar from woman to woman, no matter what her age. I have also observed *cyclic* patterns in other uniquely "female" syndromes such as irritable bowel symptoms, bladder pain or recurrent infections, vulvodynia, interstitial cystitis, and endometriosis, to name a few; and in disorders more common in women than men, such as asthma or fibromyalgia, chronic fatigue, migraines, depression or anxiety problems.

I have found a common thread in women with these disorders: low estradiol production often accompanied by low testosterone, whether or not they still make healthy levels of progesterone.

Premenstrual Syndrome ("PMS")

Most women who have menstrual periods (or remaining ovarian cycles if they have had a hysterectomy) have some physical or emotional cues that tell them that their periods are about to begin.

When these cues and physical changes become bothersome, we call them *symptoms*. About 5–10% of women have symptoms severe enough to significantly disrupt their daily lives and relationships. This is not a trivial health issue.

Because the ovarian hormones help to regulate the function of almost every system in the body, "PMS" symptoms can appear just about anywhere, from your hair to your eyes to your sinuses to your heart, lungs, intestinal tract, muscles, joints, skin, immune function, and sexual response as well as the more obvious and expected effects on the reproductive system.

In my medical practice, there are many women who have PMS symptoms severe enough to interfere with optimal function at home, at work, and in relationships. The symptom patterns fall into several main categories, shown in italics, which I have listed with sample symptoms I hear day in and day out:

1. *Brain-mood symptoms*: depression, irritability, angry outbursts, anxiety, agitation, crying spells, feeling out of control, problems with memory or word-retrieval, concentration problems, fuzzy or "foggy" thinking, insomnia.

2. *Appetite changes, food cravings*: most common—sweets or chocolate, also salty foods; food binges are common; increased desire for alcohol (for reasons similar to the hormonal-metabolic changes that trigger the sweet cravings).

3. *Physical changes*: constipation, headaches, dizziness, backaches, abdominal pain, pelvic pain, cramps; (others include racing heart beat, sweating, palpitations, nausea, tremors, shortness of breath, asthma attacks, blurred vision, more

PMS Definition
Symptoms start at ovulation or a few days later, and magically vanish with bleeding or a few days after menses begin.

Fact
Mild to moderate PMS symptoms may strike as many as 95% of women at some point in their lives.

frequent migraines), bladder pain, vulva pain, muscle and joint aches.

4. *Fluid retention:* bloating, breast fullness, swelling of hands or feet, feelings of fullness in the sinuses, ears or head.

5. *Hair-skin problems:* acne, oily skin, oily hair; more allergies, hives, urticaria, or herpes outbreaks.

6. *Changes in vitality:* low energy, fatigue, lack of motivation, desire to be alone, loss of interest in usually enjoyable activities, social withdrawal, loss of sex drive.

When women have a hysterectomy, many keep their ovaries. Yet, they still describe the body-brain markers of a residual ovary cycle. They still have cycles of breast tenderness, bloating, food cravings, and constipation, among others.

Or they describe a few days of restless, fragmented sleep, abrupt emotional shifts, crying easily, loss of energy, feeling mentally foggy," or having anxiety attacks and palpitations as they did during the first few days of bleeding, when estradiol is at its lowest.

Many physicians seem to forget the ovaries are still there and have a cycle with hormone shifts. Another cause is that ovaries decline sooner after hysterectomy due to the interruption in ovarian blood flow when arteries are tied off.

Now, do we call it PMS, or the newer term *premenstrual dysphoric disorder* (PMDD, a more severe form of PMS), *premenopause,* or *perimenopause?*

One reason this is confusing is that these terms are used in different ways among physicians, the media and scientific articles.

Generally, but not always, **Premenopause** refers to a woman *still menstruating* regularly. **Perimenopause** refers to a woman beginning to have *erratic, inconsistent periods* with changing flow-patterns (long and heavy one month, lighter and shorter the next), changing cycle lengths, a rising FSH, fewer ovulatory cycles, and skipped periods.

PMS refers to the physical and emotional *symptom cluster* occurring *between ovulation and menses,* which *then ceases* for a symptom-free interval each month.

Menopause technically means "cessation of menses" and loss of the ovary cycles. However, it is difficult to pin point the last period until a woman has gone an extended time without periods, usually at least a year. Menopausal women taking cyclic progesterone or progestin hormone therapy can have PMS-like symptoms when they start and stop the progestogen.

Post menopause refers to the years after the complete cessation of menses. Health books and articles typically write as if chronological age is the *primary* indicator of when to expect menopause changes. But this isn't always accurate.

We must know the *endocrinological* age to determine if you are menopausal or not. I have 23-year-old patients who are hormonally menopausal and women at age 54 who are not. **We must measure objective hormone levels rather than use age as the basis for whether you are "menopausal."**

Fact
PMS (and PMDD) may occur in both pre- and peri-menopause, since women still have their ovary cycles.

What Are Some of the Causes of PMS?

I think of PMS as a *neuroendocrine* disorder that begins with physiological hormonal shifts, particularly declining estradiol, which affects multiple brain centers and chemical messengers regulating functions throughout all our body systems.

The hormone shifts cause changes in chemical messengers that occur can also be aggravated by when and what we eat, what we drink or smoke, what medicines and supplements we take (or what vitamins and minerals we may be missing!), chemical exposure, sleep, and stress. It's like adding gasoline to a fire initially "lit" by hormone changes.

Relief!
PMS doesn't occur after menopause because there are no more natural cycles.

Hormonal Fluctuations: A Key Factor

A major link between hormones and mood symptoms is the *degree* **of fluctuation**, or **rate of change**, in hormone levels. Most medical studies do not address this crucial factor.

Falling estradiol decreases several mood-elevating messengers: endorphins, serotonin, and dopamine and also leads to an increase in monoamine oxidase (MAO) enzymes that break down (inactivate) the mood-lifting chemical messengers.

Ages
Chronological age doesn't always correlate with your *endocrinological* age.

These combined effects contribute to the depressed, irritable, anxious mood so typically described by millions of women during this time of the cycle. Falling estradiol may also set off a burst of norepinephrine in the brain's alarm center, activating the fight-or-flight response, and adding to the feelings of anxiety and irritability as the estradiol falls.

When progesterone falls before bleeding days, this adds to the drop in endorphins that makes you depressed and irritable. When

Effects

The more rapid the rate of fall, or rise, in any of the ovarian hormones, the greater the impact on multiple chemical messengers in the brain.

Cause

Progesterone acts like Valium by activating GABA pathways in the brain

Effects

Hormone changes can trigger mood effects as the brain's response to the *physical* hormone change.

progesterone falls, there is rebound anxiety and irritability, just as you would experience if you abruptly stopped taking Valium.

Many women describe their worst days in the cycle as the day prior to bleeding and the first day. This is exactly when estradiol falls sharply and is at the lowest point of the cycle. Progesterone has also fallen.

No wonder you feel tearful, have fragmented sleep, anxiety attacks, palpitations, and irritability. It doesn't mean you are crazy, or you have a psychiatric disorder; it means that some women are simply more sensitive to these changes than others.

PMS does not appear to be a *"deficiency"* of progesterone before menstruation, as proposed by Dr. Katharina Dalton, the British physician who popularized the use of natural progesterone (as opposed to synthetic progestins) as a PMS treatment several decades ago. Her *hypothesis* was that PMS was due to "estrogen dominance."

Dr. Dalton, and subsequent physicians who have written books based on her work, have sold a lot of progesterone products with this idea. This is a only *theory*.

None of these physicians appear to have done systematic hormone measures, by cycle phase, to confirm an *actual* deficit of progesterone and an excess of estradiol.

Everything in both the science of hormone actions and the pattern of symptoms points to a *cyclic rise* in progesterone as a major *cause* of PMS, which is *worse* if estradiol is low at this time.

Think about it. PMS doesn't occur before puberty, or after menopause or in cycles you don't ovulate (which is what causes the rise in progesterone,), or if the ovaries are removed. But as soon ovarian progesterone rises, or you take a progestin for 10–14 days a month, classic PMS symptoms return.

In fact, it is the very "PMS" symptoms in a *cyclic* HRT regimen after menopause that is one of the reasons women don't like taking hormones and stop.

Many women say to me, "*I felt great on the estrogen, but I had to give up that good feeling because I felt so horrible when the progesterone was added!*"

Mood swings, depression, irritability, bloating, breast tenderness, increased appetite, food cravings, feeling "fat" and no libido all began when progesterone was added, and *were not present during the estrogen only phase*.

In 20 years of testing hormone levels, by menstrual cycle phase, of women with PMS, I have *never* found this hypothesized condition of "estrogen dominance." In women with low levels of *progesterone* in the luteal (PMS) phase of the cycle, *I also found low estradiol levels.*

By the time women reach the stage of anovulatory cycles and low progesterone, the ovaries have already declined in production of estradiol, and testosterone has usually decreased as well.

Much of the neuroendocrine science that deals with ovarian hormones and the brain has emerged years since Dr. Dalton first proposed her theory. Dr. Dalton used high doses of progesterone suppositories, or troches, to treat PMS. She reported that many women in her program found relief from their premenstrual symptoms. Pharmacological studies show that large doses of progesterone have a Valium-like action on the brain by binding at the GABA receptors, so it stands to reason that some women would feel relief of premenstrual anxiety and tension.

The majority of PMS researchers and clinicians, however, have not found progesterone successful. In double blind, placebo-controlled studies published in recent years, progesterone treatment is not any better than placebo in relieving PMS symptoms. I tried following Dr. Dalton's progesterone recommendations, but I stopped because too many women became profoundly depressed, lethargic, and gained weight when given those high doses of progesterone.

I found that it is *estradiol* supplementation in the luteal phase of the menstrual cycle that gives the most impressive symptom relief for PMS. More recent controlled studies, such as those described by Dr. John Studd's group in London, confirm my clinical experience.

The laboratory results showed why: my patients *didn't have a deficit of progesterone.* They had unexpectedly low estradiol and quite normal progesterone levels.

Current research further shows that *progesterone decreases serotonin,* while estradiol boosts serotonin, which confirms my findings and those Dr. Studd reported.

Thus, Dr. Dalton's theory has not held up. Carefully controlled studies report very different results from those practitioners using progesterone in uncontrolled clinical settings. In the latter, progesterone is recommended to everyone for PMS, regardless of

Wisdom
Nothing in our scientific study of hormones or wisdom gained from women supports the idea that PMS is caused by a deficiency of progesterone.

The key
It's the *rise* of progesterone when estradiol is *low* that makes PMS worse!

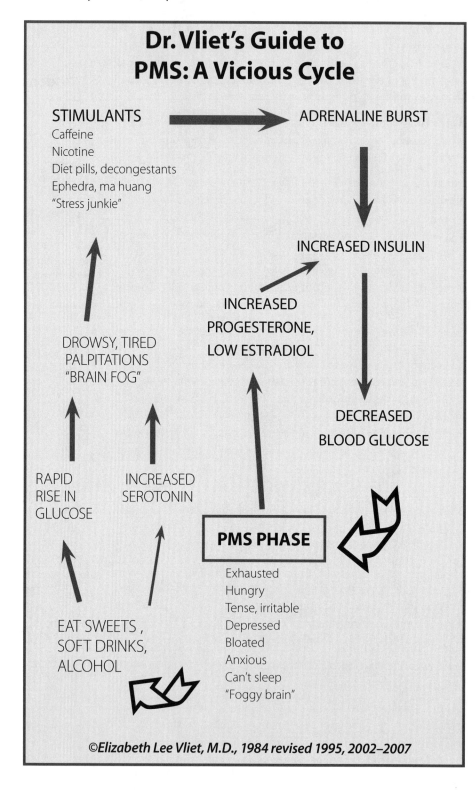

Dr. Vliet's Guide to PMS: A Vicious Cycle

STIMULANTS
Caffeine
Nicotine
Diet pills, decongestants
Ephedra, ma huang
"Stress junkie"

ADRENALINE BURST

INCREASED INSULIN

INCREASED PROGESTERONE, LOW ESTRADIOL

DROWSY, TIRED PALPITATIONS "BRAIN FOG"

DECREASED BLOOD GLUCOSE

RAPID RISE IN GLUCOSE

INCREASED SEROTONIN

PMS PHASE

Exhausted
Hungry
Tense, irritable
Depressed
Bloated
Anxious
Can't sleep
"Foggy brain"

EAT SWEETS, SOFT DRINKS, ALCOHOL

©*Elizabeth Lee Vliet, M.D., 1984 revised 1995, 2002–2007*

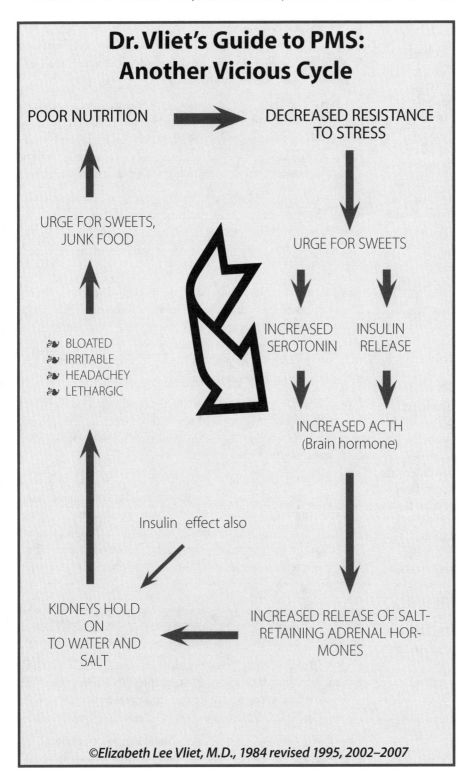

Dr. Vliet's Guide to PMS:
Another Vicious Cycle

POOR NUTRITION ➡ DECREASED RESISTANCE TO STRESS

URGE FOR SWEETS, JUNK FOOD

URGE FOR SWEETS

🍃 BLOATED
🍃 IRRITABLE
🍃 HEADACHEY
🍃 LETHARGIC

INCREASED SEROTONIN   INSULIN RELEASE

INCREASED ACTH
(Brain hormone)

Insulin effect also

KIDNEYS HOLD ON TO WATER AND SALT

INCREASED RELEASE OF SALT-RETAINING ADRENAL HORMONES

©Elizabeth Lee Vliet, M.D., 1984 revised 1995, 2002–2007

It's bad
Many women with PMS become markedly *worse* taking only progesterone. One woman even called it her "crabby cream."

whether they have documented low progesterone levels or not. So take the "progesterone gurus" with a grain of salt, and look to the more solid scientific studies, as well as your own body experiences, for sound information.

For a patient with low progesterone levels in the luteal phase and normal estradiol levels, I would use progesterone. And conversely, if there is low estradiol and relatively normal luteal phase progesterone, creating a reduced estradiol to progesterone ratio, then it only makes sense to boost estradiol back to optimal ranges as a first step.

All of the young women in the beginning of this chapter with "out of control" PMS had *below normal* estradiol levels in the second half of their menstrual cycle when symptoms were most intense.

According to the usual *age-based* definitions, these women are *too young* to be considered pre or perimenopausal. Their estradiol levels indeed reach the *endocrinological* first phase of the transition to perimenopause. Hormone testing confirms that their descriptions of symptoms matched the science, based on estradiol and progesterone levels.

So obvious?
Estradiol increases serotonin. Serotonin lifts depression, so it isn't surprising women often feel depressed when estradiol is low in relation to progesterone.

I treat these women with low-dose estradiol supplements to bring levels back into optimal menstrual cycles ranges, instead of prescribing antidepressants as is more commonly done. They consistently improve.

This fits with the results of studies by Dr. Studd, who used estradiol implants for PMS with great success. The women describe improved mood, diminished irritability, better sleep, improved libido, higher energy level, diminished food cravings (especially for sweets and chocolate), and reduced mood swings. Only a few require antidepressants once hormone levels return to healthy ranges.

Endometriosis: New Insights and Emerging Concerns About An Old Problem

Endometriosis is an enigmatic, painful disorder that is far more common than statistics convey. It manifests itself in many ways and is notoriously hard to diagnose with certainty, short of having laparoscopic surgery.

The vast majority experience its debilitating effects without explanation. For women who are properly diagnosed, it is often a long, arduous process involving multiple physicians over many years before anyone considers endometriosis.

"Endo" as it is often called, is a complex health problem; it can lead to infertility, causes severe, persistent, debilitating pain for many, and a disruption in quality of life and relationships. It is costly, to the women, their employers and their insurance carriers.

Endometriosis is on the rise today. But why? This is not simply due to better diagnostic techniques. It is related to connections I have been describing in this book: exposure to endocrine-disrupting environmental chemicals and their damaging effects to the reproductive system, the thyroid, and immune system.

There are many emerging connections between endometriosis and exposure to environmental chemicals, as well as links to thyroid disorders (particularly autoimmune forms like Hashimoto's), premature ovarian decline, mitral valve prolapse, chronic fatigue, and susceptibility to chronic infections.

Let's look at some crucial issues between environmental chemicals and this mysterious, debilitating disorder. This is an overview of critical issues. Read more in materials from The Endometriosis Association, which is conducting landmark research on links between endometriosis and organic pollutants like dioxin.

What is Endometriosis and Why is It a Problem?

Endometriosis is not a simple disease. We can describe endometriosis as tissue (*endometrium*) that should be lining the inside of the uterus but is growing somewhere else, outside the uterus.

These little blobs of endometrial tissue, medically called *endometrial implants*, or *endometriomas* if they are bigger and cystic, can cause severe pain because the endometrium outside the uterus still bleeds with our menstrual cycle hormone changes as if it were *inside* the uterus.

When the lining of the uterus is where it is supposed to be, the menstrual blood is easily released through the cervical opening, into the vagina, and out of the body.

But when the endometrial tissue lies outside the uterus, in the pelvis, the blood has no way to be released from the body and it accumulates. Endometrial implants outside the uterus also release inflammatory chemicals, such as cytokines, that *induce*

Statistics
Endometriosis affects more than 5 million women in the US alone, yet only a small percentage are accurately diagnosed.

Painful!
96% of women with endometriosis have dysmenorrhea or pain throughout the menstrual cycle

Normally

Normal
menstrual
bleeding
does not
cause pain.

more pain and inflammation. Over time, there is chronic irritation of pelvic tissues, more inflammation, causing sticky adhesions and scarring that further intensifies pain.

Newer research, discussed at the World Endometriosis Conference in February 2002, **describes another wicked way endometrial implants outside the uterus increase pain and inflammation: they produce their own estrogen (estrone and estradiol) from adrenal androgens via an enzyme system called the aromatase pathway.**

This means that even if your blood levels of estradiol are low, or you take drugs to reduce ovarian estrogen, *these little devils can still make estrogen anyway to feed their own growth!* Normal endometrial tissue *inside* the uterus does not have this "estrogen factory" pathway.

Abnormal

Blood in
the pelvis
is a major
irritant to the
other organs,
causing
inflammation
and pain.

Endometrial implants may seed almost anywhere, even beyond the pelvis. The most common sites are in the lower pelvic area called the cul de sac, on the major ligaments supporting the uterus, on the bladder, on the outside of the uterus itself, on the ovaries, on the outside of the bowel wall, or scattered along the side walls of the pelvis.

Small bits of endometrial lining have been found as far outside the pelvis as the lungs and spinal cord. Cases of periodic collapsed lung during menstruation have been reported; the women were found to have endometrial implants causing this mysterious link with the menstrual cycle.

In fact, in the studies of monkeys who developed endometriosis after dioxin exposure, the endometrial implants were scattered throughout both lungs contributing to the animals' death.

**Wicked
Trick**

Endometrial
implants
outside
the uterus
are their
own little
"estrogen
factories!"

Small endometrial implants may also migrate to the cauda equina, or "tail" of nerves at the end of the spinal cord, causing excruciating low back pain that is notoriously difficult to diagnose and treat.

Endometrial implants can burrow deep into the muscle wall of the uterus, known as *adenomyosis*. Adenomyosis implants bleed into the uterine muscle during menstruation. The menstrual "cramps" are so painful, intense, and sharp they may cause you to faint or vomit. Endometrial-type adenomyosis implants can even wedge in the connective tissue (*septum*) between the rectum and vagina, causing intense pain with bowel movements during menstrual periods.

Some women with severe pain have minimal endometrial implants in the pelvis. Other women have extensive endometriosis throughout the pelvis with little or no pain.

Most are somewhere between these extremes, and commonly experience pain with intercourse, bowel movements, or menstruation. Some of the degrees of pain may occur because of implant location rather than amount.

Discrepancies may also result from what triggers the endometriosis. For example, the monkeys exposed to dioxin had an extremely aggressive form of endometriosis and appeared to be in severe pain. Organic pollutants causing endometriosis may also damage pain-regulating pathways.

Endometriosis causes many different problems, depending on where it hides in the body and how it responds to hormone changes, and other factors. Sometimes symptoms aren't even the same from one menstrual cycle to the next. The diagnosis is first made *clinically*, based on a high index of suspicion about the classic symptoms.

Ultimately, however, the definitive diagnosis must be definitively made during exploratory surgery of the pelvis. Such surgery can be done with an instrument called a laparoscope (*laparoscopic surgery*), or the surgeon may decide to open the abdomen (*laparotomy*).

How Do I Know Whether I Might Have Endometriosis?

Infertility is one serious consequence of endometriosis, affecting some 30–40% of women with the disease according to the Endometriosis Association.

Red Flags: Clues to Endometriosis or Adenonyosis

- ❧ severe, crampy pain with your menstrual flow each month (*dysmenorrhea*),
- ❧ pain with intercourse (*dyspareunia*),
- ❧ pain with bowel movements (occurs primarily during your menstrual periods, but can occur at other times due to adhesions from endometrial implants and scarring on the outside of the bowel).

Puzzle 1
Why do some women have extensive disease yet few symptoms, while others have relatively little disease and severe or incapacitating symptoms?

Puzzle 2
The relationship between the amount of endometriosis and the degree of pain is puzzling.

Puzzle 3
The puzzling array of symptoms is one reason that it is so hard to diagnose.

Even before fertility problems are recognized, however, a woman has probably experienced pelvic and abdominal pain.

Old Theory

All women have at least some degree of backward menstrual flow, and yet *all* women clearly do not develop endometriosis.

The Endometriosis Association Research Registry shows over 96% of women with endometriosis have pain throughout the menstrual cycle, 80% report pain with bowel movements or alterations in bowel movements during menses; almost 60% of women have severe pain with intercourse. Over 82% of the women in their registry also describe fatigue and exhaustion.

I strongly suspect from my work with endometriosis patients that the low levels of estradiol and testosterone are significant causes of the low energy.

What causes it?

Endometriosis is one of the *better-studied* clinical problems for women, yet it remains one of the most mysterious. One of the oldest theories, proposed by Dr. John Sampson in the 1920s, said that endometriosis resulted from menstruation flowing backward (called *retrograde menstruation*) through the Fallopian tube into the pelvic cavity, instead of into the cervical opening, the vagina, and then out of the body.

New Theory

If this theory is correct, it means endometriosis is actually a *congenital* disorder that occurs during fetal development, and could have a number of causes.

Although this theory has never been proven, it has remained one of the most widely reported "causes" of endometriosis. One problem with Dr. Sampson's theory is that it doesn't really explain how endometriosis can be found in such far-flung spots as the lung, or along spinal nerves. The retrograde menstruation theory simply does not explain it fully.

Over the years, researchers have looked at genetic, immune, and lifestyle factors. Dr. David B. Redwine, a gynecologist in Oregon who made endometriosis a primary focus of his clinical work and research, feels that our traditional theories of cause and our traditional medical treatments with drugs have addressed only a small piece of the endometriosis picture.

Dr. Redwine proposes that **girls are born with endometriosis** rather than developing it after menstruation begins.

This view theorizes that endometriosis develops when embryonic tissue destined to migrate to the area of the uterus fails to complete the journey, landing in areas of the pelvis outside the uterine cavity. The tissue lies dormant until the hormone cycles of puberty begin, and then the outside endometrium is activated to follow the menstrual cycle pattern as is the endometrial tissue *inside* the uterus.

Dr. Redwine and others feel that endometriosis is *constant* in amount, rather than the standard medical teaching that it progressively increases with years of menstruation. This helps explain how chemicals like dioxin cause the disease: by disrupting normal fetal development of the reproductive system, and interfering with endometrial tissue development.

Pale, whitish endometrial implants, as well as other colors, can be present from birth. Researchers think their color changes over time following puberty. The darker, blackish or chocolate-colored endometrial implants are found more in women in their 30s. These are the ones surgeons see and remove more frequently because they are readily identified. The white or yellowish endometrial implants can be widespread, but more difficult to see with the usual laparoscopic techniques.

Looks are deceiving
Endometriosis can have a variety of appearances, not just the "chocolate" or a dark reddish-black color.

The theory that endometriosis is a congenital disorder actually fits well with newer research showing that dioxin, and probably many similar organic pollutants, cause endometriosis. The dioxin link was published in the fall of 1993, from the Endometriosis Association's pioneering research on monkeys.

This same connection was made earlier in a 1985 Canadian study by Dr. James Campbell, but it had been overlooked until the Endometriosis Association raised awareness of the dioxin link. Dr. Campbell's group demonstrated that another group of environmental pollutants called PCBs also caused endometriosis in monkeys.

Shocking
Researchers were stunned to find endometriosis implants in about 80% of the animals that received concentrations of dioxin compounds over the years.

PCB compounds damage the developing thyroid gland, immune system and other hormonal target tissues. Here is a way that all of these "mysterious" conditions may share a common trigger.

The first clue these chemicals caused endometriosis came from a colony of Rhesus monkeys that were part of a study to assess possible damage from the dioxin compound, "Agent Orange," a chemical defoliant used in the Viet Nam war. The endometriosis was an unexpected finding, since it is extremely rare in monkeys and apes. Animals exposed to the higher doses developed such an aggressive form of endometriosis that they died from it, also an unusual finding.

Here are two of the most frightening aspects of this research: (1) endometriosis did not develop until years after the initial exposure. In the case of dioxin it was over ten years later, so the causative link is difficult to pin down. (2) Even the highest concentrations in the studies were miniscule: 25 parts per *trillion* of dioxin in the monkeys' water supply, about *the same as the average American is exposed to in common foods contaminated with the chemical.*

Cause
The higher the concentration of dioxin, the more severe the endometriosis.

To put this in perspective, it is similar to you spitting once into an Olympic-sized swimming pool and trying to measure the effects of your saliva on the depth of the pool.

It is pretty staggering such a miniscule amount causes such profound damage, and even death, from the disease it triggers. This is one of the *silent* health crises facing women today.

Our increased exposure to these hormonally-active environmental chemicals plays a bigger role in our health than medical professionals recognize. Newer research also links dioxin exposure to insulin resistance, in both women and men, and a number of scientists have suggested that endometriosis, like PCOS, may be caused by insulin resistance. Excess insulin has been identified as a risk factor for later breast cancer.

Even with this research, we can't say with certainty what causes endometriosis, or whether there is one primary cause as once thought. The most likely explanation is that it has several causes, one of the most potent being exposure to the POPs chemicals, especially during fetal development and childhood.

Dr. Vliet's Guide to Risk Factors for Endometriosis

- Family history of endometriosis
- History of maternal exposure to DES and/or other xenoestrogens
- History of exposure to dioxin, PCBs, organochlorines in utero, in breast milk and/or early childhood
- Obesity, with excess estrone
- History of heavy and/or longer than average menstrual flow
- History of elevated thyroid antibodies
- History of recurrent, chronic yeast infections
- Presence of mitral valve prolapse

© 2003–2007 Elizabeth Lee Vliet, M.D.

Risk Factors
The more collective risk factors in your history, the more likely you will develop endometriosis.

Ovary Hormones and Your Bladder

Bladder problems are one of the least discussed of women's health issues, especially among younger women. We see the "adult diaper" commercials featuring older women and can't conceive having similar problems.

If you have premature ovarian decline and lower than optimal estradiol levels, you may experience urinary leakage, frequent urges to urinate, painful intercourse, urinary, vaginal or vulvar burning, even in your 20s.

The cells of the urinary bladder and urethra lining are sensitive to the rise and fall in estradiol levels during the monthly cycle, in pregnancy, perimenopause, as well as the loss of estradiol at menopause.

There are many changes from the decrease in estradiol: more sensitivity to the usual stimuli for the urge to urinate, loss of smooth muscle strength so you can't hold it when you have to go, decreased pain tolerance, and changes in the pressure of the bladder and urethra (urodynamics) so that the urethra can't close properly.

Together these changes cause more "leakage" problems. When your estradiol is too low, the cells lining the bladder, urethra and vagina also become fewer, thinner (*atrophic*) and are easily torn or damaged with friction (*friable*). This means urination, friction from sex, or pressure from tight clothes can hurt, and sometimes cause bleeding.

Pain threshold is higher with normal estradiol levels. When estradiol decreases, the pain threshold is lowered, the nerve endings become more sensitive, and you have more pain.

Anatomy 202
The linings of the urinary bladder, urethra and vagina all have estrogen receptors, just like other organs and tissues in the body.

The increasing pain causes more urges to urinate, more burning during urination, and more burning vaginal sensations.

There are also estrogen receptors in cells that make collagen, the major protein in the connective tissue that helps support our entire urinary and genital system.

Loss of estradiol at any age leads to decreased collagen and skin wrinkling, as well as a loss of the collagen support that holds the bladder in place and allows the urethra to close.

Bladder and vaginal problems are common for women of all ages, and it is appalling that we lack more controlled studies studying the hormonal effects on these problems.

I have heard many medical presentations on issues like interstitial cystitis, vulvodynia and other problems, but no one mentions checking hormone levels or even using hormone treatments to improve the symptoms.

Hormone connections are more likely discussed if a woman is menopausal, but are almost never taken into account for younger women who may also be suffering *the same conse-quences* of low estradiol.

Early Estrogen Decline and Vulvodynia: A Young Woman's Painful Saga

Grace was only 23 and newly married when I saw her. Her mother encouraged the consult to see if hormone factors played a role in her severe vaginal pain. She described having vaginal burning during intercourse that was so painful her husband was afraid to attempt sex. She had no vaginal lubrication with arousal and was rarely able to orgasm. She was suffering from the pain, and it threatened her new marriage.

Anatomy 203
Nerve endings contain estrogen receptors.

Her gynecologist told her she had a "hang-up" about sex and should see a sex therapist because there wasn't anything wrong physically. After such a humiliating encounter, she was embarrassed and hesitant to talk, even to a woman physician with her mother there for support.

Her vaginal pain had been getting worse since age 18. She started taking birth control pills at 16 to prevent heavy menses and painful cramps. She was taking Loestrin 1/20, a high progestin pill with one of the lowest amounts of estrogen.

Hormones do matter
Hormone-triggered changes make women much more susceptible to bladder problems.

Several significant factors in her history provided clues to the cause of her problem. She was concerned about weight gain on the pill and drastically cut down her dietary fat when she became a vegetarian. Typically vegetarian diets are high in soy, low in protein, iron and vitamin B12. Her ferritin (iron stores) was low at 8 (desirable level is about 60–100), and her B12 level was low, as expected in women with predominately plant sources of protein. The higher fiber of a vegetarian diet decreases absorption and increases elimination. She did not use alcohol or tobacco, and exercised regularly and reasonably.

Here are the important connections in the development of her vaginal pain:

- high progestin birth control pills,
- high intake of soy phytoestrogens that compete at the estrogen receptors preventing binding of estradiol,
- the low fat diet that prevents the body making enough estradiol from cholesterol,
- low B12 levels, and low ferritin.

All of these contribute to a burning type pain (*neuropathic*), because they are needed for normal nerve function and pain regulation.

Her vulvodynia pain got worse each month when she stopped the active birth control pills and took the placebo pills to have a period. Since her own ovarian estradiol was suppressed by the Loestrin, her low fat diet and the high soy intake she was especially vulnerable to the drop in estrogen when she stopped the active pills each month. Practically speaking, she had almost no estradiol during her bleeding days. No wonder she was in such pain.

I prescribed a 0.01% (0.1 mg/gm) hypoallergenic estradiol cream *without* preservatives, and told her to apply the cream on her external vulvar and clitoral area nightly to restore the tissue estradiol.

I also suggested she use low dose Vagifem estradiol tablets in the vagina to improve pH and lubrication, also reducing the dryness and burning. I also changed her birth control pill to Orthocyclen, which is higher in estrogen and lower in progestin.

At a follow-up appointment several months later, she said, *"Everything feels much better, the pain is much less. I am amazed that changing my birth control pill and finding an estrogen cream I could use could make such a dramatic difference!"*

The Premarin cream did not help her, even though it contained estrogen. All FDA-approved commercial estrogen creams, including Premarin, contain a chemical preservative that causes burning and increased pain when sensitive tissues are damaged by loss of estrogen. Many patients who cannot use commercial products are able to use an estradiol cream made for them by compounding pharmacists who can eliminate any preservatives or dyes. (See Appendix II for pharmacy resources.)

Non-hormonal Causes of Bladder or Vulvar Pain

If your estradiol is low and the nerve endings feel "on fire," the substances below will likely make the pain much worse.

Food Triggers. Many foods contain chemicals such as citric acid, salicylic acid and oxalates that intensify bladder and vulvodynia pain. Experts recommend that women avoid a long list of foods: caffeine, alcohol, tobacco (nicotine), chocolate, spices and spicy

Not again... Another specialist recommended Premarin vaginal cream, but this caused so much burning she had to stop.

Hormones 101 The loss of adequate estradiol—coupled with the negative effects of the progestin—caused the vaginal dryness, pain, and difficulty having an orgasm.

Allergy Warning

Many people allergic to aspirin are also allergic to tartrazine, but don't know it.

foods, apples, bananas, acidic foods (citrus fruits, tomatoes), Nutrasweet, saccharine, sharp cheeses, coffee, tea, carbonated beverages, chemical preservatives (in many foods and beverages), lima beans, lentils, and yogurt.

These foods produce metabolic by-products that can irritate bladder or vaginal tissue, cause pain and spasm, as well as increase the urges to urinate, in turn aggravating incontinence.

Alcohol and tobacco are potent bladder irritants, and they also significantly interfere with the metabolism and effectiveness of prescription hormone therapies.

Diets too low in fat reduce absorption of prescription hormones, while diets high in fat increase absorption if taken at mealtime. Availability of any given oral hormone therapy is affected by when it is taken in relation to a meal, the type of meal, and food additives present.

Warning

Alcohol and tobacco are potent bladder irritants

Think about the typical diet of many women "on the run" and you realize just how many "triggers" people consume. I am surprised at how many of my patients worry about chemicals in meat, yet think nothing of polluting their bodies with cola beverages that have a wide variety of chemical irritants, not to mention calories from sugar.

Keep a dietary diary and note any patterns with the foods that cause a flare-up of bladder or vulvodynia pain. Make necessary modifications and *clean up* your diet.

Bladder and Vaginal Effects of Estradiol Decline

- **Vaginal and vulvar dryness, itching, burning, stinging pain** (several disorders: vaginitis, vulvodynia, vestibulitis)
- **Pain with intercourse** (dyspareunia)
- **Recurrent bladder infections/inflammation** (cystitis)
- **Urethral infections** (urethritis)
- **Recurrent vaginal infections** (vaginitis)
- **Incontinence** (loss of urine – several types, see description)
- **Painful urination** (dysuria)
- **Urinary frequency**
- **Urinary urgency**

©Elizabeth Lee Vliet MD 1995, revised 2002–2007

Dyes. *Tartrazine-based dyes* (a common one is FD&C yellow #5, but there are many others) in medications, foods, and beverages have a molecular make-up similar to salicylate, the chemical name for aspirin.

You may not know it is in a product or food either. FD & C yellow #5 and green and red dyes based on tartrazine are ubiquitous in thousands of common products—including foods, beverages, and vitamins. They are added to herbal products, many prescription medicines, and even medications to treat asthma and allergies.

If you have bladder sensitivities and an "irritable" bladder (or bowel, or even allergies in general), try to eliminate these chemicals in your food, beverages, and medicines. Many doctors don't check these issues, so you need to know such connections exist.

If something seems to aggravate symptoms, ask your doctor to change your dose or brand of medicine to one without dyes. See what happens. You may be pleased with the results.

Preservatives. Propylene (or polyethylene) glycol (PEG) is a preservative used to prolong shelf life contained in many commercial hormone and steroid creams —prescription and over-the-counter. It is also in some antibacterial and antifungal creams used to treat vaginal infections. PEG and similar preservatives can cause itching and burning. It is also found in estrogen vaginal creams used to treat vaginal itching and burning. If you have persistent problems with vaginal or bladder burning after starting one of the creams, talk with your physician or pharmacist and check your medication for these dyes, chemical binders, and PEG.

The PDR (*Physicians Desk Reference, edited and published by Medical Economics*) is now required to list dyes and other inactive ingredients in a particular medicine. Most libraries have a PDR, or it is available for purchase at any bookstore. Many food manufacturers will furnish a complete ingredient list if you write their consumer information office.

Chronic Bladder "Infections:" Is It Really an Infection or My Hormones?

Lots of young women have problems with bladder or urinary tract infections (UTIs). Burning, frequency and urgency can have many causes. Not all are due to infections, yeast or bacte-

Pain Triggers
These dyes have metabolic breakdown products excreted in the urine that are a potent trigger for bladder and vulvar pain.

Effects
I have seen reactions from rashes and wheezing to severe bladder spasms, all traceable to dyes in medications.

Irritant
PEG can be very irritating, especially if the tissues are already inflamed and sensitive from low estradiol.

rial. I am concerned about the trend of women calling doctors' offices for help with "bladder infections" and getting repeated courses of antibiotics that merely create resistant bacteria and set you up for chronic yeast infections without correcting the underlying cause.

Wisdom
Decline in estrogen may not be the whole story, but it is a crucial piece.

Make sure you see your doctor for a vaginal exam, culture and urinalysis before you start on antibiotics. Many women with "chronic yeast" infections don't actually have yeast; the symptoms may come from a variety of causes.

It is important to check your hormone levels if you are have problems with burning, frequency, urgency, or leaking of urine. Low estradiol can be a factor in chronic bladder problems in younger women, as well as before and during menopause.

Glucose intolerance and early diabetes are two other common endocrine causes of urinary problems in women, especially if you are overweight. If you have a family history of diabetes, or an increase in craving for sweets, talk with your doctor about checking for diabetes.

In the early stages, before your *fasting* glucose remains too high, you may have frequent yeast infections, burning during urination, leaking of urine or increased frequency.

Cause
Estradiol blood levels *below* about 60 pg/ml are a significant contributing factor in persistent vaginal and urinary problems

Assess the possible hormone causes and address this problem directly, perhaps first with a vaginal estradiol cream or by using hormone therapy, rather than continuing the vicious cycle of "infection-antibiotics."

Interstitial cystitis (IC) can be excruciatingly painful. The statistics are staggering. Over 75 percent of women with IC cannot have sex due to pain, which obviously takes a toll on relationships. About 50 percent of women with IC are so affected they cannot hold down a full-time job. And about 33 percent have been abandoned by a husband or lover as a result of this disorder.

The characteristic symptoms of IC are, unfortunately, *nonspecific* and may occur in other kinds of bladder disorders: increased urination, sudden strong urges to void (urgency), intense pain becoming worse as the bladder fills up and often decreased by voiding (one woman called it "like passing fire"), pain with intercourse, urinating multiple times at night (*nocturia*).

There are many causes proposed, but no definitive answer. Some theories include over use of antibiotics; a dysfunctional bladder lining (epithelium); manifestation of an autoimmune disorder; toxic substances in the urine; or a chronic persistent infectious agent—all of which damage the bladder lining and lead to the characteristic tiny hemorrhages in the bladder wall.

The obvious connection to women's hormones is ignored. Look at some of the medical data and the startling connections that support loss of estradiol as an overlooked factor in the development of IC:

1. In a 1993 study of 374 IC patients, researchers at Scripps Institute found that the mean age of onset for IC is *42 years*, and *44 percent* of the patients *had hysterectomies prior to onset of IC*. Women in their forties are often beginning the first phase of estradiol decline leading to menopause. Following hysterectomies, even with the ovaries left in place, about 60% of women have an earlier ovarian decline of estradiol due to the effects on blood flow to the ovaries.

2. Surveys of women at any age who suffer from IC have found that flare-ups tend to occur after ovulation, just before menses, and post-partum. All are times estradiol levels fall.

3. Young women who develop IC have several common characteristics: prolonged use of high progestin-low estrogen birth control pills, ovarian suppression with low hormone levels and decreased menses (whether from diet, smoking, drug or alcohol use, excessive exercise, or any other causes).

4. IC also often begins following pregnancy, particularly with prolonged nursing, which keeps prolactin higher and suppresses return to optimal menstrual cycle levels of estradiol.

If you are suffering from persistent bladder pain and other approaches offer no relief, have your physician test blood levels of estradiol and other ovarian hormones.

If your ovarian hormone levels are low, see Chapter 16 for treatment options. To ignore hormone connections is a glaring omission. There are a number of non-hormonal treatments for IC. (See Appendix II for information on the IC Foundation, and other resources).

Cause
Low estradiol and early stages of diabetes—are the most frequent *unrecognized* causes of persistent urinary problems.

Abysmal!
About 1 in every 250 women suffers from some form of IC, yet *fewer than 1 out of 5 have been properly diagnosed.*

Shocking
For women late in life, incontinence carries an additional significance: loss of bladder control is one of the most frequent causes for nursing home admission.

"Leaky Bladders"—Young Women Can Be Affected Too

Continence is the ability to hold urine in the bladder and control urine flow. After toilet training, most of us control urination urges unconsciously as we go about our daily activities.

Accidental loss of urine, or difficulty controlling the start and stop of urine flow, is called **incontinence**. A widespread misconception is that urinary incontinence is inevitable as we get older. Not true.

Nor is it true that it "can't" happen to younger women. Grace, the 23-year-old newly-wed who had vulvodynia, was having urinary "leaks" when she laughed, jogged, and had sex, likely the result of the low estrogen-high progestin birth control pills.

There's Help
Never think incontinence is something you just have to "put up with."

Younger women can also develop incontinence from damage to the pelvic floor muscles and nerves following difficult vaginal deliveries of large babies or pelvic surgery. For perimenopausal and menopausal women, the loss of estradiol causes loss of muscle tone and elasticity of connective tissue that leads to incontinence.

There are several types of incontinence, with different characteristics and causes.

Stress incontinence is one you hear often, and patients are frequently confused about it. "Stress incontinence" does NOT refer to emotional factors causing loss of urine. It means loss of bladder control due to the physical stress of increased pressure in the abdomen from activities such as laughing, coughing, sneezing, orgasm, jogging, or straining to have a bowel movement.

Fact
Estradiol plays a role to help prevent chronic bladder problems in younger women, as well as during and after menopause.

This type of incontinence is not caused by bladder spasms; it results from weakness or loss of tone in the bladder muscles from many causes: damage to the bladder muscles in childbirth; ligaments and muscles weakened by age; or loss of hormone or nutritional components necessary for healthy tissue.

35 to 40 percent of women experience post-partum stress incontinence for as long as 6 to 12 weeks after childbirth. This is due to trauma to the bladder muscles and the sudden drop in hormone levels after delivery. Stress incontinence is not usually associated with urinary frequency and urgency.

Urge (urgency) Incontinence is the sudden urge to urinate and the inability to hold your urine long enough to reach the bathroom. It is usually caused by bladder spasms. It can also be caused by medical conditions such as herniated intervertebral disks, bladder infections, fibroids exerting pressure on the bladder, or loss of normal estradiol effect on urinary and reproductive tissues.

See a physician for a thorough evaluation since bladder cancer also may cause urge incontinence and should be considered before treatment starts. Many cases of urge incontinence do not have a clear-cut physical cause, but still respond to treatment.

Overflow Incontinence is the accidental loss of urine from a chronically full bladder. A common cause is a *cystocoele*, a vaginal hernia or bulge due to weakened vaginal muscles. It occurs after childbirth, hysterectomy or menopause. The bulge from the cystocoele makes a mechanical obstruction and prevents complete emptying of the bladder. A woman then loses small quantities of urine when she stands, sits, or bends.

Loss of adequate estradiol and diabetes damage the muscles and nerves that control the bladder and cause overflow incontinence.

It can also occur from a herniated lumbar disc. This happened to me at 28, before I was correctly diagnosed with a herniated disc. I certainly relate to the embarrassment of incontinence episodes and the frustration of getting help. In my situation, removal of the herniated disc, which took the pressure off the spinal nerves, restored normal nerve function and the incontinence resolved.

Overflow incontinence is treated by identifying and resolving the underlying cause. Pessaries, a device inserted into the vagina as a supportive structure, is sometimes be used to lift the bladder away from the obstructed outlet, or bladder surgery can repair a cystocoele.

Distinguish which type of incontinence you have because effective treatments are different. For example, stress incontinence is often relieved by bladder surgery, but urge incontinence is not.

Loss of urine at night can result from a combination of continence dysfunctions. Some are responsive to hormone therapy with estradiol creams, rings or vaginal tablets that restore the estrogen effects on bladder lining, smooth muscle of the bladder and urethral, and the connective tissues supporting the bladder. Explore these factors with your doctor.

Warning
Urge incontinence is also aggravated by increased urine formation from excessive fluid intake, alcohol, diuretics ("water pills"), caffeine, and/or tobacco.

Good News
An estradiol-releasing vaginal ring (Estring) provides both mechanical and hormonal support that can help incontinence.

In Summary

PMS, endometriosis, vulvodynia, bladder pain.

All have the potential to significantly disrupt your life.

All have important, overlooked hormone triggers that need to be checked.

All are treatable, and generally respond well to the kinds of approaches I mentioned here, and in Chapters 16 and 18.

There is also good news about incontinence. Regardless of your age, it is also a treatable problem, with a variety of medications or surgery, as well as alternative approaches that include everything from biofeedback to magnets.

With current knowledge about causes, and variety of diagnostic and treatment options, not always drugs and surgery,) more than 50 percent of incontinence patients are cured, another 35 percent markedly improve, and the remaining 15 percent are more comfortable.

See a knowledgeable, caring and competent physician, or contact one of the resources in Appendix II to locate an appropriate professional near you.

Don't sit home and suffer in silence.

Chapter 12
Ovarian Hormones and the Brain

You hit age thirty, your health is good, you exercise three or four times a week, and wham! Out of the blue, you are anxious; have an upset stomach and clammy skin. Or you suddenly have palpitations and pounding sensations as if your heart was going to literally jump out of your chest.

"What's going on? Am I having a panic attack? A heart attack, I'm too young for that!"

The family doctor examines you and diagnoses Panic Disorder (PD). Or, he says you have Generalized Anxiety Disorder (GAD), and need to relax and reduce stress.

You leave the doctor's office, wondering just how to "relax and reduce stress." You go about your daily routine and then, a few weeks later, just as your period begins, it happens again. *What is this?*

PPD. PMDD. MDD. MDI. BPD. OCD. GAD. PD. ADD. ADHD. There is a veritable alphabet soup of psychiatric disorders common in women of reproductive age, especially in their thirties and forties.

Over the last three decades, there have been enormous advances in scientific findings about the biological basis of these disorders, as well as the role of serotonin, norepinephrine, dopamine and the brain's other chemical messengers and receptor actions.

But science has not paid enough attention to the essence of women's biology…ovarian hormones, and how they trigger mood and anxiety problems. The *application* of current brain science has not yet filtered down to the general medical settings where women receive treatment. Most of these clinical syndromes are

Ancient history

Ancient Greeks thought women's moods resulted from a "wandering uterus" (the Greek word was *hyster…*), the origin of the word "hysteria."

still viewed as "only" psychiatric disorders, and treatment is almost inevitably a prescription of antidepressants.

From ancient Greece onward, we find a long history of inadequate study and incorrect conclusions about women's emotional life and causes of "abnormal" emotions.

First of all, the definition of *"abnormal"* was based on what was considered *"normal" for males*, not considering that "normal" for women's emotional expression may be quite different. *Hysteria* has had a negative connotation as in *emotional, excitable, anxious women*, overwrought about their health.

And physicians still have not recognized the hormone connection in mood syndromes in women, even after a few thousand years of observation.

During the Middle Ages women healers, who deal with psychological problems, relieved illness and suffering with herbs, were considered to be witches, and burned at the stake.

Some five hundred years later Freud erroneously concluded that women's psychological disturbances were due to "penis envy."

Sad…

The obvious *hormone link* has been overlooked or dismissed.

American psychiatry in the 1940s and 1950s labeled all psychoses "schizophrenia," failing to recognize that mania or depression *or endocrine disorders* could also produce the same abnormal thought patterns, hallucinations or delusions.

In the 1980s and 1990s, American psychiatry focused on the "serotonin connection" and developed "serotonin boosting" medicines that are now prescribed like candy for women of all ages, in numbers far greater than for men.

Fact

Hormones have many actions and sites in the nerve cells to modify the ways nerves function.

British psychiatrists and gynecologists presented different explanations for such mood problems in women *decades* before these concepts made it across the ocean to the United States.

In Britain, Manic-depressive illness (MDI) and major depressive disorder (MDD) were recognized as distinct from schizophrenia even though all of these mood disorders, in their severe forms, can cause delusions and hallucinations.

Several leading gynecologists and menopause researchers in Great Britain, such as Drs. Campbell, Whitehead and Studd, described Post-partum Depression (PPD), PMS, PMDD, and perimenopausal depression caused by the *abrupt drop or decline in estradiol*. They did not simply focus on serotonin imbalance as a primary cause.

Dr. Studd's group successfully treated women with estradiol implants or patches for years, yet few psychiatrists or gynecologists in the U.S. use that option. Women in the U.S. are given more expensive serotonin drugs that also have more side effects.

Ovarian Hormones and the Brain

Estradiol, progesterone, and testosterone receptor sites exist throughout key areas of our brain, spinal cord and peripheral nerves. In the brain, these hormone receptors are concentrated in the cortex and the limbic system areas. There are multiple connections between the limbic system and all the other parts of the brain and spinal cord.

The rise and fall of estradiol, progesterone, and testosterone increases or decreases chemical messengers such as serotonin, norepinephrine, endorphins, and others that give directions to the limbic system areas regulating changes in mood, sleep, memory, pain, and appetite.

Hormone levels affect the number of neurotransmitters produced as well as the sensitivity of neurotransmitter receptors. The changing hormone levels at puberty, during our menstrual cycle, in pregnancy, after delivery, and at menopause, all can affect many body systems.

First, let's clarify some terms: **Mood symptom** usually refers to a brief period of mood change not severe enough or long-lasting enough to qualify for a formal diagnosis of mood disorder.

Mood disorder generally refers to a group of physical and emotional changes severe enough and sustained enough to indicate an illness, based on criteria agreed upon by researchers, that needs evaluation and treatment.

For example, about 90% of women in many different cultures experience mood changes or symptoms with their menstrual periods, post-partum and during perimenopause. About 5 to 10%, on average, experience symptoms severe enough to be considered a *disorder*, requiring more comprehensive treatment.

Effect

The brain clearly responds to withdrawal, or absence, of our ovarian hormones with a variety of physical and "psychological" effects.

Dangers

Low estradiol effects to reduce serotonin activity are made worse if women smoke, or don't eat well.

Effect

Low brain levels of 5-hydroxy-indoleacetic acid (5-HIAA), a serotonin breakdown product, are found in women and men who attempt or commit suicide.

The same is true with anxiety, a widely-used term, which has many meanings. Some people use it to mean a mood: "I'm feeling anxious." Others use it to describe a characteristic or trait: "She's always anxious and uptight." It can mean a brief symptom: "I had an anxiety attack over my bounced check." It can also mean a sustained pattern of physical and emotional changes called Generalized Anxiety Disorder, or Panic Disorder.

Good! Estradiol has multiple effects on the brain that together act as a natural antidepressant and nerve growth promoter.

In these chapters, I am generally referring to fairly short-lived, episodic anxiety symptoms that occur in relation to changes in physiological variables such as levels of glucose, thyroid hormones, estradiol, testosterone, and progesterone.

Estrogen Effects

There has been an explosion of research interest and exciting new findings about how hormones affect the brain. Estradiol, produced by the ovary, has wide-ranging effects on brain function through many different pathways and mechanisms that I summarized in the chart that follows.

One effect of estradiol is its role in serotonin production, which influences such diverse problems as mood changes, insomnia, anxiety, appetite, pain, and headaches.

Serotonin decline— Many causes Aging, stress, cigarette smoking, alcohol excess, cocaine use, pesticides, dietary deficits, loss of E2, rise in progesterone, low thyroid, etc.

In women of any age, declining estradiol is a cause of *reduced* serotonin production, *reduced* serotonin receptor density, and changes in serotonin activity at receptor sites.

A rise in progesterone also decreases serotonin. Loss of usual serotonin activity in the brain helps explain why depressed, irritable, anxious moods occur in many women before their periods or during perimenopause.

The hormone connection in younger women's problems—PMS, postpartum depression, insomnia, headaches, and anxiety symptoms—make even more sense when you consider all the dietary, environmental, and lifestyle factors I described earlier that can cause premature decrease in estradiol and also decrease serotonin.

Numerous worldwide studies over the past two decades show reduced serotonin levels as a primary cause of depressed mood, increased irritability, increased anxiety, increased pain sensitivity, eating disorders, obsessive-compulsive disorders and disruption of normal sleep cycles.

In fact, decreases in other measures of serotonin activity in perimenopausal women correlate with a peak of suicide in this age range. This *peak of suicide is not seen in men.*

Many factors affect serotonin balance, but the loss or decline in estradiol appears to be a critical gender difference that contributes to greater rates of depression, anxiety syndromes and suicide in women.

Loss of estradiol decreases serotonin and also affects endorphins, our body's natural painkillers, and mood-elevators. Endorphin production is highest when estradiol peaks at mid-cycle, or during the last stage of pregnancy. Endorphins fall sharply when the placenta is delivered after the birth of a baby, causing both estradiol and progesterone levels to plummet.

Endorphin withdrawal produces effects similar to heroin or morphine withdrawal: irritability, tearfulness, anxiety, stomach upset, diarrhea, and sweating.

Smile
Estradiol plays a major mood-lifting role, maintains our sense of well being and helps boost our energy level.

Dr. Vliet's Guide: Estradiol and Your Brain

- Increases production and/or prolongs action of serotonin
- Enhances CNS availability of norepinephrine and dopamine
- Inhibits the monoamine oxidase (MAO) enzymes, which prolongs the mood-lifting actions of serotonin, dopamine, and norepinephrine
- Increases production of the enzyme needed to make acetylcholine, a crucial memory-enhancing neurotransmitter
- Increases blood flow to the brain
- Regulates contractility of blood vessels (vasomotor tone)
- Regulates sleep centers
- Regulates body temperature
- Raises pain threshold, which improves pain tolerance
- Increases dendrite connections between nerve cells in memory centers, which improves memory function
- Enhances attention and concentration mechanisms, increases sensory perception for fine touch, olfactory, and visual stimuli
- Involved in Growth Hormone release at night
- Prolongs neuron responses to excitatory amino acids in the cerebral cortex, cerebellum, hippocampus, hypothalamus, midbrain, and pons may alter seizure threshold (direction of change is dependent upon type of seizure)
- Acts as antioxidant, vasodilator, and nerve growth promoter

© Elizabeth Lee Vliet, M.D., 1995 revised 2001, 2007

Ahhh!
EEG brain wave studies show that testosterone has a general activating or stimulating effect on brain pathways much like the antidepressant imipramine or the stimulant amphetamine.

The drop in endorphins that occur with declining levels of estradiol during the menstrual cycle, perimenopause, postpartum, and at menopause, plays a contributing, if not a causative, role in anxiety, insomnia, depressed mood, headaches and pain symptoms that many women describe.

Testosterone Effects

Testosterone is also a "woman's hormone," made by the ovary before menopause, and to a much lesser extent, the adrenal gland (see Chapter 2). Testosterone receptors are found in several areas of the brain. This hormone is crucial for sex drive because it activates the brain's "sexual circuits" in both women and men. These effects are one way testosterone improves a woman's sense of well-being and energy level.

Lose your optimal testosterone, and you lose more than your sex drive—you feel sluggish, tired…"blah."

Tough stuff
Progesterone is one of the most potent naturally occurring "androgen-blockers," of all the ones yet identified.

Too much testosterone, however, can cause nervousness, agitation, anxiety attacks, insomnia and restlessness in the same way amphetamines do, even before you see it cause excess facial hair or acne.

A certain level of estradiol must be present in our brain for testosterone to function properly because the brain testosterone receptor appears to be created by the presence of estradiol. Without enough estradiol to "prime the pump," testosterone, also produced by the ovary, cannot attach or function properly in brain centers to stimulate sexual arousal.

Sex?
It isn't surprising that sex drive plummets the premenstrual week when progesterone is naturally high, or when you take high-progestin birth control pills or large doses of progesterone for PMS.

In women who have had breast cancer, and are not taking estradiol, studies show that providing supplemental testosterone may only partially improve their sexual desire and ability to have an orgasm.

No matter what your age, if testosterone is lower than normal, its impact is enormous. It is rewarding to hear patients describe how they feel with natural testosterone supplementation: "*Gosh, I feel like I have my old self again. I have my energy back. I'm interested in sex again.*" (See Chapter 16 for more information on natural testosterone).

Progesterone Effects

Progesterone has interesting effects on the brain, acting as an estrogen "blocker" to reduce estradiol binding at receptors. This action is similar to Tamoxifen, the anti-estrogen breast cancer drug headlined in the news.

Progesterone decreases testosterone effects by several other mechanisms, including a decrease of estradiol and testosterone receptor activity in the brain, called "down-regulation."

Progesterone competes with testosterone passing from the blood into the brain, competes for binding at testosterone receptors, and also decreases the conversion of testosterone into its most active form.

Women taking menopausal hormone therapy also describe loss of libido during the progestin or progesterone phase of their therapy. Low estradiol further intensifies the libido-blocking and depressant effects of progesterone.

Both estradiol and testosterone have mood-elevating effects, so it's easy to see why you feel grumpy, irritable, or tearful whenever progesterone decreases the binding of estradiol and testosterone at brain receptors.

Progesterone can cause mood changes in other ways. There are several important progesterone breakdown compounds that attach to the brain's GABA receptors just like the anti-anxiety medicines (Xanax, Valium, Ativan, Klonopin, and other benzodiazepines).

Our brain makes it's own natural anxiety-relieving chemical , called endozapine which normally attaches to the GABA receptors to help alleviate anxiety.

If you don't make enough endozapine, prescription medicines like Valium or Xanax can help replace it, and thereby relieve anxiety symptoms. Taking benzodiazepine medicine to replace endozapine is similar in concept to replacing lost thyroid hormone with thyroid medicine.

Several progesterone metabolites act like endozapine at GABA receptors to produce a calming, sleepy sensation. But for some women, this GABA effect causes depressed mood, just as we see with the depressant effects of benzodiazepines, leading to low energy, blunted sex drive, and decreased memory and concentration.

Experiments show that it isn't just women who experience these sedative and depressant effects of progesterone, *men given progesterone experience them too.*

Moody
Progesterone effects are more inhibitory than excitatory; so its combined effects on the brain are depressant.

Fact
Studies show women with one post-partum depressive episode are at high risk for a recurrence with the next pregnancy.

Pregnancy High
Estradiol levels in the last trimester are in the 20,000 pg/ml range.

Post-partum Anxiety, Depression, Memory and Sleep Problems

The "crash"

A few days after delivery, estradiol plummets to about 100 pg/ml.

Physicians since the time of Hippocrates have described post-partum depression as being triggered by the abrupt fall in hormones that occurs with delivery of the placenta after the baby is born.

Our "modern" medical model has been slow to accept endocrine causes, focusing instead on serotonin and other neurotransmitter imbalances as primary causes.

The clinical syndrome of post-partum depression has symptoms like other types of depression, so doctors often overlook hormone changes as triggers of depression that may need hormone treatment. This problem is aggravated by researchers who receive funding from the manufacturers of antidepressants, and *only* study these drugs, *not hormones*.

Not here?

Hormone treatment of post-partum depression has been widely studied and used in England for many years

Women experience drops in estradiol with every menstrual cycle, but the drop when the placenta is delivered is over 2,000 times greater. And that's only one of many hormone changes after delivery. Talk about falling off a hormone cliff!

Women who experience post-partum depression are quick to connect the rapidly falling hormones to their profound depressed-anxious mood and fragmented sleep. The problem that faces women in the U.S. is finding a doctor who considers these hormone connections important, and who will use hormonal treatment approaches.

Treating the patient with antidepressants is more convenient, and easier, but doesn't really address the underlying cause. Sometimes, as you see in the women's stories I share, the consequences of over-looking the hormone issues can be serious.

Overload

She had a lot of *metabolic-hormonal issues* that were not getting addressed.

Following the birth of her daughter, *Leslie* developed severe anxiety, insomnia, scattered thinking, and trouble focusing on her work. She was told she had a "generalized anxiety disorder" and was treated with Klonopin.

No one did an endocrine work-up to test for hormonal changes that could also cause such symptoms. She struggled through each day, feeling sleepy and tired on the Klonopin, but at least it kept her anxiety symptoms under control so she could return to work.

A few years later the marriage crumbled. Her husband filed for divorce, seeking custody of their daughter, claiming that Leslie was on the "addictive" medicine Klonopin and unable to care for the child. She wanted to get off the Klonopin to thwart her husband's tactic of using a psychiatric disorder as grounds for custody.

She saw a naturopath who unfortunately prescribed progesterone cream and DHEA supplements that further aggravated her underlying low estradiol and excess free testosterone, making her anxiety, fatigue and headaches much worse.

Bad Formula
Excess DHEA + stress + progesterone + being too thin + thyroid excess + low E2 = hormone disaster!

Taking daily progesterone also prevented return of her normal ovarian estradiol production and further contributed to depressed mood and lack of energy. The naturopath also recommended multiple soy isoflavone supplements that also interfered with estradiol and progesterone production. She was in a horrible downward spiral.

She came for a comprehensive hormone evaluation. When I saw her, the anxiety symptoms were clearly cyclic, and worse when her estradiol dropped abruptly with ovulation.

The blood tests confirmed that her estradiol was *less than one-third of a normal healthy level for a woman her age.*

Cause
Her anxiety symptoms began in the post-partum phase when her estradiol plummeted after delivery.

My evaluation found two other overlooked hormonal imbalances that can cause marked anxiety and insomnia: *excess thyroid activity* (hyperthyroid), and *excess free, active testosterone* relative to her low estradiol.

When there is too much thyroid or testosterone, it over-stimulates brain pathways that mimic the physical and emotional experiences we call "anxiety."

She also had a very high level of NTx that indicates excess bone breakdown; additional evidence that estradiol was far too low and thyroid too active. Leslie also had a B12 and iron deficiency that further added to the anxiety, insomnia and fatigue.

Cause/ Effect
Several primary medical conditions triggered her secondary psychological (anxiety) symptoms.

Her prematurely low estradiol was easily remedied with an estradiol patch, along with 12 days of natural progesterone every other month and vitamin B and iron supplements.

It is unfortunate that Leslie was misdiagnosed as having a *primary* anxiety disorder when the proper medical/endocrine evaluation for such syndromes was not done.

Good News
With the foundation of proper hormone management women need lower doses of anti-depressants, often only half the usual dose or even less.

Without this complete evaluation, important hormonal problems were not getting proper treatment. Her anxiety and insomnia symptoms were relieved by hormone therapy. She was finally able to taper off Klonopin and eliminate the medicine that caused daytime tiredness and difficulty concentrating.

Leslie won full custody of her daughter when she showed medical documentation of her abnormal hormone levels, the revised diagnosis based on objective laboratory studies, and her new hormone treatment that relieved her symptoms.

Getting proper treatment with estradiol, instead of the "band-aid" approach to symptoms with Klonopin, also stopped her excess bone breakdown, helping to reduce later risk of osteoporosis. See why it is crucial to check hormone levels?

Where Are We Now?

I have worked with post-partum hormone connections for many years and have successfully used a variety of hormone approaches for women suffering significant post-partum depression, anxiety, and sleep disruption.

As with Leslie, many women do not need antidepressants when hormone balance is restored. Some do still need antidepressants or anxiety-relieving medicines, so we combine these with hormone approaches tailored to each woman.

Patients often say that my clinical observations and their obvious improvements are discounted by other doctors, citing no "proof" that the hormones play a role in mood symptoms or recovery. Recent objective studies have, however, provide "hard data" on this hormone connection that may convince skeptical physicians. The next section describes some of the key studies on the hormone-mood connection.

Proof
"The proof lies in how well I feel and that I have tapered off other medicines that cause side effects."

Hormone Crashes and Withdrawal: More Profound Than You Realize

When there is a tremendous drop in estradiol, from pre-delivery to post-partum levels, it is like your brain falling off a cliff to the rocks below. Such a precipitous fall in estradiol creates an *"estradiol withdrawal syndrome"* that appears to be a critical factor in setting off brain changes that lead to post-partum psychosis and/or major depression. Keeping estradiol steady after delivery helps blunt the dramatic decrease in mood-lifting serotonin and endorphins and the surges of anxiety-provoking norepinephrine.

Drs. Block and Schmidt did an interesting study to support, or "prove," that the "estrogen withdrawal state" can trigger mood or psychotic changes. They mimicked the high hormone levels of pregnancy in a group of women, and then put them into a "hormone withdrawal" creating the same response in the brain and body as with the delivery of a baby.

Gently now
An estradiol patch is like having a parachute that lets you glide gently and safely to the ground to prevent this drastic fall in estradiol.

They found over 60% of the women with a history of post-partum depression developed significant increases in depressive symptoms when hormones were withdrawn, but none of the control group did.

Here, the "controls" were women who did not have past history of post-partum depression. Their conclusion states quite clearly: *"The data provide direct evidence in support of the involvement of the reproductive hormones estrogen and progesterone in the development of postpartum depression in a subgroup of women."* Exactly what I see in my patients.

In 1996 Dr. John Studd led a pivotal double-blind, placebo-controlled study in England investigating the effectiveness of transdermal estradiol for women with severe postpartum depression. Sixty one women with a major depression that began within 3 months of childbirth were randomly assigned either placebo treatment or an active treatment with transdermal 17-beta estradiol using 200 micrograms daily for 3 months followed by 3 months of estradiol with added cyclical progestin at a dose of 10mg daily for 12 days each month.

The women were assessed monthly by self-ratings of depressive symptoms and by a clinical psychiatric interview. Based on the objective rating scale scores, the women in both groups were severely depressed at the pre-treatment evaluations.

During the first month of therapy the women receiving estradiol improved faster, and to a significantly greater extent, than those receiving placebo patches. The control group improved over time but, on average, their improvement was much slower: their scores did not fall below the major depression threshold level for at least 4 months.

Most of the women with the estradiol patches did not need anti-depressant medication. Dr. Studd and his team concluded that transdermal estradiol is an effective treatment for postpartum

That's Results!
During the first week on the 17-beta estradiol treatment, psychiatric symptoms decreased greatly, with mean scores dropping from 78.3 to 18.8, a remarkable change!

More proof
Dr. Ahokas' group concluded that boosting the low estradiol levels led to complete reversal of the psychiatric symptoms in all patients.

depression, recommending further research studies on dosage and duration of treatment.

Finnish researchers, led by Dr. Antti Ahokas, used an open trial of 17 beta-estradiol to treat women who met diagnostic criteria for post-partum psychosis, the most severe form of post-partum psychiatric disorders.

Serum estradiol levels were measured at baseline and weekly for six weeks. The baseline estradiol levels for these patients were lower than the threshold we use to indicate ovarian failure. All of the patients exhibited high scores on the psychiatric symptom scale.

The researchers used doses of estradiol designed to restore healthy menstrual cycle levels. By the end of the second week serum estradiol concentrations rose to approximately the values normally found during the follicular phase of the menstrual cycle. At these higher levels of estradiol, the patients became virtually free of psychiatric symptoms. The one woman who then discontinued her estradiol suffered a recurrence of psychotic symptoms.

In 2001 Dr. Ahokas' group evaluated the effect of sublingual 17-beta estradiol for the treatment of women with post-partum depression. They again found that the severe depressive symptoms were quickly alleviated by estradiol therapy in women with post-partum depression who have low estradiol levels at the outset. Dr. Ahokas said, **"In spite of multiple contacts with health providers, women with postpartum depression often remain unrecognized and untreated."**

In the United States, internists, family medicine doctors, and Ob/Gyns are the highest prescribers of anti-depressants in the country—and *none of these physicians routinely do hormone tests*, nor do most psychiatrists. This helps you understand why it is so difficult for U.S. women to get hormonal treatments for post-partum depression.

Dr. Ahokas' study found that women's depressive symptoms diminished significantly within the first week of the 8-week treatment period, which is a far more rapid response than with the standard antidepressant therapies. By the end of the second week, the researchers found that the scores on standard depression ratings were compatible with complete recovery in

19 of the 23 patients. These are remarkable statistics, *better than anti-depressants recovery rates.*

Correcting the hormonal balance with bio-identical forms of 17-beta estradiol, creates a rapid, positive effect on mood and sleep for these mothers, many of whom did not respond to traditional antidepressant treatments. If a new mother's mood and sleep patterns are improved quickly, it obviously helps mom, dad, and baby!

Another study from the University of Zimbabwe was published in 1999 and pharmacists reported, *"Estradiol patches are now being used in the prevention and treatment of post-partum depression."* If estradiol patches can be used to treat post-partum depression in Africa, you'd think we could do a better job in the United States!

The Finnish researchers described *one drawback to sublingual estradiol:* this form of delivery causes extremely *rapid absorption,* and the *effects only last a short time* because of rapid metabolism. The patch is a significant improvement over the roller coaster effect of sublingual estradiol.

A Massachusetts General Hospital Clinical Psychopharmacology Unit study, published in 1995, described high-dose oral estrogen treatment of seven women with histories of postpartum psychosis and four with histories of postpartum major depression.

None had histories of depression or psychosis during non-post-partum times, and all were free of mood symptoms throughout their current pregnancy. These women were at high risk for a recurrent episode of depression or psychosis post partum due to their past history. Estrogen treatment was begun immediately after delivery.

With the estrogen, only one woman developed a relapse of her postpartum mood disorder. All others remained well and required no antidepressants or other psychotropic medications during the one-year follow-up.

With all of the scientific evidence now available, it is *not sufficient* to tell a woman who is significantly depressed or anxious following her delivery that she's "just stressed" as a new mother, or she feels conflicts about being a mother, or that she just needs a serotonin booster medicine.

My proof
The results matched the positive results I see in my own practice when using estradiol patches in this manner.

Too rapid
Sublingual estradiol must be given several times a day to maintain stable blood levels

More natural
A transdermal patch gives more gradual delivery, keeping estradiol steadier over a few days.

Physicians in all specialties treating women with post-partum depression must do complete laboratory tests of the ovarian, thyroid, adrenal and pituitary hormones, and then incorporate treatment approaches that correct the imbalances.

Your Rhythms
Noticed where in the menstrual cycle these palpitations or panicky episodes occur?

Other Brain Effects: Hormone Triggers of Anxiety, Racing Heart, Flutters, and Palpitations

Many women are puzzled about hormone shifts that cause brain symptoms such as anxiety, or heart symptoms such as palpitations, flutters, and rapid heart beat.

There is a simple straightforward connection: hormone levels rising or falling too fast trigger a burst of norepinephrine that sets off the central alarm center in the brain's limbic system.

Falling estradiol, for example, is like someone pulling the cord on a hotel fire alarm; the signal is relayed to the central alarm center that sends the warning to all the rooms of the hotel. The brain's alarm center, called the locus ceruleus, does the same thing. The flood of norepinephrine makes you feel "anxious," and sends a signal to the heart to pump faster and get the body ready for an emergency. This causes the heart pounding, skipping or fluttering sensation.

Signals are sent to other parts of the body to either shut down (bowel) or speed up (metabolism) and get you ready to "fight or flee." If you are sleeping, this surge of norepinephrine bolts you awake; it is also the trigger for the "hot flash" and sweats that can hit at the same time as the anxiousness and racing heartbeat.

Warning
Fluctuating hormone levels cause these same heart-related symptoms.

This cascade of events spreads over the body from the simple hormone-triggered release of brain chemicals.

If your physical symptoms (heart flutters, heart racing or pounding, feeling queasy or nauseous, sweating, feeling anxious for no apparent reason) come at times of the menstrual cycle when estradiol is low or falling (around ovulation, a day or so before your period starts, or the first two or three days of bleeding), they are likely the hormone-triggered brain-body reactions.

If you are someone who is very sensitive to the rate of hormonal changes, this same "alarm" response can occur with a rapidly rising level of estradiol or progesterone, as in pregnancy, or when starting hormone therapy or birth control pills.

Hot flashes used to be considered psychological, a figment of your imagination. We now know this is a physiological reaction when low or falling estradiol triggers reactions in the brain and blood vessels that fire off norepinephrine (NE) in the limbic system, disrupting normal function of the heat-regulating center in the hypothalamus, signaling the arteries to dissipate excess heat.

Dilation of blood vessels is accompanied by sweating. The body temperature begins to drop, and a chilly sensation sweeps over you. If it happens at night you wake up, often soaked in sweat, each time it happens. If estradiol falls abruptly, this same series of events occurs in younger women, just as happens with menopause.

Women "get" it
While it is true that the chemical changes originate "in your head," it is not your imagination. It is very real.

Serotonin helps maintain sleep and decrease anxiety, so a drop in this chemical messenger also adds to night-time awakenings, and aggravates adrenaline-induced feelings of irritability, tension, palpitations, and chest discomfort. Low estradiol causes decreased serotonin, compounding the problem.

It is wise to have palpitations and chest pain evaluated to rule out underlying cardiac disease, especially if you have several risk factors, but if the cardiologist tells you "nothing is wrong," that simply means you don't have cardiovascular disease. It doesn't mean you are imagining these sensations.

Don't jump to the conclusion that if it isn't cardiovascular disease, it must be "just stress," as many doctors tell women.

As you get older and estradiol production declines, a fall in this key hormone before menses triggers an even more pronounced physical response. It's a new, more intense feeling that makes you sit up and take notice.

Women say they know "its a physical, chemical kind of thing," but are told "it's just stress, it's all in your head," as if they are imagining it. *These sensations are physical reactions of hormone changes hitting brain centers.*

Understanding Hormonally-triggered Migraines

Migraine connection
60–70% of women with migraine have one triggered by falling estradiol at onset of menses.

Women are all too often told that hormones don't cause headaches! For women susceptible to migraine or other vascular headaches, the *monthly fall in estradiol* can set off spasms in the blood vessels and changes in serotonin that trigger the headache at predictable times in the cycle.

Estradiol falls sharply around ovulation and again rather dramatically about day 22 to 24 of your cycle and reaches its lowest point on days 1 to 3 of bleeding. The estradiol level remains low for the first 4–5 days of bleeding, a reason for the increase in migraines during the early days of menstrual flow.

Female migraine sufferers more likely to be affected by hormone triggers the week they stop birth control pills to have a period, or post-partum, when estradiol, serotonin, and endorphin levels drop sharply.

Proven
The migraine attack was triggered by the premenstrual drop in estradiol, not progesterone.

The high frequency of migraines occurring at the onset of menses has been observed for several thousand years. It wasn't known which hormone was the primary cause until the mid-1970s when Dr. B.W. Somerville did a series of studies that clearly demonstrated that estrogen and progesterone have very different effects on migraines.

For menopausal women on hormone therapy, headaches can be set off by stopping estrogen for days 25–30, or by starting the progestin phase of HRT.

It's true that there is a genetic predisposition for migraines. Most doctors, and most migraine sufferers, also recognize the usual classic migraine triggers such as red wines, aged cheeses, foods with MSG and nitrites or sulfites, histamine, alcohol, caffeine, chocolate, barometric pressure weather changes, stress, "rebound" from pain medication, and sometimes dairy products.

But the fall in estradiol as a migraine trigger continues to be overlooked in almost 99 percent of women with migraines, even though this hormone trigger can be alleviated in fairly simple ways. (See Chapter 16.)

Migraine headaches often include a number of phenomena, such as aura, visual changes, sensitivity to light and sound, nausea or vomiting, numbness or tingling of face and arms, along with the throbbing head pain.

Doctors used to think all these phenomena were due to circulation changes: blood vessels becoming first constricted (vasoconstriction) and then dilated (vasodilatation).

Research shows migraine is a state of central nervous system "hyperexcitability," making you more susceptible to episodes of spontaneous firing (depolarization) of neurons, followed by dampening down of neuron function, which then causes changes in blood flow. Hormones affect all these pathways.

Whole textbooks are devoted to the subject of migraine head-ache, so *my focus is on the important hormone connections* that can set off the migraine cascade.

The following table summarizes some of the ways falling estra-diol can set off migraines, particularly if added to dietary, stress, weather, and medication triggers.

Dr. Vliet's Guide to Mechanisms of Estrogen Effects on Headaches

- Falling estrogen decreases the amount of available serotonin (5-HT), as well as the number of certain 5-HT receptors, important in decreasing migraine pain. The drop in serotonin levels causes cranial blood vessels to spasm painfully. Adding estrogen to serotonin-boosting medications has a synergistic effect to boost serotonin.
- Falling estrogen causes a decrease in the pain-relieving beta-endorphins in the brain, spinal cord, and body tissues.
- Estrogen withdrawal (either naturally in the cycle or by stopping hormone-containing medication) causes a rebound in dopamine (DA) that can intensify pain.
- Estrogen decline causes vasoconstriction by contracting the muscles in the artery walls, aggravating pain of vascular headaches.
- Falling estrogen causes a burst of norepinephrine (NE) release in the brain's locus ceruleus, which increases vasoconstriction and diminishes blood flow to the area of the brain involved in vision, thus producing the aura.
- Increased NE release further intensifies pain.
- At the same time, a decrease in estradiol lowers the pain threshold, making nerve endings more sensitive to painful stimuli.

© Elizabeth Lee Vliet, 1995, revised 2002–2007

The Role of Progesterone and Progestins

Studies show that synthetic progestins in birth control pills or hormone therapy regimens can increase the frequency and severity of migraine, vascular and muscle-tension headaches for some women.

In my clinical experience, progestin-only types of contraceptives like Norplant and Depo-Provera are among the worst offenders.

Causes
Progesterone,
even though
it is a natural
hormone, has
mixed effects
in headache
syndromes.

Warning!
Progesterone
withdrawal
can cause
throbbing
headaches
that can be
mistaken for
migraines.

**Not
good...**
Overall, I have
found that
progesterone
in high doses
does not
help prevent
migraines.

These products without any estrogen have a high rate of causing daily tension headaches as well as vascular headaches like migraines, even in women who did not have headaches prior to using these contraceptives.

Combination birth control pills with both estrogen and progestin aggravate or cause headaches *if the pills are higher in progestin and lower in estrogen.*

If I prescribe an oral contraceptive in a woman with migraines, I use a pill such as Ovcon 35, Ortho-Cyclen, or Yasmin that have better estrogen but have a lower dose of progestin that is still enough to decrease heavy bleeding and provide contraception. This approach often decreases menstrual migraine frequency quite significantly.

Progesterone may be both positive and negative, so its role is more difficult to define. A normal effect of progesterone is to retain fluid and constrict blood vessels. In headache-prone women, these effects can combine to trigger a migraine when progesterone is rising. This is especially true if estradiol is lower than optimal.

In other women, progesterone's calming effects relax muscles in the head and neck that tense with stress, so some women may have fewer headaches in the progesterone phase of the cycle.

Progesterone also acts as an anesthetic when levels are high (as in the last trimester of pregnancy). Like the benzodiazepines, high doses of progesterone have anticonvulsant and sedative effects at brain centers that can decrease headaches for some women.

There are several possible explanations why progesterone may make headaches worse in some women. Progesterone stimulates the production of prostaglandins that cause spasm of the smooth muscle lining the artery walls, another migraine trigger. *If stopped abruptly, progesterone produces withdrawal symptoms* similar to those of benzodiazepines, barbiturates, and alcohol.

You need to decrease progesterone gradually if you are taking it for PMS or for hormone therapy at menopause, especially if taking more than 200 mg a day (based on oral dose).

I use progesterone in migraine sufferers as I do other therapies: I pay attention to what each woman says about her headache pattern in relation to hormone cycles. I integrate observations with hormone pharmacology and we work together to identify the best hormone and other medication options.

Since progesterone effects can differ so much from one woman to the next, it's a good idea to track your personal cycle pattern to see when headaches occur and whether hormone changes appear to aggravate your headaches. Then you can work with your physician to find the most appropriate hormone options for you.

In women who still have headaches when taking natural progesterone, I use the lowest dose that will protect the uterine lining (see Chapter 16), and divide the total daily amount into smaller portions given several times a day.

I also find that for some women the non-oral forms of progesterone, such as Prochieve vaginal cream, or injectable progesterone in oil, also reduce headache frequency better than oral progesterone.

Cause
Progesterone *decreases estradiol binding* at serotonin receptors, *creating a "low-estradiol" headache trigger.*

Pregnancy Effects on Migraine

The dramatic hormone shifts and high levels in pregnancy can affect migraine headaches in several ways. Some women develop migraines for the first time during pregnancy. Women who have migraines with aura often find their migraines intensify with pregnancy. Still other women experience headaches different in quality and intensity from those prior to pregnancy.

Women whose migraines get worse typically report that this occurs during the first trimester when both estrogen and progesterone are rising rapidly and the placenta produces hormones independently of the ovaries.

Timing
The pattern is variable and depends, to some extent, upon the phase of pregnancy.

Women who experience relief show improvement most often after the first trimester, when progesterone levels have dropped and estradiol levels are higher and more stable.

Since migraines tend to be worse with fluctuating estradiol levels, you can see how migraines may improve during pregnancy with the absence of a cyclic hormonal "up-and-down" pattern and the increased levels of estradiol and endorphins.

These same effects explain women's reports of enhanced mood and feelings of well-being in pregnancy, which appear to be related to the mood-elevating effects of the high estradiol levels augmenting serotonin and endorphins.

Oral Contraceptives, Migraine, and Stroke

Until recently, it was thought that women with migraine headaches who used birth control pills had a slight increase in risk of stroke. However, early studies from around the world were done in women who took the older, high dose oral contraceptives, rather than today's lower dose pills.

Interesting
70% of women who have migraines without aura report relief of migraines when they are pregnant.

The international Collaborative Group for the Study of Stroke in Young Women re-analyzed these earlier data and *did not confirm the initial reports* that migraine headaches might increase the risk of stroke in young women using oral contraceptives. *This risk increased only in smokers taking birth control pills.*

Physicians have also been taught that oral contraceptives aggravate migraines, but this is an *incorrect generalization*. Current studies, and my clinical experience, have shown many women actually achieve relief of menstrual migraines IF they have the right hormone ratio in an oral contraceptive and if they do not stop the pill to have a period each month, which allows continuous, stable hormone levels.

Old idea
Some physicians still think women with migraines should not use oral contraceptives, but this belief has not been supported by recent international data analyses.

Earlier studies, concluding OCs increased migraines, did not look carefully at when in the pill cycle the headaches occurred. For example, researchers often did not ask whether the headache occurred while on the active hormone-containing pills (which would likely mean the pill did make the headaches worse), or whether the headaches occurred in the placebo cycle (which would indicate hormone-withdrawal as the cause).

Forty to sixty percent of women with migraines who take oral contraceptives experience headaches in the last seven days of the pill pack during "placebo" pills, which supports rapidly falling estradiol levels as the trigger.

Danger
Cigarette smoking was the primary risk for stroke in women with migraines also taking BCP.

In four double-blind placebo-controlled studies there were no differences in headache frequency between women on the birth control pills and those taking placebo. Dr. Stephen Silberstein, a well-known migraine specialist, emphasized in an article *Neurology*, 15 years ago: "*Estrogens and OCs are not contraindicated in migraine patients. In fact, they may actually be indicated for certain women.*"

The variation in birth control pill effects summarized in the table on the next page is another indication of the crucial need for individualized therapy.

Dr. Vliet's Guide to Potential Birth

Control Pill Effects on Migraines

1. **Headaches can increase.** This is typically seen with pills having varying hormone content, such as Tri-Levlen, Ortho Tri-Cyclen, Triphasil. Increased headaches are also seen with high progestin pills such as Loestrin, Alesse, Mircette, and with progestin-only contraceptives such as Norplant, Depo-Provera, or the pills Micronor, Nor-QD and Ovrette—if they not prescribed with estradiol to balance the progestin.

2. **Headaches can be eliminated or significantly decreased.** This is more common with monophasic (constant dose) pills with lower progestin content, such as Ovcon 35, Modicon, Necon, Ortho-Cyclen, Yasmin, Diane 35, particularly if taken continuously with no break for menses. Studies show as much as 60 to 80 percent improvement in migraines when women use steady dose combined estrogen-progestin contraceptives taken continuously.

3. **Birth control pills can contribute to the first appearance of a migraine, usually in women with a significant family history.** This response suggests that the progestin is too high, and a pill with a better hormone balance should be found. If the headaches continue, then I would not use BCP and would look for other options.

4. **New or different symptoms, such as aura or visual changes, can occur.** This change is potentially serious and should be discussed immediately with your physician. It usually means you should stop right away.

There is no one right answer for all women. You must work closely with knowledgeable specialists to make best use of available products to find the right balance of estrogen and progestin for you. (See Chapter 16 for more information.)

Hormones and Seizures

Over the years, I have encountered women with seizures that were clearly affected by their menstrual cycle. This letter from a young woman's brother in Illinois, and illustrates many important points.

"Dear Dr. Vliet,

I am writing to you in response to a (newspaper) wire article about you and your practice. The problem is with my sister. Back in January of this year (1996), while she was on her job as a nanny, she had what appeared to be a black-out. She became disoriented about the date, time and place. She left the child on the floor, and left the house. They found her later that day but she did not remember anything that happened. She scheduled an appointment with a doctor (I assume an internist) who ran a battery of tests and found nothing. She was released with a perfect bill of health. The very next month she had another episode while visiting Tucson. She became disoriented and was putting salt and pepper on her cereal. Again, she remembered nothing. This time she went to see a neurologist who also performed a battery of tests and found nothing. She was released again. Shortly after this, the association was made with the fact that the episodes were occurring at the beginning of her period. She made an appointment with an ObGyn who gave her a checkup and released her with a clean bill of health. We were worried but did not know what to do."

"Well, on Memorial Day, it happened again and this time she was not as lucky. She was driving my father-in-law, who incidentally happens to be a D.O. (Doctor of Osteopathy) physician in Arizona. According to my father-in-law, she began to have a seizure while approaching a red light. She was frozen solid with her foot on the gas. He tried to remove the key but could not. She sustained minor injuries from the impact but the car was totaled and my father-in-law is in the hospital in Illinois awaiting neck surgery for two ruptured disks and replacement of most muscles and ligaments of the area. My sister had wandered away from the accident but was taken to the emergency room after she was found. She did not feel any pain and had no memory of the accident. Another battery of tests was done and the doctor was told of the relationship to her period. She was released with minor injuries

2 + 2 = Answers

Sometimes finding the right treatment just takes a little common sense, some thinking "outside the box," tracking patterns with the menstrual cycle and listening to observations from patients and their families.

related to the accident,. This time she was in and out of a prolonged spell that lasted two days. My parents took her to the University of Chicago Hospital where yet another battery tests were performed. They said nothing was wrong and she had to be released. She is currently awaiting an appointment with another neurologist at the University of Chicago. This is why I am appealing to you. We have come close to exhausting all avenues and the doctors say she is fine. The fact is, if she were fine, my father-in-law would not be in intensive care. They were extremely lucky that the accident was not fatal. If nothing can be done, she would have to remain in the constant care of my parents indefinitely. The doctors seem to be ignoring the fact that it must be related to her periods. Can you offer any help?"

Essential
Estradiol has a significant role in preserving normal nerve cell growth, repair, and memory function

My office staff responded, and described our approach to evaluating the hormone triggers of such episodes. Her family decided to send her for our evaluation. We discussed the abrupt fall in her estradiol and progesterone at the onset of her periods as one trigger of her seizures.

Her EEG did not show seizure activity, which wasn't surprising since the test was not done *during her menses*, the *only* time she had seizures.

Her neurologist started her on the anticonvulsant, Tegretol, but even with this medicine her family reported that she was still having seizures with onset of her periods.

I prescribed a trial on a steady dose birth control pill to suppress ovarian cycles, stop the rise and fall in ovarian hormones, and give a steady estrogen-progestin amount each day. She took the pills steadily for 4–6 packs, which reduced the number of times her hormones fell if she stopped the pills to have a period.

Fact
Dementia is not one disease; it is a group of brain diseases, with a hundred or more different causes.

I also prescribed a Climara patch to keep the blood level of estradiol steady during her period, which eliminated the estrogen drop that appeared to precipitate her seizures. She has done well on this regimen for almost 10 years, without any further menstrual seizures. She is cleared to drive again.

Hormones and Memory: "Now What Was It I Was Going to Do?"

"Where did I put my keys? What did I come in here to do? I feel like I am losing my mind." I hear these comments every day from women, young and old. It isn't just at menopause that you can't think of words or you forget where you put your "To Do" list, much less what was on it!

You feel scattered in your thinking, and can't focus like you used to. You worry about Alzheimer's. Familiar? Don't worry, you aren't alone, nor are you imagining it.

Abnormal

Dementia is not a normal part of aging. It is an illness that affects about 10 percent of the population.

You probably don't have "attention deficit, more likely you are experiencing a subtle decline in the important ovarian, and possibly thyroid, hormones that oversee the brain's memory centers. Science shows the ways estradiol and testosterone oversee normal memory function.

Dementia means generalized loss of the brain's ability to retain, perceive, integrate, retrieve, and act appropriately on information. Collectively, we call these tasks cognitive function. Some types of dementia are treatable, and reversible if the cause is caught early. For example, untreated hypothyroidism or B12 deficit can lead to marked impairment of cognitive function or even full-blown dementia.

Alzheimer's Disease is a different type of irreversible dementia with no known cure that leads to inexorable loss of all brain function, then death. Some medications, including estradiol, may delay the progression of brain damage. In women who already have Alzheimer's disease, recent studies show that estradiol may slow the progression by as much as two years.

Effects

Estrogen deficiency plays an important role in causing memory loss and even some dementias.

In women who do not have the disease, studies from several countries show that estradiol can reduce later risk of developing Alzheimer's disease by 40 to 50%. Horse-derived Premarin and Prempro appear to *increase* the risk of dementia in older women, unlike what we see with 17-beta estradiol, the primary *human* estrogen.

Milder forms of memory changes that women describe during post-partum, pre and perimenopause, and after menopause are generally not the more serious illness of dementia.

If hormonal decline is one contributing factor that helps explain memory loss in women, physicians must consider and address this before permanent damage to nerve cells occurs.

Some Basics About How Memory Works

The complex components of our memory system were only recently delineated. Memory functions are primarily in the limbic system that includes the hippocampus, mammillary bodies, septal region, and part of the thalamus. There is much still to clarify about how memory processes work, but so far, it appears to be a system of "storage centers," located in both hemispheres of the brain.

Having storage centers in different areas of the brain is like back up for your computer. Memory is not completely lost if one hemisphere of the brain is damaged or injured. Memory function differs from other brain functions; most have specific locations in one hemisphere or the other, not both.

Most people think of verbal memory, but the brain has mechanisms for remembering specific types of sensory memories as well: sound (auditory), sight (visual), touch (kinesthetic), smell (olfactory), and other sensory perceptions. These sensory memory centers are also widely distributed throughout the brain.

Since memory is so crucial to survival, it makes sense that the brain has evolved multiple areas for memory storage of all kinds of information needed to keep the organism alive and functioning.

To simplify, memory is either short-term or long term. We use short-term memory in day-to-day situations. For example you hear a telephone number or a name and remember it just long enough to use it.

When the name or number or piece of information is something you want to remember longer, you convert it to long-term memory. The hippocampus and mammillary bodies are the primary centers involved in converting short-term to long-term memory.

This conversion involves an actual physical change in the brain with the creation of new connections between nerve cells. Estradiol stimulates growth of these sprouts, called dendrites, to make more new connections between neurons, and this helps memory. This physical change can also involve the creation of actual "memory molecules" that contain specific codes for information.

Short-term memory is affected first by memory robbers such as estradiol decline, nutritional deficits, or dementia-type illnesses. Later, with more damage, long-term memories are lost.

Advances in Neuroscience: Estrogen Effects on Memory

Positive effects!
The positive changes disappeared after estrogen therapy stopped, strongly suggesting estrogen's major influence on cognitive functions.

Dr. Barbara Sherwin, at McGill University in Canada, has spent almost three decades researching estrogen effects on the brain.

Dr. Sherwin's studies show improvements specifically in verbal memory in healthy postmenopausal women on estrogen compared to those who are not.

Dr. Sherwin and her colleagues also evaluated surgically menopausal women and found those treated with estrogen did significantly better on several measures of cognitive function than those given a placebo. Other studies of surgically menopausal women show that taking estradiol specifically enhances short-term verbal memory.

None of these women had any type of dementia; they were all healthy and were considered impaired in their memory abilities. Yet, the improved performance in women on estrogen therapy was statistically significant and fits with what patients say when their hormone levels are restored to optimal levels.

In an ongoing study of 8,879 female residents of a retirement community in California, researchers found that estrogen users had a 40% lower risk of dementia (or only about 60 percent of the risk of Alzheimer's) than seen in women who did not take estrogen. These preliminary results were published in 1998.

Window of opportunity
The key is to keep estradiol optimal BEFORE damage occurs.

The USC investigators further found that the higher the dose of the estrogen, the lower the risk of Alzheimer's. The risk of dementia also decreased more the longer women took estrogen: Women who took estrogen 7 years or more had a 50 percent lower risk of dementia than those not taking ERT.

In 1994, Japanese researchers showed ERT gave measurable improvement on measures of recent memory, distant memory, attention, orientation, personality, mood, sleeping and eating behaviors in women with documented Alzheimer's.

Serum estradiol levels with ERT matched those of healthy, younger women right before ovulation. These results suggest that the estradiol and serum levels achieved with therapy must reach a certain threshold or minimum level to reap the benefits on memory and other cognitive functions. At the end of the

Dr. Vliet's Guide to Estrogen Effects on Memory and Cognitive Pathways

🔊 17-beta estradiol, the primary estrogen produced by the ovary before meno-pause, has specific receptor binding sites in many different areas of the brain. These receptor sites appear to be quite specific for the native human form of the molecule. (All of my clinical work with patients strongly supports these basic scientific findings in animal models and studies of human brain cells in tissue cultures)

🔊 Estradiol *promotes growth* of new dendrites between nerve cells, making more synaptic connections. More synapse connections mean nerve cells can handle more incoming signals.

🔊 Progesterone *breaks down* the nerve cell connections.

🔊 When estradiol declines, synapse density in the hippocampus (memory and learning center) decreases as well. Denser synapses allow better cell-to-cell information flow, and better "multi-tasking."

🔊 Estradiol enhances nerve cells' ability absorb nerve growth factor (NGF). In animals without ovaries, those who did not receive estrogen had a marked (56 percent) decline in the number of nerve cells; the animals given estrogen had only a slight decrease in nerve cells.

🔊 Estrogens regulate memory-regulating (cholinergic) nerve cells in the basal forebrain of rodents. The basil forebrain is one of the regions of the brain involved in cognitive function and one of the areas that degenerates in hu-mans with Alzheimer's disease.

🔊 Estrogens increase the production of choline acetyltransferase, an enzyme needed to make acetylcholine (ACh). Estrogen thereby prevents the marked loss of ACh found in patients with Alzheimer's. ACh is the brain's most impor-tant chemical messenger for storing new memories in the brain, regulating memory retrieval and cognition. Loss of the cholinergic nerves and chemical messengers is the most marked brain change in Alzheimer's disease.

©Elizabeth Lee Vliet MD, 1995, revised 2002–2007

study, the families of these patients saw the improvement and requested that estrogen therapy continue long-term.

In 1999, Yale researchers found that even a three-week course of ERT changed brain activity in postmenopausal women performing memory tasks in a randomized double-blind placebo controlled clinical trial.

On a humorous note

When someone in my office forgets something, another staff will often ask (based on experience), "Did you forget your patch this morning?"

Brain activity changes in the ERT group, documented on MRI, mimicked brain activation patterns typically seen in younger women.

Dr. Karl Mortel found that among women with cardiovascular disease (CVD), those taking estrogen showed improved blood flow to the brain and improved cognitive function. His work fits with other research showing estradiol's relaxing effect on arteries, leading to increased dilation and better blood flow to all organs in the body.

Worldwide research and my own clinical experience shows clearly that the brain is a target organ for estradiol action in women. But the crucial point we now know is that estradiol has to be maintained at normal levels *before* damage occurs. There is a *"window of opportunity" to prevent brain cell death...* after that damage can't be reversed.

Regardless of age, we must consider the effects of estradiol decline on memory and thinking when we are evaluating women. Psychological symptoms, like memory changes, are not only caused by stress; they also have physical, endocrine causes as well as.

We don't yet know the entire spectrum of estrogen's effects on memory and cognitive pathways, there are a number of intriguing hypotheses about how it works, summarized in the table.

Gender matters

MS involves important gender-related hormone issues.

Multiple Sclerosis: New Insights on Hormone Connections

MS is the most common non-traumatic neurological disease of young adults. It is an immune-mediated disorder that targets the central nervous system causing inflammation, loss of the myelin protective coatings around nerve cells (demyelination), death of axons, and formation of scar tissue. The cause of MS is unknown, but it appears to involve a variety of genetic, hormonal, immune system, and environmental factors, such as excitotoxins, chemical pollutants, and/or infectious agents.

Multiple sclerosis (MS), hits young women hard, much harder than men. Approximately 75% of MS sufferers are women, most between the ages of 15 and 50, with an average age of onset at 28–30 years.

With these patterns, it has long been suspected that there are important hormonal factors contributing directly or indirectly to MS.

MS causes puzzling symptoms that come and go. At first, you wonder if you are imaging the visual changes, muscle weakness, loss of bladder control, numbness or tingling of hands, feet, legs or arms that can be fleeting in the initial stages of the illness.

These same symptoms can have a hundred or more different causes, including hypothyroidism, menopausal loss of estradiol, diabetes, and a variety of vitamin deficiencies, to name a few.

If symptoms disappear and don't return for months or years, people do not realize there could be the potentially serious problem of MS.

The brain abnormalities of MS are more widespread than once thought, causing problems like memory loss, difficulty with concentration, focus and attention, all of which may also be mistaken for other disorders.

There are important links between the endocrine, nervous and immune systems that are played out in both the onset and progression of MS. MS patterns during pregnancy have led to important clues.

Pregnancy has a short-term, favorable effect on MS, followed typically by a serious relapse in the immediate postpartum period for about 65–70% of women, as hormone levels fall sharply after delivery. This observation suggests *that ovarian hormone loss plays a role in the relapse.* Breast-feeding, which also suppresses estradiol production, also seems to affect the progression and severity of symptoms of MS.

There is a much higher incidence of cognitive impairment in menopausal women with MS compared to men of the same age with MS. This points to estradiol and possibly testosterone having a stabilizing effect.

Some studies show that higher estrogen levels protect against some of the progression of CNS damage. Other data suggests that times of low estradiol and progesterone during bleeding days

Wisdom
Since estradiol is well-documented to improve memory and other brain functions, current research suggests that hormone therapy for menopausal women with MS can help reduce cognitive loss.

of the menstrual cycle, and during menopause, are times women are more likely to have MS flares, with about 25–30% of women experiencing more intense MS symptoms at these times.

Osteoporosis is another medical issue for women with MS. There are several reasons for risk of bone loss to increase: from corticosteroids used to treat MS; from decreased physical exercise resulting from fatigue and loss of muscle strength; reduced heat tolerance keeps many MS sufferers from getting sun, which in turn means a possible vitamin D deficiency.

Why?
Only 1% of the women with MS took medications like Fosamax or Actonel to preserve bone.

Women with MS are not screened with DEXA tests for bone density, nor are they offered treatments with bone building medications. One survey conducted at Mt. Sinai in New York found that 80–85 % of women with MS were not tested for bone density, whether they were menopausal or not.

In all areas of MS management, there are unique issues that affect women. Women often have a harder time getting a correct early diagnosis, in part related to many studies showing doctors have a stereotype of women as "hypochondriacs" and think women have more stress-related problems or "just" depression.

Tragic
I find it tragic that there is such widespread failure to diagnose and treat bone loss in MS.

This deeply ensconced physician attitude leads to greater possibility of the diagnosis of MS in women being missed in its early stages.

Once MS is diagnosed, medications for management of symptoms and to modify the course of the disease have potentially more adverse effects for women than men.

Hormone therapy, when used, can have different effects and benefits depending on what forms are used. The approaches for women with MS need to take into account types and routes of hormones most likely to avoid side effects that could aggravate symptoms of the disease.

There are many challenges for MS sufferers, and we need to make significant improvement in the approaches tailored for women's unique needs.

Hormonal Decline: An Unrecognized Cause of Fatigue

Chronic Fatigue Syndrome (CFS), a more severe degree of fatigue, has many causes and contributing factors. Ovarian hormone levels play an important, overlooked role, even if this is not the only factor involved. Milder forms of fatigue and loss of vitality, or "zest," are even more dramatically affected by decreases in ovarian hormones.

Losing optimal estradiol and testosterone, which are key metabolic hormones, makes you tired, lethargic and sluggish, even if you don't have full-blown CFS.

Fatigue that makes it hard to get through the day is described by 70–80% of women experiencing such hormone changes, whether they are adolescents with Polycystic Ovary Syndrome, post-partum women with low ovarian hormones from suppression by nursing, women infertile from premature loss of ovarian hormones, or perimenopausal and menopausal women with naturally declining ovary hormone levels.

What about *ovarian* hormones?
60–70% of patients with CFS are women.

Sleep disruption comes with low estradiol and is another connection between ovarian hormones and persistent fatigue. These sleep changes can begin eight to ten years before you stop menstruating.

Sleep deprivation robs you of normal daytime energy, contributes to persistent fatigue, and also causes suppression of the immune system that makes you more susceptible to infections that make you tired.

A wide variety of endocrine disruptor compounds can further interfere with normal function of your ovarian and thyroid hormones, leading to fatigue and low energy. (See Chapter 5.)

Most physicians check the adrenal and basic thyroid hormones in people with CFS, but do not check women's ovarian hormone levels, even though there is an enormous female preponderance in the incidence of CFS. In all of the medical articles I have read on CFS, however, I have not seen one that adequately addresses this issue.

Timeline
The average age of onset is 41.9 years. This is the same time frame that ovarian decline commonly begins.

Another study found that 90 percent of patients with fibromyalgia were female, with an average age of 44.0 years, again the perimenopausal stage. Nothing was mentioned about hormones in either study. The amazing thing is that there were two female physician investigators in one of these studies. Not one comment about checking women's hormones was made!

CFS appears to be one of a cluster of neuroendocrine disorders that includes Fibromyalgia (FMS) and Multiple Chemical Sensitivities (MCS). There are many theories about causal factors in these conditions. Many physicians are skeptical that CFS is a "real" disorder, and the condition is controversial. Researchers have been unable to identify a cause, predict a course, or find effective treatments.

Cause

One theory has been that viral infections like Epstein Barr, Cytomeglovirus, herpes, and others can lead to a viral infiltration of the thyroid gland (thyroiditis), ovary (oophoritis), or adrenal gland (adrenalitis) creating a subsequent decline in the optimal functioning of these hormone-producing organs.

Thyroid hormone dysfunction is another common hormonal cause of fatigue and loss of vitality.

Viral illnesses are known to trigger later development of auto-immune disorders affecting many endocrine organs, another potential link between a viral illness and subsequent appearance of CFS, FMS or MCS.

Viral-induced loss of endocrine gland function can lead to subtle forms of hypothyroidism or adrenal decline causing fatigue, and subtle forms of ovarian decline that cause infertility and fatigue syndromes. These types of viral syndromes (thyroiditis, oophoritis, adrenalitis) are commonly overlooked in most medical settings, especially for women.

Alert

Other stressors to the body's immune system are implicated in CFS. Persistent low-grade infections such as Mycoplasma (a cause of "walking pneumonia") can lead to CFS symptoms, but are hard to detect unless a clinician tests for Mycoplasma.

Estradiol and testosterone have significant activating or stimulating effects on energy level.

Environmental pollutants (such as "sick building syndrome"), toxic chemicals ("Persian Gulf" syndrome, insecticide toxicity, DES exposure in utero), and even low grade toxic effects from chronic use of common household chemicals can lead to immune suppression causing symptoms of CFS.

Some of these common chemicals also damage endocrine tissues like the thyroid gland, ovaries in women, and testicles in men, causing disruption in hormone production.

Prolonged stressful situations also suppress the ovaries, and can lead to the neuroendocrine changes associated with CFS, FMS, and MCS. Illnesses like depression and generalized anxiety stress the immune system and play a role in CFS. We also know that declines in both thyroid and ovarian hormones can affect the onset of these mood symptoms.

Louise was 37, and developed a severe, persistent fatigue in the post-partum phase. She said,

"I've had a horrible struggle with total exhaustion and hormonal problems since the birth of my daughter 8 years ago. I had pre-eclampsia (toxemia of pregnancy) and then a severe hemorrhage after the placenta came out. I was healthy before all that. Now I am totally exhausted all the time. My doctors told me I had chronic fatigue but they said there wasn't anything to do about it. I live in a constant brain fog, my memory is terrible. I don't sleep well and I don't have the energy to exercise. I am still having periods, so my doctor said it couldn't be hormonal. I can feel the ovulation twinge most of the time, but my periods have changed in that they aren't as long and the cycles changed from short to long. I just know it is connected to my hormones somehow."

Her blood pressure was very good at 110/68, so I didn't think hypotension was a cause of her fatigue. She was not overweight, her cholesterol profile was very good, and her thyroid tests, including antibodies, were all negative for evidence of thyroid disease. Her 8 AM cortisol was slightly *higher* than desirable at 25 as a "stress" response, so she certainly didn't have "adrenal insufficiency." Her serum ferritin, a measure of iron stores, was lower than optimal, but not so low that it was a major factor in her fatigue.

While her adrenal and thyroid hormones were checked numerous times, *none of her physicians ever checked her ovarian hormone levels.* A pharmacist gave her a progesterone skin cream to use twice a day, but she had to stop this because it made her fatigue markedly worse.

This wasn't surprising, in light of progesterone effects on the brain that I described above. When I checked the more reliable serum hormone levels, the primary cause of her fatigue became clear. Her estradiol on Day 1 was significantly low at 27 pg/ml, and her Day 20 estradiol low at 61 pg/ml (it should be about 200-250 pg/ml or so).

Like many younger women with this pattern of low estradiol, she still had a healthy luteal phase ovulatory rise in progesterone, (15.2). Her N-telopeptide level was too high at 65, indicating rapid bone break-down, even though she was only 37. This further confirmed that her estradiol level was lower than optimal.

No wonder she was so tired. She didn't have enough estradiol to provide the metabolic fuel for her muscles, brain and body! After eight years of struggling, she finally had some test results that made sense in understanding her symptoms.

Interesting
The viral theory offers one possible connection that could explain the marked female preponderance of cases.

So... Test!
Proper testing can identify many of these potential overlooked causes for fatigue and immune changes.

Her ovarian hormone production had not "bounced back" following pregnancy and the post-partum hemorrhage. She was not clinically depressed. The continued loss of these vital hormones had caused her fatigue and other neuroendocrine symptoms.

Where have we heard this before?
A pharmacist checked saliva levels of her hormones and told her she was "estrogen dominant and deficient in progesterone." NOT CORRECT!

I took a fairly simple approach and suggested a steady dose, estrogen dominant birth control pill using Ortho-Cyclen. At each of her 3-month follow-up appointments, she described feeling more and more like her old self.

At her one-year appointment, her fatigue symptoms had completely resolved, along with the brain fog.

Margie was 20 years old when I first saw her, and she was struggling with severe fatigue, confused and fuzzy thinking, mood swings, night sweats and PMS since age 17. She was a professional ballet dancer, and having difficulty with her training schedule because of her profound fatigue. *"I am too young to feel so old!"*

She didn't eat well, restricting calories to keep her weight down, causing loss of her regular menstrual periods.

Her ovarian hormone levels showed disturbing results: an estradiol less than 10 pg/ml on day 2, and only 60 pg/ml on day 20; a testosterone level of 10 ng/dl; all far too low for optimal energy, normal muscle growth and repair, and bone preservation.

It was clear why her dancing suffered. Her low bone density was consistent with the hormone findings.

By putting her on the Ovcon birth control pill and improving the quality of her nutrition, she had better hormone and food fuel.

Six months later
Annette was jubilant: "I have my energy back, that awful fatigue is gone, and I am able to work fulltime."

Her energy returned, her PMS was controlled, her mood stabilized, and her bone density is building appropriately again for a young woman her age. She now longer needs the antidepressants that a previous physician prescribed, which had made her fatigue worse.

At 46, *Annette* had been having restless sleep, low sex drive, marked fatigue, premenstrual sweet cravings and depressed mood for the last five years. The fatigue and insomnia had gotten so bad she had difficulty working fulltime. Her doctor had started her on *Mircette, a low estrogen-high progestin contraceptive pill*, to help regulate her periods. Her fatigue, mood and sleep problems got worse the longer she was on it, although it did help reduce her cramps and heavy periods.

Then she saw her family physician who started her on Zoloft for the depressed mood, but this made her even more tired during the day, so she stopped this and the Mircette.

She consulted an alternative practitioner who told her she had "adrenal exhaustion" and recommended adrenal hormones, even though her 8 AM serum cortisol was in the *high*, not low.

Annette's comprehensive hormone evaluation revealed several causes of her problems: extremely low estradiol, low testosterone, and elevated thyroid antibodies that suggested the beginning of Hashimoto's thyroiditis. Her low bone density and high NTx indicated she likely had low estradiol for awhile.

I suggested Yasmin, a pill with a better ratio of estrogen and progestin that would help keep the cramps and heavy bleeding under control but not cause the unwanted side effects she had with Mircette.

I also suggested she start a low dose of thyroid hormone to slow down the progression of her thyroiditis.

The full syndrome of CFS requires severe, persistent fatigue plus four of the following eight symptoms: myalgia (muscle pain), arthralgia, sore throat, headache, sleep disruption, malaise following exercise, tender neck, and cognitive difficulty (memory, concentration, focus difficulties).

Decline in women's ovarian hormones may not explain *all* cases of CFS, or why CFS occurs in males, but if some 70 percent of the patients with CFS are women, it makes sense to check ovarian hormones.

I think we should also check the major hormone levels in men with CFS, although I have not seen a formal study of that connection. The male patients I have evaluated for CFS had low testosterone and/or DHEA.

Finally
Once we had reliable hormone levels to clarify the cause of her problems, it became a straight-forward approach to helping her get better.

Definition
However we define the disorder of CFS, many of these same symptoms are a result of declining ovary or thyroid hormones.

Summary

Doctors treating women seem to ignore the basic science advances in understanding of the many metabolic effects of the ovarian hormones on every organ system in the body.

Everywhere in medicine, clinicians have blinders on when it comes to incorporating an awareness of the key hormones that make a woman's body different from a man's.

If you have "brain" symptoms, you need a careful evaluation of the endocrine, nutritional, and metabolic factors that can cause such symptoms before you allow health professionals to write off your problems as "stress" or a "psychiatric" disorder.

Antidepressants are fine, if biological depression is truly what you have.

But if hormone loss, such as estradiol, is causing your mood changes, fatigue, memory loss, and insomnia, then antidepressants won't be the answer.

So, take into account the connections described here. Have your hormones checked before you simply pop a Prozac, Paxil, or Effexor pill.

Links
Hormones and brain. Brain and body. These are inextricably linked.

Chapter 13
The Perils of PCOS, Obesity, Syndrome X, and Diabetes

Most doctors *still* do not take an aggressive approach to diagnosis and treatment of PCOS, Syndrome X, or Diabetes, particularly in young women. These serious metabolic syndromes lead to obesity and rob you of your health.

Not just because PCOS, Syndrome X and Diabetes affect your fertility. Not just because they cause short-term concerns like acne, excess facial hair and excess weight.

Because PCOS, Syndrome X and Diabetes are *deadly diseases*. All three cause heart attacks and premature death in women in their 30s- and 40s.

They increase risk of serious depression.

They increase risk of uterine cancer.

They increase risk of early breast cancer.

They increase risk of early stroke.

You may say, "I'll skip this…I'm too young to worry about diabetes!" Well don't.

What was called *adult*-onset diabetes has become a serious health crisis in *children* in the United States.

PCOS is clearly on the rise in this country, in large part for the very endocrine-disrupting reasons discussed throughout this book. I am shocked at the number of calls from mothers of girls as young and 9 and 10, asking for a hormone evaluation because of their daughter's ominous body changes, even before menses start.

Plan ahead
Reduce your risks while you are young, before diabetes develops.

Too late
I see more and more obese adolescent girls who are already diabetic.

Too sad
Women in their 20s, eager to start a family, find out the hard way that obesity can cause infertility.

Misleading
The name "polycystic ovarian syndrome," is seriously misleading however. It is a multi-system, complex endocrine disorder.

I am convinced the rise in PCOS, diabetes and obesity represent an overlooked part of the spectrum of the endocrine system damage from environmental pollutants and chemical additives in foods that affect us from the womb onward.

Polycystic Ovary Syndrome (PCOS): Hormonal Havoc That Devastates Health

Polycystic ovary syndrome (PCOS) has begun to get attention in women's magazines and physician offices. In the past, it was "an infertility problem," meaning it is only a concern if a woman is trying to get pregnant.

PCOS is far more dangerous, and potentially deadly. And, it is on the increase in young women today, PCOS was first described in 1935 and called *Stein-Leventhal Syndrome*, named for the doctors who first described the characteristic body changes and tiny cysts covering the ovaries. That label is woefully inadequate.

At that time, doctors thought it was a disorder that just affected the ovaries, causing excess body hair, irregular menses, infrequent ovulation, and follicles that become multiple tiny cysts instead of developing properly to become an egg.

PCOS is *the most common* endocrine disorder affecting young women in their childbearing years, affecting more than 6 percent of premenopausal women, *including teenagers and pre-pubescent girls.*

Six percent of women may not sound like much. But stop for a moment: 6% means *millions* of women. And that statistic *doesn't include* girls who have budding PCOS no one has yet recognized.

The hormonal imbalance of PCOS leads to a *metabolic syndrome* with widespread effects that can wreak havoc throughout the brain and body. PCOS dramatically increases your risk of many serious health problems, beginning in your early teens.

By age 30, 50% of women with PCOS have either impaired glucose tolerance, significant insulin resistance, or overt diabetes. Newer studies report that women from 39 to 49 years old with PCOS have a heart attack risk that is *four times* that of women without PCOS in this age group. Women with

PCOS also have a higher risk, at younger ages, of uterine and breast cancers.

Today, we know these diverse complications of PCOS are caused primarily by several critical hormone imbalances, which I describe shortly.

The combination of elevated androgens and elevated insulin causes rapid waistline weight gain that often feels totally out of control. The fatter you get, the more insulin resistant you become, and the more abnormal your hormone ratio becomes, the more fat you gain.

Effects

Women with PCOS have an *eleven-fold increased* risk of cardiovascular disease that can appear as early as the 20s and 30s.

What are the symptoms of PCOS?

The most obvious ones are your body changes:

Marked weight gain

The *pattern* of weight gain holds clues to the presence of PCOS:

Statistics

About 1 in every 17 women suffer from the devastating serious endocrine imbalances.

1. **The *weight gain is usually rapid,* often without change in food intake.** Many of my patients say it feels like the cookie monster running amuck inside them. The pounds pack on faster than they can shop for new clothes. They diet, they exercise, and nothing seems to halt this inexorable growth in girth. They are puzzled and frightened.

2. **The *excess fat is typically deposited around the waist, upper body, shoulders and arms,* rather than hips and thighs.** Women tell me they feel like a fireplug or a barrel. Breasts get larger, fat sticks like glue under and around the arms and upper chest. Waistline? It disappears.

   The hormone imbalances of PCOS create the damaging male pattern apple-shaped body. Weight gain from overeating is usually more symmetrical and distributes in a woman's pear shape.

3. *Weight gain is commonly accompanied by acne and excess face and body hair, and thinning scalp hair.* Weight gain from simply *over* eating and *under* exercising doesn't usually come with these other problems.

4. *The weight gain doesn't respond normally to diets.* The metabolic abnormalities of PCOS make it almost impossible for a woman to lose weight by simply eating less. The endocrine imbalances *must* be treated first.

A 16-year-old young woman I saw recently had severe hormonal imbalance typical of PCOS, with a very high level of free testosterone, and low estradiol. She had gained 50 pounds over six months in spite of a healthy diet and exercise regimen. She had PCOS, but her gynecologist had not recognized it. He saw her as simply a teenager obsessed with weight gain and complaining of PMS. His advice was to "just eat less, and you'll lose weight." It is not that simple when someone has PCOS.

Being thin is not immune
PCOS can also occur in thin women. It doesn't always cause weight gain.

Excess facial and body hair

This excess hair growth is called *hirsutism*. Hirsutism itself is not a disease; it is a *symptom* of an underlying hormonal imbalance. Androgen excess in PCOS causes hair that is often dark and coarse to grow on the chin, cheeks, upper lip, chest, around the nipples, on the stomach and inner thigh, back and buttocks.

In PCOS, the primary culprits for the excess hair are excess androgens (testosterone, DHEA, androstenedione). There is also over-activity of an enzyme called *5-alpha reductase* that converts testosterone to a more potent form called *dihydrotestosterone* (DHT) in the hair follicle, causing increased male-type hair growth.

Thinning scalp hair, or hair loss

The changes in hair texture, thickness, and pattern of loss in PCOS are related to the excess androgens and are similar to menopausal women with higher androgens relative to their estradiol.

Hair is thinner overall with loss of hair on the top of the head and around the forehead. The PCOS pattern is similar to male-pattern baldness, again related to excess androgens.

Acne
In PCOS the acne doesn't always confine itself to your face; you can have cystic acne outbreaks on your chest, back, arms, and legs.

Severe acne

The acne in PCOS is typically far worse than just simple adolescent "zits" the week before your period. The acne can be large, painful, inflamed cysts that look and feel like boils.

One young woman had become severely disfigured from the cystic acne, but had never been checked for possible PCOS despite the telltale signs. It took six months of aggressive hormonal management for her acne to resolve.

For more information and a more complete description of the causes, effects and more specific treatment of cyclic acne, see my book, *The Savvy Woman's Guide to PCOS*.

Irregular menstrual cycles

The menstrual cycle can be affected in many different ways. Sometimes women with PCOS go months without a period, other times periods are fairly regular. Some PCOS sufferers have very heavy bleeding; others have periods that are barely there. Some women may ovulate, others don't.

Difficulty getting pregnant, or frequent miscarriages

Excess levels of male hormones combined with excess body fat lead to increased conversion of androstenedione, an androgen found in high concentration in body fat, to the estrone form of estrogen.

Excess production of estrone feeds back to the brain and alters the pituitary secretion of FSH and LH, which in turn means the menstrual cycle follicle progression gets disrupted.

Follicles become cysts and ovulation is less likely. If there is no ovulation, progesterone isn't produced, so bleeding becomes unpredictable.

High prolactin, found in about 60% of women with PCOS, also suppresses the normal menstrual cycle hormone production.

There are several factors that combine to increase the problem of infertility: decreased ovulation, lower levels of both estradiol and progesterone, high levels of *estrone* and prolactin, excess androgens, and excess insulin and cortisol, to name a few.

Hormone Havoc: *Serious* Imbalances

The invisible changes *inside* the body, however, are even more ominous. These rob you of energy, fertility, mood stability, and health. Here are the primary abnormal findings in PCOS:

- High androgen (male hormone) levels (testosterone—both free and total, DHEA-S, DHEA, androstenedione). This is the most consistent hormone abnormality in PCOS, seen in more than 70–80% of sufferers. High androgens can also cause irritability, anxiety, insomnia and agitated depressed moods, and scattered thinking.
- High estrone (E1) to estradiol (E2) ratio, also a consistent finding in the majority of PCOS sufferers, and the same cause of similar symptoms seen around menopause in women who don't have PCOS.
- High LH to FSH ratio (the reverse of normal); common, but not *always* present

Warning
Miscarriages are more likely in women with PCOS because the estradiol and progesterone levels are lower than needed to sustain early pregnancy until the placenta can take over production.

Warning!
Estradiol, our most important and active form of estrogen, is actually *lower than expected* in women with PCOS.

so does not differentiate from hypo

Mistake

Doctors still mistakenly think there must be cysts to qualify for PCOS. Not so.

Hiding

PCOS is a master of disguise. Not all women with this disorder have all these symptoms or lab abnormalities.

≈ Lower than normal SHBG, which means more male hormones are "free" and therefore more active, causing more of the adverse body changes listed above

≈ Glucose intolerance, leading to "blood sugar swings" that disrupt memory, concentration, mood, sleep patterns and cause weight gain

≈ Insulin resistance, usually with excess insulin production, that makes you get fatter and fatter, even if you are eating less and exercising more

≈ High cholesterol and triglycerides with low HDL ("good") and high LDL ("bad") cholesterol

≈ High blood pressure

≈ Elevated prolactin, with or without nipple discharge (*galactorrhea*), in about 60% of PCOS women

≈ Recurrent ovarian cysts that come and go. The classic PCOS cysts on the ovary appear on ultrasound like a "string of pearls." Not every woman with PCOS has visible cysts, however, because many times cysts are so tiny they can't be seen on ultrasound and are only found during surgery, often done for other reasons. Or, since the cysts are not present all the time, they may elude detection on ultrasound.

Master of Disguise

The variability in *how* PCOS presents itself makes it difficult to create a specific criteria for diagnosis. This is different from diabetes for example, where we have national standards for glucose levels that clearly alert doctors to diabetes or the milder glucose intolerance.

Tragically, many physicians see PCOS as a "cosmetic" problem when young women complain of excess face or body hair, and weight gain.

In a number of studies, women with abnormal ovaries on ultrasound *overlapped* with those who had abnormal hormone levels. Whether cysts are present on ultrasound does not, however, have much predictive value in determining who has the abnormal hormone levels characteristic of PCOS.

PCOS is *both* an elevated estrogen and an elevated androgen syndrome, but don't be misled. The terms "elevated estrogen" or "excess estrogen" or "estrogen dominance" or "hyperestrogenic and hyperandrogenic" that some health writers use to describe PCOS refer to the elevated form of "estrogen" as a result of excess body fat.

Among my PCOS patients, women have a much *lower* than optimal estradiol level, and *have symptoms of estradiol decline,* even with higher estrone levels. Estradiol has a dramatically different effect in your body from estrone.

My research found only one report of polycystic ovarian disease with significantly elevated estradiol levels. In this case the plasma estradiol was so massively elevated, it suggested the presence of an estrogen-producing tumor, which is extremely rare.

The bottom line is that all estrogens are not alike. A thorough diagnostic evaluation, including detailed hormone testing of all ovarian hormones, is crucial.

Why PCOS Is Often Missed

Many physicians do not realize that PCOS has far-reaching and potentially devastating consequences, or causes early onset diabetes or heart disease.

Another reason PCOS is overlooked is that gynecologists have traditionally been taught lack of menstruation (called *amenorrhea*) is a hallmark of PCOS. If a woman is still having periods, she could not have PCOS.

We now know this is not correct.

Many women with PCOS still have periods, but they are irregular and don't produce optimal levels or the normal balance of ovarian hormones.

Infertility is the most common reason women with PCOS see a physician. But what if you are not trying to become pregnant?

Especially if you still have menstrual periods, you are likely to be overlooked in our current, fragmented approach to women's health, even though you may have all the *other* metabolic changes of PCOS.

Another difficulty is that traditionally, endocrinologists in this country haven't focused on the ovary, since this endocrine organ is the "turf" of gynecologists.

In the United States, endocrinologists focus on other endocrine disorders like thyroid and diabetes management. They rarely check ovarian hormones, especially estrogen levels.

Gynecologists, on the other hand, are trained as surgeons, and don't routinely check hormone levels. They aren't concerned about

Turf wars
This "split" of women's endocrine system meant different doctors addressed different body parts, which obviously makes it hard for a woman with PCOS to get properly diagnosed.

Not my problem
The problems caused by PCOS just haven't seemed as important in a busy obstetrical-surgical practice.

Just "moods"
The *brain* symptoms resulting from PCOS *hormone imbalances* are missed.

Treatments

that improve symptoms and help you feel better are similar, regardless of whether you have all or some of the findings.

Dismissed

Women with this very serious disorder are often discounted and simply told to "not worry, everybody misses periods sometimes" or "just go exercise and lose weight and your periods will come back. You'll be fine," or "just take this antidepressant or mood-stabilizer and you'll get better."

problems they perceive as being "just cosmetic" (waistline weight gain and excess facial hair).

The surgical training of gynecologists focuses on pregnancy and birth, on surgical approaches to correct gynecological problems like fibroids, endometriosis, and cancers.

PCOS also causes severe mood problems, typically evaluated and treated by psychiatrists. But in this country, psychiatrists are not taught much about the brain effects of ovarian hormone, and rarely check *any* hormone levels, much less the ovarian ones. Even worse, some of the commonly used "mood-stabilizer" medicines aggravate the hormone imbalances of PCOS.

So, what happens when all these specialty groups overlook the underlying metabolic changes in PCOS? Women with this very serious disorder are often discounted. This happened to a 35-year-old patient who then went on to have 3 heart attacks by the time she was 38, and almost died with the third one before I showed her the serious hormone imbalances from PCOS that had caused the problems.

I have another concern about PCOS: the very treatment of PCOS-induced infertility may itself cause more problems. International specialists in the field of climacteric (menopause) medicine have studies showing that drug treatments such as clomiphene citrate (Clomid) to stimulate ovulation, as well as laparoscopic ovarian treatments to remove cysts, can cause premature menopause and a higher risk of ovarian cancer later. Women with PCOS have a *double whammy*—they often need specialized treatment to get pregnant, and some of those treatments can lead to serious hormone imbalances later.

Do I Have PCOS? Getting Tested

Doctors who specialize in researching and treating PCOS are the first to tell you there is "no consensus" about tests and criteria to confirm the diagnosis.

But even if doctors can't agree on "diagnostic criteria," for the full-blown disorder, the abnormal findings can still wreak havoc on your hormone balance and health. Even mild forms of PCOS can cause a lot of damage.

I think that sometimes in medicine we get so hung up on "proof" of a diagnosis that we forget to focus on the *person* who is suffering and what we can do to help alleviate the suffering.

My point is that if you have the symptom and body changes, you need thorough testing and appropriate treatment. Here are the tests I think are important to do for a baseline evaluation to decide whether you may have PCOS:

Dr. Vliet's Guide to Laboratory Studies to Check for PCOS

- FSH, LH ratio (abnormal if shifted toward LH)
- Estradiol, estrone
- Free and total testosterone
- DHEA, DHEA-S
- Androstenedione
- SHBG
- 8 AM cortisol, and if elevated, 4 PM free cortisol or a 24 hour urinary free cortisol
- 17-OH progesterone—(to identify Congenital Adrenal Hyperplasia (CAH) or 21-hydroxylase deficiency).
- Prolactin
- IGF-1 (insulin-like growth factor—1, a marker for growth hormone)
- Fasting, two and three hour post-prandial glucose and insulin; or a 5 hour insulin response to glucose test
- Thyroid profile, including thyroid antibodies
- Comprehensive Metabolic Profile that includes tests of liver and kidney function, lipids (cholesterol, HDL, LDL, TG), complete blood counts, calcium, magnesium, iron and ferritin.

© 2001–2007 Elizabeth Lee Vliet, M.D.

Causes of PCOS

No one is certain what causes PCOS, but there are many proposed explanations, and we will likely find multiple causes that produce the same metabolic syndrome and disruption of normal hormone production.

- *genetic* factors
- *environmental* factors—endocrine disrupters like dioxin, PCBs, and many others (see Chapter 5)
- *autoimmune disorders—ovarian, adrenal, pancreatic and thyroid*
- *excess insulin production related to obesity-induced insulin resistance*
- *excess intake of substances such as excitatory amino acids* (see Chapter 4)
- *medications that increase prolactin*—such as serotonin boosters and others

I have discussed these in depth in my book, *The Savvy Woman's Guide to PCOS, The Many Faces of a 21st Century Epidemic…And What You Can Do About It.*

Look at Some Examples of Labs:

Characteristic abnormal hormone levels in PCOS are illustrated by some results from the 16-year old young woman I mentioned earlier. Her doctor told her to "just eat less and you'll lose weight." These are her lab values, with my observations:

Hormone Levels of 16 year-old PCOS patient:

Total testosterone 81 (ng/dl). Optimal for women is the 40–60 ng/dl range, but some women start excess hair growth at levels over 50, especially if DHEA is also too high.

No wonder
She didn't have a "female" hormone profile!

- **Free testosterone** 20 ng/dl; optimal is about 4 to 6 if total testosterone is in the desirable range
- **Free plus weakly bound testosterone** 37; optimal is about 10–15 if total testosterone is in the desirable range
- **DHEA** 1093; optimal about 200–400 for women
- **Estradiol** 32 (day 19); at this time of the menstrual cycle, estradiol should be about 200–250 pg/ml. This is seriously low especially in the face of such high levels of her androgens
- **8 AM cortisol** 25; healthy ranges at that time of day would be about 10–18.
- **NTx** (N-telopeptide, a marker of bone breakdown) 131: high, even for an adolescent, and this reflects her very low estradiol.

Her TSH, free T3, free T4, and thyroid antibodies were all excellent, so I did not think she had a thyroid disorder.

Sadly
Even mild forms of PCOS can cause a lot of damage.

When you see how severely out of balance her androgen/estradiol ratio is, it isn't hard to understand why she had severe cystic acne (face, chest, back, arms), marked facial and body hair, severe mood swings, irritability (excess testosterone can do that!), and severe insomnia.

I started her on Ovcon-35, a birth control pill that suppresses the ovaries' abnormal hormone production and also increases the SHBG that "binds up" excess free androgens. I also suggested spironolactone to help block androgen effects and also recommended a diet of 35% complex carbs, 35% protein and 30% fat, emphasizing more of the healthy vegetable oils, such as olive oil, instead of saturated fats.

Three months later, her total testosterone dropped to 25 ng/dl, free and weakly bound testosterone was 11, and free testosterone of 6. Her DHEA had come down to 400, and her 8 AM cortisol was now normal at 15. Since she was on the birth control pill that suppresses estradiol, I did not re-check estradiol at her first follow-up. I primarily wanted her androgens down to normal ranges.

Her acne cleared up nicely, her excess facial hair growth de-creased, and she described her mood as more stable. Her weight was no longer on the up escalator, and she felt like her body responding more normally to exercise and diet.

Individualization is critical. Effective overall management of the serious medical aspects of PCOS requires integrated treatment to restore hormone balance, reduce health risks, and improve how you feel.

Getting Help for PCOS: What Are Some Treatments?

I see a lot of women with PCOS and they are all ages, from menopausal women with complications from unrecognized PCOS when younger, to young girls only 10 or 11 but already developing body changes that suggest PCOS.

Most treatments are a process of fine-tuning various therapeutic ap-proaches. Sometimes this accomplished in a few months; for other women, it takes a year or more to find the right combination.

Appropriate treatment for PCOS depends on many variables. Some include age, whether you are trying to get pregnant now or want to preserve fertility for the future, whether you have other medical or gynecological problems, whether you have insulin resistance, or diabetes, and whether you have serious mood disturbances.

I do not provide specific evaluation or treatment for infertility in my office, although some of our patients have gone on to become pregnant once we addressed their metabolic and hor-monal imbalances. The subject of infertility is quite complex; see Chapter 14 for additional information.

Here are some general principles of medical and non-medical treatments to discuss with your own physicians.

Medication Approaches

Wisdom
Pills that have a steady dose formula every day (monophasic) typically have fewer adverse effects, especially on moods, than pills with varying hormone content (triphasic).

[handwritten margin note: Cancer nursing see p. 429]

Oral Contraceptives, or birth control pills (BCP)

BCP are one of the foundations of treatment, helping with several problems in PCOS. They suppress the abnormal cycling of the ovaries and help prevent cysts from forming. They improve the balance of estrogen and androgens by increasing SHBG, which then keeps more of the androgens in the bound, less active form, and decreases hirsutism and acne. They provide daily progestin that prevents excess thickening of the lining of the uterus from estrone (the estrogen in body fat) stimulation.

Over time, such thickening, called hyperplasia, can lead to an increased risk of uterine cancer. Taking the birth control pills can help preserve future fertility by preventing ovulation or loss of follicles at a time when you are not trying to get pregnant.

BCP also help prevent multiple cysts from forming, and damaging the ovaries further. I find that patients with PCOS do better using pills that have higher estrogen to progestin ratios, such as Ovcon 35, Modicon, Ortho-Cyclen, Yasmin, or Diane 35.

In my experience, high progestin pills with less estrogen (Loestrin, Alesse, Mircette) cause more of the negative progestin effects (weight gain, low libido, hair loss, acne, lethargy, headaches, depressed mood, abnormal glucose/insulin, high cholesterol and high triglycerides) that are already common in PCOS.

Warning!
Women with undiagnosed PCOS who take DHEA will commonly have more acne, facial and body hair, scalp hair loss, and weight gain.
Don't take DHEA!

[handwritten margin note: too much ... or + say ... no ...]

Ovarian Hormone Replacement Therapy

(See Chapter 16 for more about this). As a general comment now, I find the FDA-approved *bioidentical* forms of ovarian hormones, such as 17-beta estradiol or progesterone, cause fewer side effects, and yield more positive responses on the abnormal measures in PCOS. Women with PCOS already have higher than normal androgens (testosterone, DHEA, etc.), and generally do not need this added for therapy. *[handwritten note: See p. 429 ... use ... prog]*

Insulin-sensitizing Medication

Medicines that lower insulin and improve insulin response are effective in PCOS, both to address the metabolic imbalances, and also to help restore ovulatory cycles and fertility. Glucophage (metformin) and the glitazones Actos and Avandia are medicines approved for the treatment of diabetes that are commonly used in PCOS. Although none has yet been approved by the FDA specifically for PCOS, studies are underway and physicians report success using these medications in an integrated treatment program.

In a 1998 study published in *The New England Journal of Medicine*, 90 percent of the women who took metformin either ovulated spontaneously or with help from the fertility drug Clomid. Only 12 percent of the women taking a placebo pill had ovulatory cycles, even if they also took Clomid.

The Challenge
It is often quite a challenge to find the right combination of hormone and non-hormonal approaches to restore balance.

We still need more studies on the safety of these medications on a developing fetus, and women trying to get pregnant should discuss taking metformin with a fertility specialist. There was an encouraging study published in March 2002 in *Fertility and Sterility*. Researchers found a *10-fold* reduction in risk of gestational diabetes in women with PCOS who took metformin throughout pregnancy. This is a remarkable reduction in risk.

I use metformin successfully for many PCOS patients, and have found that it works well to reduce insulin resistance (and its complications) and facilitate weight loss in women who are not trying to become pregnant. Weight loss decreases many risk factors for both diabetes and heart disease.

Androgen-blocking Medications

Excess androgens cause a lot of unwanted effects in PCOS, so if this hormone imbalance doesn't respond to the medicines above, there are a number of other effective androgen blockers: *spironolactone* (50 to 200 mg daily), *flutamide* (125–500 mg daily), *finasteride* 5 mg daily, *cyproterone* acetate (2–50 mg daily).

Sometimes leuprolide, dexamethasone, or ketoconazole may be necessary, all of which suppress androgen production in the ovaries and adrenal glands.

These medicines have potentially serious side effects, so I generally use only if a woman hasn't responded to any other options. Since leuprolide (Lupron) suppresses estrogen, you need to replace estradiol to avoid menopausal symptoms.

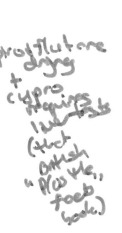

Mood-managing Medicines: Anxiolytics, Antidepressants, Anticonvulsants

The hormone imbalances of PCOS have many mood-disrupting effects, and can even mimic bipolar disorder, panic disorder or major depression. Look at all the brain effects of the ovarian hormones (see Chapter 12), and you quickly see how the hormone problems in PCOS can cause such serious mood symptoms. If you have significant mood symptoms, and body changes to suggest you have PCOS, have your hormones checked and PCOS treated before concluding that you have a psychiatric disorder and need "mood managing" medicines.

Caution
Excess testosterone can cause anxiety and agitation that is often mistaken for a psychiatric disorder.

For women with PCOS who are struggling with weight gain I do not recommend tricyclic antidepressants (Elavil, Pamelor, etc.), Remeron or Zyprexa, because these medicines stimulate appetite, cause weight gain, and increase the likelihood of insulin resistance and later diabetes. SSRIs can also cause weight gain if used in high doses over a long period of time.

A word of caution about Depakote (valproic acid). This medicine is used as a "mood-stabilizer" more and more often in younger women. I do not recommend this medication for women with possible PCOS, since recent studies report that it can actually cause PCOS in 40–50% of female patients treated with it, likely from its side effect of increasing prolactin production. It is not clear at this time whether other anticonvulsants (Tegretol, Dilantin, Neurontin, Lamictal, Topamax, etc.) have similar effects.

Feeling "blue"
Low estradiol can contribute to significant depression, and also anxiety.

Non-medication Approaches

The best success for getting PCOS under control and feeling your best is to incorporate a number of strategies: dietary balance, physical activity, stress management, vitamins and supplements.

These, working in concert with medicines to restore hormonal balance, help reduce your long-term health risks and improve energy level and mood.

Reducing foods that quickly turn to glucose (sweets, simple carbs like pastas and breads, etc.) will minimize the adverse effects of excess insulin and glucose intolerance.

Exercise improves insulin sensitivity and glucose control, so it is a critical component to reverse hormone imbalances.

I don't recommend herbs for hormone-related symptoms if you have PCOS. First, they aren't adequate to restore hormone balance. Second, many herbs act as phytoestrogens and can further impair the function of ovaries and thyroid.

Statistics show that women with PCOS often take multiple prescription medications, and *most herbs have the potential for significant drug-herb interactions* with oral contraceptives, menopausal hormone prescription medications, antidepressants, antianxiety medications, anticonvulsants, antibiotics and others.

For example, St. John's wort can decrease the effectiveness of birth control pills by 50% because of the herb's ability to increase metabolic breakdown of the hormones in the liver.

Adequate sleep and stress management are important parts of PCOS treatment. If insomnia persists talk to your doctor about sleep studies. Sleep apnea increases in women with PCOS because of the decline in estradiol levels and the increased body weight, especially in the upper abdomen, that impairs respiration at night.

Psychological support is also crucial. Women with PCOS often describe concerns about weight, body hair, mood changes, and other physical-psychological effects of PCOS that are not taken seriously in the usual health care settings.

I find women with PCOS often have intense feelings of anger about being ignored, about the diagnosis being missed, frustration with body changes feeling out of control, and feelings of grief if pregnancy is desired but unfulfilled. Support groups and individual therapy are helpful and provide an outlet for intense feelings.

You are more than just body; you are mind and spirit. Your physical and emotional needs are important and valid. You need physicians and health professionals who are competent, and also empathic, and caring. If you don't feel support from your current health professionals, seek new ones! You have the power, and right, to choose health partnerships that are mutually beneficial and helpful.

The Poignancy of PCOS: Women's Stories

Antonia illustrates over-medication when PCOS isn't diagnosed and treated as the metabolic-endocrine disorder it is. When she first came in, she was 27 years old, severely obese, with painful acne. She was so self-conscious that she rarely looked up when talking.

For several years, she was ballooning up and frightened by a body out of control. Her acne was impossible to control no matter what

Stop! If you have PCOS, and smoke cigarettes, STOP! PCOS alone can cause early heart attacks. If you add the damage from cigarette smoking, it is like gasoline on a fire.

Big picture PCOS can affect all dimensions of your life. *You are a person, not just a pelvis with reproductive problems.*

Diagnoses are imperfect

My view has always been that ultimately it doesn't really matter who is "right" and who is "wrong" with a diagnostic label. What matters is whether the medicines make someone better, or whether they aggravate underlying problems and make people worse.

Downward spiral

Her medication costs were astronomical, but even more frightening, many of the medicines were making her weight gain and hormone imbalances worse.

she tried. She had other troubling symptoms for someone so young: hot flashes, insomnia, fibromyalgia-type muscle pain, anxiety that became worse with her periods, daily tension headaches, migraine episodes, severe fatigue, daytime sleepiness—especially after meals, inability to concentrate, and shortness of breath that made her fear a lung problem.

When I saw her, she was being treated by multiple specialists: a primary care physician, a neurologist for the migraines, a pain specialist for the daily headaches, a rheumatologist for the muscle pain, a psychiatrist for the anxiety, a pulmonary specialist to check for asthma, and her gynecologist who said her pelvic and Pap smears were normal, and she didn't have a hormone imbalance —she just needed to lose weight.

No hormone levels were checked by anyone.

When I checked the levels, *the results were staggering.* Her estradiol was markedly low; all of the androgens were seriously elevated, especially the free testosterone; her cortisol was elevated (another factor adding to her weight gain); her fasting and two-hour insulin and glucose levels were both elevated; and she had a high LH to FSH ratio.

In short, she had all the classic indicators of PCOS. I felt sad that no one, out of all those doctors, had ever considered or checked her hormone levels, especially since her body shape and symptoms were such strong warning signals of PCOS, and such risk factors for diabetes.

By the time of her appointment with me, Antonia took **thirteen** medicines every day: a sleeping pill, two muscle relaxants, several pain meds, two mood-stabilizers, Prozac and a tricyclic antidepressant, two anti-anxiety medicines, and a beta blocker.

Tricyclics, added to use of SSRIs, can increase appetite, especially for carbs, which then increases insulin resistance. Beta-blockers make the insulin resistance worse as well, and can contribute to shortness of breath from effects on lungs and heart. Beta-blockers also interfere with normal thyroid function, contributing to weight gain, low energy, and depressed mood.

Klonopin for anxiety and insomnia make her tired and sleepy during the day. *It was a medication nightmare.*

Turning this around would be a long struggle, because it could take a year or more to improve the hormonal balance and see which medicines could be gradually tapered off. Sadly, I only saw her a few times and never got to help her turn it around, because she was told by so many other professionals that her problems were not hormonal, and that I was wrong.

Nightmare She was trapped in the hormonal quicksand of PCOS and the quagmire of medication side effects.

In her case, she wasn't getting better on all those medicines, and each had effects well-documented in the medical literature. Her headaches weren't controlled, she still had trouble sleeping, and she was still gaining weight and suffering from acne and excess facial hair.

Jodie was 39 when I first saw her. Her hormone evaluation showed abnormal levels characteristic of PCOS. We worked with her over a number of months to restore a healthier hormone balance.

But there is a part of her story *before* I saw her that gives me goosebumps every time I think about it. If you think people are silly to believe in God and guardian angels, her experience may convince you otherwise.

Her first heart attack was at age 36. She was 39 when I saw her, she had already suffered *three* serious heart attacks and almost died during the third one.

In fact, the cardiologist had told her husband she would not likely come out of the coma because her heart simply wasn't pumping enough blood, she wasn't responding to medications, and there was nothing else to try.

What happened next was quite touching, and very meaningful to me. Two friends of Jodie's, one a patient of mine, took a copy of my previous book that described the effects of estradiol on the heart to Jodie's husband at the hospital where she was in ICU, in a coma. The doctors had told Jodie's family that it was "only a matter of time" before she died.

Jodie's husband said, *"She always thought her heart attacks had something to do with her hormones, and asked many doctors about it, but they always told her it couldn't be. This is amazing."*

But Jodie and her friends had discussed something that no one thought important: Jodie's heart attacks always happened at the start of her menstrual period, a time when estradiol drops sharply, which can cause spasm and reduced blood flow in the coronary arteries to the heart.

The two women showed the page in *Screaming to Be Heard* to Jodie's husband. Right away, they went to the cardiologist and showed him the page describing estradiol's effect on the arteries to improve blood flow. They asked if he would be willing to put an estradiol patch on Jodie. The cardiologist read the material

Remarkable

I was amazed at the progress after her near-death experience.

and said, *"Nothing else is working, we have nothing to lose. We may as well try it. It certainly won't hurt her."*

To everyone's surprise and relief, including the doctor's, Jodie's condition improved. Her "ejection fraction" (a measure of the blood being pumped by the heart) was critically low and not improving on the other medicines.

Within a few hours after the Climara estradiol patch was put on, the ejection fraction began increasing significantly. Slowly she came out of the coma as her heart function improved. Her doctor continued the estradiol patch during the rest of her hospitalization, amazed at the changes. She was finally discharged, though she still had a long recovery from the damage to her heart. She wrote her story as she scheduled her first consult with me.

Jodie's legacy

"I want to help other women understand PCOS and get proper evaluation before someone else goes through what I did."

I reviewed her serum hormone levels and showed her *why* the estradiol patch had helped so much. Her own menstrual Day 1 estradiol was barely detectable, and her free and total testosterone and DHEA were all quite high, as were her total and LDL cholesterol, triglycerides and insulin. The low estradiol, coupled with high androgens, high cholesterol with a high LDL and low HDL and her high insulin, set her up for heart attacks. I explained that our goal was to keep her estradiol as steady as possible using an estradiol patch during bleeding days, and then decrease the androgens, improve her cholesterol profile, and decrease the excess insulin.

She did exceptionally well on her hormone and dietary plan for another 7 years, able to be an active mom and involved with her children and her life again. She lost weight and returned to moderate exercise. She became an avid spokesperson in Internet support groups for PCOS.

Heart Attack!

Low estradiol leads to coronary vasospasm that can seriously decrease blood flow to the heart muscle.

Sadly, she died at 47, a sudden heart attack from all the earlier damage. Her family, while deeply saddened, said they were so grateful for the gift of an extra 7 years, so she could live long enough to see her children graduate from high school.

Body Fat Promoters: Glucose Intolerance/Hypoglycemia, Insulin Resistance, and Diabetes

If you have sudden, inexplicable weight gain or "creeping corpulence," feel so tired and draggy you can't get through the day, are overcome by sleep attacks after lunch, or have wicked mood swings, you may have one of the metabolic problems that often accompany ovarian hormone imbalances.

"Syndrome X" is the name most often given to this cluster of insulin-glucose imbalances that occur in women with greater frequency as their estradiol declines. Syndrome X is a metabolic-endocrine syndrome with many similarities to PCOS, and may actually share some of the root causes.

Syndrome X-type findings in young girls is another ominous sign of environmental and dietary endocrine disruptors that are now more of a problem for infants and children. These chemicals that I talked about earlier serve to set the stage for abnormal weight gain in childhood and then at puberty for girls, an increased production of androgens that make the metabolic effects even worse.

What are these conditions, and what can you do about them? Let's explore these questions.

How Glucose is Regulated: The See-Saw of Insulin and Glucagon

Glucose and oxygen are such critical fuels for the brain's survival that the body keeps tight control on levels. Glucose changes can have severe consequences so the body has ways to keep glucose from "swinging" to dangerous extremes, high or low. Insulin and glucagon are the two major regulators of the glucose to keep it in healthy ranges.

When these two hormones work normally, insulin keeps blood glucose levels from rising too high (*hyperglycemia*), and glucagon prevents blood glucose from dropping too low (*hypoglycemia*).

Insulin serves to lower glucose levels by moving it from the blood into muscle cells where it burns to provide immediate energy, and by moving it into fat cells where it is stored as fat for future energy needs.

Glucagon has the opposite effect: it stimulates the liver and muscle cells to break down stored glycogen and send the glucose molecules rushing out of the cell into the bloodstream to raise blood sugar when levels drop too low.

In addition to actual high or low blood glucose levels, the rate of rise and fall in glucose is a crucial factor that can also lead to the hypoglycemic symptoms, and trigger insulin and glucagon release.

Natural see-saw Insulin and glucagon are called the "counter-regulatory hormones," acting in opposite ways, much like a see-saw.

As we get fatter, however, insulin and glucagon don't work as well, so our body has difficulty keeping blood sugar in the healthy range. We develop problems like hypoglycemia (low blood sugar), glucose intolerance (rapid rises and abrupt falls), insulin resistance (excess insulin and decreased sensitivity to insulin), and Diabetes Mellitus (sustained high blood glucose).

How do these relate to weight gain, middle spread, mood swings, and flagging energy for girls and women of any age?

Cause

The *rate* of fall is more important in triggering symptoms than is the actual blood level.

Hypoglycemia and Glucose Intolerance

Hypoglycemia, or "low blood sugar," usually goes hand in hand with something called *glucose intolerance*, the body's difficulty handling glucose and other sugars normally. Both are common in the early stages before diabetes develops.

Hypoglycemia is officially defined as a blood glucose level below 50 mg/dl, but you can have *symptoms* of hypoglycemia at levels above that if glucose falls rapidly.

It's similar to a smoke detector that doesn't distinguish between the serious smoke of a fire and the expected smoke of cooking. It sends out an alarm for both. If the steak on the stove sends up smoke faster, it will set off the alarm before a smoldering couch fire does.

Steps to Disaster

Think of each of these "conditions" as steps along a path from normal to diabetic.

Since glucose is so critical for brain cell survival, our brain has sensors that warn us of a dip in adequate glucose supplies, from either a rapidly *falling* glucose or an actual low level.

This is why diabetics sometimes check blood sugar when they have symptoms of hypoglycemia, only to find that the level is high. They have likely experienced a high glucose level that falls and sets off the brain alarm, even though the actual level is still *above* normal.

This is also the same way you experience symptoms of hypoglycemia only a short while after eating. Too much insulin, triggered by too much simple or refined carbohydrate food, causes glucose levels to fall too fast, even though glucose may not drop below 50, the magic number for a hypoglycemia "diagnosis."

Many physicians don't realize that a rapidly falling glucose can trigger a hypoglycemic "fight-or-flight" reaction, even though the glucose doesn't drop below 50.

This problem is common in glucose intolerance and insulin resistance when you have a tendency to "swing" between blood sugar levels being too high after you eat, followed by rapidly falling or low levels 2–4 hours later.

It is an early warning of problems regulating glucose. You could be on the way to developing diabetes. This situation should be a clue that you need to have glucose-insulin levels checked after eating (*post prandial*) as well as fasting.

Falling glucose can cause food cravings and anxious, panicky feelings.

Insulin Resistance, or Syndrome X

Insulin is a major *anabolic* (tissue-building) hormone of metabolism, governing many aspects of glucose regulation, body fat storage and many other functions. Unlike the anabolic effects of testosterone that build muscle and bone, insulin is an anabolic hormone that *builds fat.*

Insulin actually works to increase the *ratio of fat to muscle*, so the more insulin stimulation you have, the lower the ratio of your *fat-burning* muscle cells.

You must have some insulin to get the glucose from the bloodstream to the cells that must have it as fuel to live. Glucose must also get to the fat cells to be stored as triglycerides for your body's later energy needs. This is why diabetics who don't make insulin must take it as shots, or in an insulin pump or new nasal spray. But too much insulin isn't good.

Insulin balance Excess insulin is a serious problem, but lack of insulin can lead to death.

The excess insulin makes your body excel at storing excess fat, and less effective at allowing fat stores to convert to energy for muscles and the rest of the body. Each day this pattern repeats. You get fatter, and fatter and fatter while you eat less and less and less.

Normally, when glucose is rising, insulin is produced in order to move the glucose out of the bloodstream for use by muscle or storage as fat. Insulin levels are supposed to then quickly drop back down to baseline after it has done its job.

Early warning In case you've been told you don't have these problems because your glucose is "normal," that's not always true.

But as we gain body fat, the insulin receptors don't work as well. The cells become distorted in shape and size and this causes the receptor site (like a lock) for insulin, to get out of proper alignment. As a result, the insulin molecule "key" no longer fits easily into the receptor "lock." This impairs insulin response.

When this happens, glucose levels remain high after you eat because the insulin, even though present, isn't working well. Your brain sensors detect continuing high glucose levels, and signals

Fat promoter
Insulin is a potent promoter of fat storage (lipogenesis) and a potent inhibitor of fat breakdown (lipolysis).

the pancreas to release even *more* insulin to bring glucose down. Your bloodstream and cells become flooded with insulin.

Then suddenly, when all this insulin starts working, the glucose rushes into the cells, and your blood glucose level plummets.

We call this response "*reactive hypoglycemia*" (low blood sugar), and when it happens you feel ravenously hungry and also tend to feel shaky, sweaty, nauseous, lightheaded, experience fuzzy thinking and heart palpitations along with racing pulse.

Such a drop in blood sugar creates intense food cravings, especially for sweets. As soon as you give in, however, the whole cycle starts over.

A rapid rise in glucose makes you lethargic, sleepy, and unfocused. Then when the glucose falls too fast from the excess insulin, you feel sweaty, anxious, irritable, weepy, and foggy brained. *Menstrual cycle hormone changes accentuate this pattern.*

A hit to the brain
Rate of *fall* in glucose is more critical in triggering symptoms than is the actual *blood levels*.

Insulin resistance refers to this entire pattern—high levels of both insulin and glucose in the bloodstream and excess insulin causing glucose to be stored as fat instead of used for immediate energy.

Since the insulin isn't working properly to deliver a steady supply of glucose to working muscle cells, the effect is the same as not getting enough food. The cells are not getting their fuel, so you get hunger signals and eat more, even though plenty of fuel (glucose) is circulating in the bloodstream. What's worse is that your fat cells are also screaming for more food.

Insulin resistance's host of body-wrecking effects:

- ૐ impaired immune function making you more susceptible to infections
- ૐ increased build-up of the smooth muscle in artery walls that narrows the passage for blood flow, leading to reduced flow to critical organs

Prevention
Our natural estradiol helps prevent excess platelet "stickiness" and lowers risk of serious blood clots.

- ૐ plaque build-up in the arteries also narrows the passage for blood flow, leading to strokes and heart attacks, even in younger women (as we see in PCOS)
- ૐ more platelet stickiness leading to increased risk of clots
- ૐ later, increased risk of breast cancer

With all these damaging effects on the blood vessels, excess insulin is now considered a risk factor for heart disease and early heart attacks, particularly when estradiol is too low.

With optimal levels of estradiol, we are less likely to have problems with insulin resistance because the estradiol improves insulin response in the cells.

Tank seems empty! It's like you have a leak in a gas line. You keep filling the tank (eating), the fuel never gets to the engine so it can work.

But estradiol loss is not the only way our ovaries are involved in this insulin pathway. Researchers have found insulin receptors in the ovary. Insulin acts at the ovarian receptors to change the enzymes so they make more *androgens* rather than the normal estradiol-estrone balance.

Higher androgens then feed back to the glucose regulating hormones and cause more insulin production. Higher insulin levels stimulate more androgen production in the ovary. This is a major cause of the marked weight gain in young women with PCOS or Syndrome X.

A milder form of this imbalance occurs in perimenopausal women who are losing estradiol and "unmasking" the effects of their androgens (DHEA, testosterone, androstenedione). As you shift toward more androgen effects and away from the normal estradiol balance, more body fat builds around your waist and deep inside the abdomen (visceral fat), similar to males.

Listen up, Doc! PCOS rarely gets treated as early as it should.

Low fat, high carbohydrate diets stimulate more insulin production by the pancreas and make this worse. More insulin pushes the body to store more abdominal fat. More abdominal fat then makes more insulin resistance.

Dr. Vliet's Guide to Causes of Excess Insulin

Excess insulin can happen no matter what your age. Here are some of the most crucial ones for women:

- constant dieting with the wrong kind of foods, eating more high carbohydrate foods, and/or eating big meals late in the day
- increased stress with high cortisol
- loss of estradiol, excess progesterone
- high free testosterone relative to estradiol
- high levels of DHEA
- disrupted sleep and/or altered sleep-wake cycles, such as getting up at noon and staying up until 2:00 or 3:00 in the morning
- declining thyroid function
- less physical activity

© 2001-2007 Elizabeth Lee Vliet, M.D.

Diabetes Mellitus

Diabetes is the third leading cause of death in the US, as well as the third most expensive to treat. More importantly, diabetes disproportionately affects women in over 50% of the cases, with some 8 million women of all ages suffering its ravages. Diabetes is alarmingly more common as Americans get fatter, and is a woefully under-recognized medical problem, especially in younger women. Yet, most women fear breast cancer more.

Gender "thing"
Type 2 diabetes, caused by excess body fat, is far more common in women.

Diabetes robs you of your energy, memory, sight, and kidney function. It can cause nerve damage, severe pain in the hands and feet, depression, dementia, amputation of limbs, loss of sexual response, and early heart attacks, strokes and premature death. Diabetes attacks the tiny end arteries throughout the body that provide blood to cells. This is the reason complications of diabetes are diverse and affect many different organs. Diabetes must be treated early, and aggressively to prevent these complications.

Wise brain
Your brain and body haven't read textbook definitions, they just know what they need!

In the past, most diabetes began in adulthood as an outgrowth of obesity. That's why it used to be called adult-onset diabetes. That name is no longer valid. This form is now called non-insulin dependent diabetes mellitus (NIDDM) or Type II diabetes to distinguish it from insulin dependent or Type I diabetes, previously called juvenile onset diabetes.

Diabetes is a greater problem for women than men for two reasons: (1) more women of all ages get diabetes, and (2) women tend to have more severe and more frequent diabetic complications. Women have smaller arteries than men, so diabetes damages arteries throughout the body faster.

Tragic
Today we see a truly alarming rise in "adult form" diabetes in children and teenagers.

Depression is also more common in women, and in women with diabetes, depression occurs three times more frequently.

Women get another hit: certain antidepressants, such as tricyclics, can cause even higher blood sugars, memory loss, a marked increase in carbohydrate craving, and more weight gain—all making the diabetes worse.

The *wrong* choice of birth control pill (e.g. high progestin pills) or the wrong type of hormone therapy can aggravate weight gain, impair glucose control, and cause more yeast infections that are already more prevalent in women with diabetes.

Osteopenia and osteoporosis are also more common in diabetics because high levels of glucose lead to decreased bone-building, decreased response to the parathyroid hormone, and decreased response to a type of vitamin D needed to build healthy bone.

Loss of optimal estradiol, for whatever cause, at whatever age, is one more factor that increases the risk of diabetes. Estradiol actually *improves* our sensitivity to insulin, and makes us *less likely* to become glucose intolerant and insulin resistant. Estradiol also prevents the excess androgen effects that aggravate insulin resistance, and estradiol acts as an antioxidant to prevent the cell-damaging effects of excess glucose.

Optimal estradiol also counteracts the dangerous effects of excess glucose on blood platelets. Excess glucose makes platelets stickier and more likely to clot. When you lose estradiol, and also have elevated glucose, both factors increase platelet "stickiness" and clumping that may lead to clots and stroke.

Eating a high carbohydrate diet makes this problem even worse: one Harvard study found that women aged 38–63 who ate a diet high in refined (simple) carbohydrates had a 40% greater risk of heart attack or stroke than did women with a diet lower in refined carbohydrate.

Diabetes complications can begin years before the disease is actually diagnosed, so you must watch for early signs of glucose intolerance, get tested and treated. See Chapter 17 for suggested tests and treatment approaches.

Caution
These may sound like problems for older women, but believe me, young women are not immune. Remember, Jodie was in her 30s.

In Summary

Insulin resistance, PCOS, Syndrome X, and Diabetes all disrupt normal ovarian hormone balance, affect millions of women, causing untold pain and suffering, disability and early death.

These conditions must be recognized and treated when you are younger, *before* you have developed serious disease or permanent complications.

The good news is that PCOS and all the disorders in this chapter are treatable problems *if recognized* and treated early with an *integrated* approach.

PCOS and Syndrome X desperately need careful attention by you and your physicians. If you have body changes like I have

No more! About 80—90 percent of the time when women have irregular periods, increased body/face hair, abnormal weight gain and elevated androgens, PCOS is the overlooked culprit.

described, or suspect an imbalance in any of these hormone systems, get evaluated properly.

Seek out a physician who is experienced in these problems disorder and will help you get answers. You do not have to put up with feeling lousy and missing out on your life.

If you are not satisfied with your physician's evaluation, don't hesitate to get a second opinion. Addressing these hormonal imbalances in young women prevents many of the chronic weight and health problems commonly seen today. There are answers and help available.

There is no need to wait another 10 or 15 years to address the situation, as *Noel*, a 28-year-old patient with PCOS and insulin resistance happily found out.

With a change in her birth control pill and the addition of Glucophage, spironolactone and a higher protein meal plan, she exclaimed,

"I didn't realize how messed up I was until I got better. I had adapted to all those symptoms and didn't realize how bad it was. I am eating better, I don't crave carbohydrates like I did, my body is reshaping, I am less heavy on top, I see my waist coming back, my headaches are almost gone, and I am not as depressed and foggy-brained as I was. I feel so encouraged, Finally I have hope for a healthier future."

Chapter 14
The Many Faces of Infertility: Overlooked Factors

There are few things more poignant and painful than a couple who fervently want a child, only to find that they cannot conceive. Advances in assisted reproductive technologies can solve the problem of infertility for some. Yet it is an expensive, challenging, and emotional hormonal roller coaster for those who take this route. It has, unfortunately, a lower success rate than we would like.

I am not a fertility specialist, and do not evaluate or treat infertility. Infertility is a huge, complex subject; an in-depth discussion of is far beyond both the space available and my expertise.

In the course of my hormone work over the years, however, I have identified subtle imbalances in ovarian, thyroid and adrenal hormones that contribute to infertility. Once restored to healthy hormone levels, a number of my patients conceived without further treatments.

From my clinical experiences, I will share some common, often overlooked, causes of infertility that you can discuss with your own physicians. Some are overlooked in traditional fertility centers because the standard medical school curriculum doesn't teach future physicians these connections. Others are lifestyle factors that doctors sometimes forget to address, or assume that most women know.

The three major areas that intersect my hormone work with infertility are (1) Subtle imbalances in ovarian hormones, (2) subclinical thyroid imbalances, and (3) "endocrine disruptors" in herbs, supplements, our environment, lifestyles and eating habits. (See Chapters in Section II for more information).

Subtle saboteurs
Watch for hidden "fertility "disruptors" in your food, drink and lifestyle.

Fact
Even when you are given a "diagnosis" to explain infertility, you can still have other factors that *also* contribute to the problem.

Since fertility declines significantly beginning about age 27, the older you are, the more important all of these other fertility "saboteurs" become.

Alert

With something as complex as infertility, you must thoroughly eliminate or reduce as many "disruptors" as possible.

The factors discussed here, coupled with those identified by your physician, have an *additive* effect to lower your fertility. Identify as many as possible and remember that some of the same factors for women may also cause lower than normal testosterone levels, sperm counts and/or sperm viability for men.

This is particularly true of the chemicals discussed in chapter five, as well as the adverse effects of alcohol, cigarette or marijuana use. If you have any fertility saboteurs, and the man's sperm is also less than optimal, the combined effect means your fertility as a couple is even lower than either one of you alone.

Subclinical Thyroid Fertility Saboteurs

The thyroid has a crucial role in regulating normal ovarian function and hormone production, so healthy thyroid function is critical to fertility. This section highlights key thyroid issues related specifically to infertility. (See Chapter 9 and 17 for more information on the thyroid).

Undiagnosed Thyroiditis

Women have far higher rates of thyroiditis than do men, and a telltale symptom is often "unexplained" infertility. Most fertility centers check for clinically evident hypothyroidism with a TSH and the standard tests of total T3 and T4 hormones.

Fact

If the TSH is "normal," meaning anywhere between 0.5 to 5.0, testing for thyroid antibodies is rarely done.

Therein lies two problems. One is that "normal" TSH for women trying to conceive is actually between 0.5 to 2.0; women with TSH in the higher end of normal range may have enough impairment of thyroid that they don't become pregnant.

The second problem is that TSH can be normal, but the antibodies are markedly elevated and interfere with thyroid function at the cellular level.

Studies report elevated antibodies in the range of 10–50% in patients with various "vague" clinical symptoms, including infertility, even though TSH is still normal.

For women, elevated thyroid antibodies lead to subclinical thyroid dysfunction—hypo or hyper—and can disrupt the extraordinary precision of the brain-ovarian pathways just enough to impair fertility, even before the TSH has reached the standard, arbitrary, cutoff points that "officially" diagnose hypothyroidism or hyperthyroidism.

You must have a test of the two primary thyroid antibodies, antithyroglobulin and antimicrosomal (also called anti-thyroidperoxidase or anti-TPO), to detect the early subclinical stage of autoimmune thyroiditis.

Suboptimal Thyroid Hormone Replacement

A corollary of the first thyroid "saboteur" of fertility is diagnosing a hypothyroid condition, and then not giving quite enough thyroid medication to return to an optimal range for fertility.

Also keep in mind, excess thyroid hormone can also impair fertility. When treating thyroid conditions in women who are trying to conceive, I adjust the dose until TSH is in the range of about 0.5 to 2.0 for optimal, safe thyroid hormone replacement. (See Chapter 17 for further discussion).

Alert
Recent studies show that TSH levels above 2.0 indicate less than optimal thyroid replacement for fertility in women.

Foods and Medicines that Diminish Thyroid Function

There are a number of medications commonly prescribed for women that can decrease T4 conversion to the more active form of thyroid hormone, T3. Examples are glucocorticoids (such as Prednisone) used for asthma or autoimmune disorders and beta-blockers (such as Inderal or propanolol) used in younger women for migraine headache prevention or to treat palpitations from mitral valve prolapse.

Soy isoflavones, the current darling of supplements for women with menstrual, PMS or menopause problems also block T4 to T3 conversion.

Warning
Many medicines can affect thyroid balance, and in turn affect fertility.

Red clover isoflavones, such as found in Promensil and other over-the-counter products, have similar adverse thyroid effects, as do foods high in phytates.

Coumestrol, a phytoestrogen found in many fruits, grains, and coffee, is associated with reduced ovulation and increased early pregnancy loss of the embryos in mice when fed amounts even as low as 100 parts per billion.

High phytoestrogen exposure in sheep caused cycle abnormalities, infertility, and early embryo loss; phytoestrogens also cause reproductive abnormalities in rats.

Action
If you take any of the medicines I listed, talk with your doctor about checking the *free* T3 and *free* T4.

Some medications increase the amount of thyroid binding globulin (TBG), the thyroid hormone carrier protein in the bloodstream, which in turn means less thyroid hormone in the free, and therefore active, portion.

If you are taking thyroid hormones, these medication factors must be taken into account in adjusting the dose up or down as needed.

For example, birth control pills increase TBG and decrease the free active hormone, which means you might need a slight dose increase of thyroid to eliminate hypothyroid symptoms.

Heroin or methadone use also increases TBG and may aggravate hypothyroidism as well as impair fertility in other ways. TBG is also increased by tamoxifen, 5-flurouracil, clofibrate, and perphenazine.

Excess androgens (such as testosterone or DHEA) and high cortisol (stress, remember?) both decrease TBG, as do corticosteroids such as prednisone. When taking these hormones, you may actually become a little hyperthyroid from the increase in free thyroid hormones and your doctor may need to slightly decrease your dose to stay in the desirable range.

Salicylates (found in aspirin and many foods) and non-steroidal anti-inflammatory medicines (common ones are Advil, Aleve, Motrin and many others) may decrease the binding of T4 to thyroid binding globulin, which also means *more T4 in the free, active phase.*

Other common, often overlooked, factors can affect thyroid balance, which in turn affects ovaries, so pay close attention to all of these if you are trying to conceive. See Chapters 9 & 17 for more information.

Dieting Disruptors of Your Thyroid

Diets either too low in protein or too low in carbohydrate, as well as too low in total calories, also impair the thyroid gland's ability to make T3 from T4. Dieting causes the body to prepare for famine rather than pregnancy, so it shifts more of the active, free thyroid hormones into the "stored," inactive protein-bound form.

This shift makes you *functionally* hypothyroid, even if all the tests appear "normal." These changes are the body's protective responses against having too little fuel to run its systems. (See Chapter 7 for more detail.)

Iodine deficiency is another dietary contributor to subtle thyroid dysfunction. We are taught that iodine deficiency doesn't exist in the United States any longer, since the advent of iodized salt. But let's look closer.

More and more women today completely cut out added salt in their diet and eat more low salt foods, especially those in their reproductive years who are watching their weight or making dietary changes to relieve PMS.

In addition, most of the mid-western states make up the "goiter belt," so called because of high rates of hypothyroidism due to iodine-deficient soils. If the soil doesn't contain enough iodine, that means vegetables grown in the soil can't absorb adequate iodine either.

The thyroid gland is critically dependent upon the right balance of iodine to function normally. This is true even if you take thyroid medication.

Many good multivitamins contain iodine, but far too many women in their reproductive years still don't take a multivitamin every day. And if you are significantly deficient, even a multivitamin may not be adequate.

Ovarian Hormone Imbalances

Premature decline in estradiol

Once again, young women can have less than optimal estradiol due to many causes, even when progesterone levels are still in the healthy, normal range.

Optimal levels of estradiol are needed in the first half of the menstrual cycle to "prime" the ovary for a healthy "egg" at ovulation in the second half of the cycle. Optimal estradiol is needed to prime the endometrial lining of the uterus to create a receptive "nest" for the fertilized egg to implant and grow.

Alert!
If your TSH is in the target range and you still have symptoms of hypo-thyroidism, check to see that your iodine intake is optimal.

Tip
"Hostile" mucus is caused by a number of factors, but insufficient estradiol is a fairly simple one to correct.

Estradiol is also needed to produce enough, and the right type, of cervical mucus around ovulation, creating a favorable environment for sperm. With the optimal rise in estradiol in the first half of your cycle, cervical mucus increases over tenfold, and changes to a clear, stretchy, more liquid, and alkaline make-up so sperm survive during their journey from vagina to Fallopian tube to penetrate the egg.

Fact

PCOS is the number one cause of infertility in women and the most common endocrine disorder in women of reproductive age.

Some fertility specialists suggest that if follicular phase estradiol levels are too low, women can wear a low dose estradiol patch (usually 0.025 to 0.05 mg) for cycle days 10 to 14 to improve cervical mucus and growth of the uterine lining. You need to know your serum hormone levels to determine treatments that may be helpful.

After ovulation, the rise in progesterone once again changes the cervical mucus to become thicker and more viscous, which provides a barrier to bacteria that might harm a developing fertilized egg. Once pregnant, you need optimal levels of both estradiol and progesterone to maintain the early part before the placenta form and takes over its hormone-producing role.

Blood levels of estradiol and progesterone can be checked and your fertility doctor can suggest options to keep the hormone levels optimal.

Overlooking PCOS and Excess Androgens

PCOS is also most overlooked, under-diagnosed endocrine disorder in younger women. See Chapter 13, or my book, *The Savvy Woman's Guide to PCOS,* for detailed information.

Warning!

Don't use OTC progesterone or wild yam creams if you are trying to get pregnant. They can disrupt cycles even more.

PCOS wrecks havoc with your entire endocrine system; causing excess production of testosterone, DHEA and estrone along with lower than optimal levels of estradiol and progesterone. These imbalances lead to erratic or non-existent ovulation and irregular cycles.

Women with PCOS have excess insulin and cortisol levels that interfere with fertility by many different pathways, including adverse effects on the thyroid. About 60% of PCOS patients also have elevated prolactin, which suppresses fertility. If women's hormone levels aren't checked completely, PCOS and other causes of excess androgens that impair fertility are often missed.

Progesterone excess, use of OTC progesterone creams

This may surprise you. After all, doesn't progesterone help pregnancy? Yes. But there's a catch. Progesterone helps pregnancy only *in the right balance* with estradiol. Over-the-counter progesterone cream for "improving fertility" may be treating the wrong problem. Many types of hormone imbalances create symptoms similar to those often listed in popular media as caused by "progesterone-deficiency/estrogen dominance."

Some progesterone creams available over the counter actually have so much progesterone that regular use can actually suppress ovaries and lead to even less production of estradiol.

Don't "self-medicate" with these widely touted progesterone creams if you are trying to get pregnant. If you need hormones, do it under the guidance of a reputable specialist who can oversee an integrated approach to infertility, after checking hormone levels properly.

Endocrine Disruptors in Your Lifestyle and Habits

Dieting, especially extremely low fat diets, high soy diets

Overly restrictive dieting is so basic, and yet so often overlooked as a factor contributing to ovarian suppression and infertility. All of our ovarian sex hormones and adrenal steroid hormones are made from the building block cholesterol. If you cut back fat to below about 20% of your total daily calories, there is not enough for the liver to make cholesterol to then be turned into critical hormones.

If you are trying to get pregnant, you need about 25–30% of your daily calories from fat, preferably the healthy, unsaturated vegetable oils.

You'd have to be a hermit to miss all the ads exclaiming soy's fabulous phytoestrogen load—**but did you realize that all these phytoestrogens compete with your own ovarian hormones at receptor sites and prevent your own hormones from working properly?**

A number of current studies have shown that a diet high in soy caused decreases from 20–50% in ovarian production of both estradiol and progesterone. This is a critical overlooked point in all the media hype about soy today. This effect of soy on hormone production explains why vegetarians have a higher frequency of

Warning

Avoid high intake of flaxseed, soy, herbs and other phyto-estrogens if you are trying to get pregnant.

Caution

Vegetarians with a high intake of phyto-estrogens have more irregular menstrual cycles, lower ovarian hormone levels, and decreased frequency of ovulation.

irregular menstrual cycles than women who eat animal sources of protein. You can easily control these fertility disruptors in your diet. See Chapter 4 and 18 for more detail.

Yes!
You *can* be *too thin* to become pregnant.

Excessive Thinness

You have heard the saying that you can never be too rich or too thin. When it comes to fertility, you can definitely be too thin. The rail-thin bodies of today's celebrities are emulated by young women, yet worldwide studies in various ethnic groups show that women's fertility is impaired when body fat drops below 20–22% of total body mass. Mother Nature meant for women to have extra fat as fuel stores to support a pregnancy in case of food scarcity, so our fertility suffers if we lose too much fat. Keep your weight and body fat in a healthy range.

Obesity

Yes
Obesity can *also* cause infertility.

Obesity also impairs fertility, in part from insulin resistance, and in part from increased production of androgens and estrone in the body fat, as well as other pathways. The more obese a woman, the less likelihood of her becoming pregnant and the higher her chances of miscarriage. Although I certainly empathize with the difficulties of losing excess weight, it is worth the time, energy and effort to invest in a healthy weight loss program if trying to get pregnant. Weight loss provides a more optimal hormonal environment of the body to sustain a pregnancy. See Chapter 13.

Too much exercise

Excess exercise suppresses ovarian cycles, hormone production and can impair fertility (see Chapter 8). If you have trouble getting pregnant, talk with your physician or exercise physiologist about decreasing the frequency and intensity of your exercise workouts to a lower level, such as 3–4 days a week.

Walk briskly for 20–40 minutes rather than a high intensity stair-climbing for 90 minutes or jogging 5 or more miles a day six days a week!

Excess stress, and sleep deprivation

Women burn the candle at both ends today, living hectic lives that cause increased cortisol, reduced ovarian function, decreased deep sleep at night, and decreased Growth Hormone production at night. And these are just a *few* of the adverse metabolic effects.

See Chapter 7 for more in-depth explanations about the effects of stress and how to avoid it.

Excitotoxins in soft drinks, snacks, and convenience foods

Excitatory amino acids, like glutamate and aspartate, are ubiquitous in our foods and soft drinks today. They can disrupt the pituitary pathways that regulate ovarian function. This is a factor not addressed in most medical settings that treat infertility.

Vital
Read labels
carefully!

Even if excitatory amino acids have not been found to cause obvious birth defects, there is some evidence that they can adversely affect subtle neurobehavioral and neuroendocrine pathways in a developing baby.

You can control what you eat and drink. Even if there are other "diagnoses" for your infertility, you will only help the situation if you eliminate these endocrine disruptors. See Chapter 4 for more details.

Cigarettes, alcohol, marijuana, excess caffeine and stimulant use

There are many pathways where these substances disrupt the ovary hormone production in women (and testicular function in men). A *teratogen* is a drug or chemical that causes damage to the fetus ("birth defects"). Teratogen exposure is another factor contributing to early pregnancy loss, before you are even sure you are pregnant, as well as to recurrent miscarriages later on.

Warning!
Caffeine,
cigarette
smoking,
cocaine and
marijuana
are *suspected*
teratogens
for the
developing
embryo.

Each one of these "endocrine disruptors" alone can interfere with fertility; using more on a regular basis has even more impact. Do a basic "housecleaning" and get rid of these fertility robbers before you spend thousands of dollars in infertility testing and treatment, especially if you *are* in such a program now.

Your efforts will give *you* a healthier body, a better chance of becoming pregnant, and are definitely better for your baby. (See Chapter 6.)

Chemical exposure at home or work

Serious endocrine disruptors such as pesticides, PCBs, Bisphenol A, organic solvents and others described in Chapter 5 have far more damaging effects on fertility—for men and women—than you realize.

Several thousand animal and human studies show truly alarming effects on reproductive pathways, as well as ways these same chemicals disrupt important thyroid pathways. And, as mentioned earlier, if your thyroid isn't working right, there's a high probability that your ovaries aren't either. See Appendix II for these studies.

There are some practical steps you to reduce your exposure to these chemicals. Keep in mind, however, if you question most physicians, they may not answer definitively because past studies on the toxicity of these compounds have primarily focused on cancer-causing effects, rather than effects on fertility, sustaining a pregnancy, or the impact on a developing embryo.

Doctors simply may not know future effects possible with some of these hormonally active agents. It was not long ago that DES was given to pregnant women in the mistaken belief that it helped sustain a healthy pregnancy; we now know otherwise. DES and similar hormone-disruptors during pregnancy cause serious abnormalities in both male and female embryos, as well as recurrent miscarriage rates in DES daughters and diminished quality of sperm in DES sons.

Remember, medicine is slow to accept new connections and even slower to change. Doctors want *scientific proof* before they act. While that's a plus in many ways, physicians need to heed the warnings from biologists reporting serious reproductive and neurological problems in animals.

Just in case the environmental scientists are really right, I encourage you to take the time to eliminate these endocrine disruptors from your home and work environment. (See Chapters 5 & 18 for more information.)

Herbs That Sabotage Your Fertility

Long before the development of modern contraceptives, women in ancient cultures used plant medicines to control their fertility. Women healers around the world knew which herbs prevented pregnancy and could induce abortions. Healers' use of herbs as contraception was in violation of church doctrine, one of the reasons so many were burned at the stake as "witches" in Europe during the Middle Ages.

In all the extensive marketing of herbs as "more natural" and "safer" options than prescription medicines, we have lost sight of our ancestors knowledge of how powerful herbs are.

You don't want to inadvertently have a miscarriage, or cause birth defects in your baby just because ads tell you various herbs are "natural" and "safe."

Women are not the only ones who should use caution with herbs. Men's sperm can be affected too. A March 1999 study published in *Fertility and Sterility*, described adverse effects on male sperm viability and ability to fertilize an egg from four commonly used herbs—*St. John's wort, Echinacea purpura, Gingko biloba and saw palmetto.*

> **Warning**
> If you are in your reproductive years, *avoid using herbs when you are trying to conceive.*

Saw palmetto made sperm less viable, and the other three herbs decreased viability and affected the sperm's ability to penetrate the egg for fertilization.

More ominously, *sperm exposed to St. John's wort developed a mutation of the tumor suppressor gene, BRCA1, a shocking finding.*

As you have probably seen in the news, mutations in this gene significantly increase the risk of both breast and ovarian cancers in women who inherit the altered gene.

> **Warning**
> Men's sperm can be damaged by herbs, too.

Manufacturers of many vitamin and mineral supplements today add a variety of herbs to sell more products to consumers enthusiastic about "natural medicines."

Dr. Vliet's Guide to Herbs That Can Cause Infertility and Problems with Pregnancy

The following herbs can cause infertility, spontaneous abortions/miscarriage, birth defects, or premature labor:

- black cohosh
- blue cohosh
- cat's claw
- chaste tree
- dong quai
- feverfew, ginseng
- gotu kola
- ma huang (ephedra)
- passionflower
- evening primrose
- red clover
- St. John's wort
- Vitex
- wild yam

Adverse effects on sperm: *St. John's wort, Echinacea purpura, Gingko biloba and saw palmetto.*

© *2001-2007 Elizabeth Lee Vliet, M.D.*

In Summary

Just Do It!
Clean up
your diet,
and get rid
of these
fertility
saboteurs.

Fertility is a delicate balance of many interconnected facets: age, hormone levels, body fat, what you eat, what you drink, how much you exercise, what medicines you take, what supplements you take, what's present in your environment, your vitamins and minerals, your genetic makeup, your immune function, your mental outlook, how much stress you live with, just to name some major ones.

Problems in one of these *add* to problems in other facets. The more fertility robbers you have, the less likely you are to be able to conceive.

Follow the recommendations of your fertility specialist, but also work on getting rid of these other fertility disruptors that I have described here.

You and your baby will be healthier!

Chapter 15
Your Ovaries—Effects on All Your Body Systems

Our ovaries are marvelous, magnificent organs that month after month, year after year, produce hormones that interact with every cell, tissue and organ in our bodies, providing metabolic power for our cellular engines.

Eyes, hair, skin, bones, muscles, joints, heart, lungs, brain and nerves, ears and hearing, vocal cords, digestive tract, kidney, pancreas, bladder, and immune system.

There isn't a single part of the body that isn't affected by estradiol, and to a lesser degree, testosterone. In our reproductive years, progesterone also affects many of these systems—often blocking estradiol actions and producing effects that we may not always like, such as PMS and insulin resistance.

Fact
Ovarian hormones have major effects on the function of all our systems, not just our ability to become pregnant, carry a child, nurse and menstruate.

Your Ovaries Are Connected to Your Eyes, Skin, Hair, Eyes, Voice, and More

Estrogen and Your Eyes

So you hit thirty, and your eyes feel dry and scratchy. Your contact lens aren't as comfortable. Or, maybe you started birth control pills and can't wear contacts at all. Your skin is dry and itchy, your hair thinner. As one 34-year-old mother of three said *"I'm getting pimples again like a teenager, my hair is falling out, and I have all these wrinkles. What is going on?"*

Mucus membranes from skin, scalp, eyes, mouth and nose to intestinal tract, bladder and vagina are all affected by increasing dryness as estradiol declines and we are left with an excess of estrone and androgens.

To fit properly, contact lenses "float" over the eye on a thin film of water. If the surface isn't moist, contact lenses don't have their "floating pad," and feel scratchy or burning.

Too dry?
Remember, estrogen is Mother Nature's moisturizer.

Other eye problems are triggered by low estradiol: age related macular degeneration (ARMD), glaucoma, cataracts, decreased visual sharpness, and decreased visual coordination. Research shows that estradiol helps reduce all of these adverse changes to the eyes.

For example, one study of perimenopausal women with eye problems found that one third had dryness, tearing, decreased visual acuity, decreased visual coordination, red and swollen lids, or a sensation of a foreign object in the eye. The authors reported that all improved with estradiol therapy, including a topical ophthalmic solution applied directly to the eye. Objective tests by eye specialists confirmed the improvement.

Dry eyes?
Dry eyes result from loss of optimal estradiol effects that moisturize the tissue on the eyeball.

Other studies support these positive effects of hormones on the eye. Some studies go back many years, making it surprising that this information is not more widely used in medical settings when women describe these symptoms.

A 1971 study showed better hydration of the cornea during the highest estrogen phase of the menstrual cycle.

Another group reported in 1981 that corneal sensitivity decreased toward the end of pregnancy and during the preovulatory peak of estradiol in the menstrual cycle, both normal times of high estradiol levels. Recent research has confirmed these findings.

Dry eyes 2
Testosterone also maintains secretions from the mebothian glands that moisturize the eye.

Specialists think that low estrogen makes the eyes more susceptible to deficiencies in aqueous formation and decreases the formation of the lipid layer of the eye. Both changes make us vulnerable to "dry eye" or *keratoconjunctivitis sicca (KCS)*.

Testosterone adds to estradiol effects on eye moisture by improving function of the mebothian glands in the eyelid. Testosterone and estradiol ophthalmic solutions are already being studied by eye specialists in Europe as a treatment of *"dry eye syndrome."*

Progesterone, on the other hand, has a number of effects that make your vision less sharp, or even blurred. Progesterone rises during the second half of the cycle and during pregnancy causing mebothian glands to increase production of a fatty material creating an oily film and deposits on the eye's surface, leading to blurred vision and reduced wearing time with contact lenses.

Rising progesterone also affects how the brain processes visual information. During women's "PMS" week, visual perception skills are decreased; research shows less visual sensitivity as well as *diminished* detection and discrimination abilities.

Estrogen and Your Skin

You can tell dry skin by its look and feel. Just looking at the skin, however, doesn't readily reveal the loss of *collagen*, which gives skin its elasticity and firmness. The loss of collagen gives the leathery, wrinkled, sagging appearance associated with aging.

Skin collagen decreases markedly after age 40 in most women as estradiol declines. It decreases in younger women who lose estradiol for other reasons. *The decrease in collagen is greater in women who have a surgical menopause.*

No one dies of "old age of the skin," so it isn't surprising estradiol effects on skin aging haven't been studied as much as effects on more critical body systems, such as heart, bone and brain.

A 1992 study from Spain evaluating the effects of different estrogen regimens on skin collagen content shows that *estrogen replacement prevented decrease in skin collagen.*

The amount of collagen benefit varied depending on type of therapy used. Transdermal patches using 17-beta estradiol show the greatest degree of collagen preservation. Oral conjugated equine estrogens (Premarin) with a low amount of 17-beta estradiol were not as effective.

Other changes in the skin related to loss of optimal estradiol are more unusual. *Dermatographia* refers to an atypical type of allergic reaction in the skin that causes a reddened, raised line where you "write" or draw a shape on the skin with a fingernail or other sharp object.

One 31-year-old woman I treated developed a severe form of this after being on Loestrin for three years, with its high progestin–low estradiol content. Even touching her skin caused raised red welts that persisted for hours. The dermatographia

Poor eyesight You aren't imagining it if your vision seems less "sharp" the week before your period, or if you started Depo-Provera or high progestin birth control pills!

Dry skin As estradiol declines, so does collagen formation.

Dermato-graphia occurs more often when estradiol is low, with normal or high progesterone.

Formication
a sensation of something crawling inside or on the skin, is a skin change caused by low estradiol.

resolved with a birth control pill containing a higher estradiol ratio.

Formication may cause itching, crawling, or feelings like little twitches just under the skin. It may even feel like hordes of ants traveling in your skin. It can be very unpleasant!

Women say they think they are going crazy. A feeling exacerbated by their doctors saying they never heard of such a thing!

This "crawly, itchy feeling" has been described for decades as part of the menopausal changes, and is likely due to nerves endings that are "hypersensitive" from loss of estradiol.

More than a bad hair day
When your hormones are out of kilter your hair shows it. Losing hair (alopecia) is one of the more common problems women report.

Many doctors don't recognize that it can occur in younger women who have low estradiol levels. Formication resolves quickly when the right balance of estradiol is restored.

Hormones and Your Hair

Thinning, brittle, dry hair is not life threatening, but it certainly is a source of major distress to many women. I'm not talking about the occasional "bad hair" day.

Declining estradiol, excess testosterone as well as low testosterone, excess DHEA, hypo and hyperthyroidism, *low* or *excess* cortisol, several vitamin or mineral deficiencies, vitamin A excess, and low ferritin are common causes for women to lose hair.

Dermatologists often tell my patients they have "menopausal alopecia," which certainly implies a hormone cause. Then they usually prescribe Rogaine without even suggesting hormone levels be checked!

Bad hair, bad hormones
The visible changes in hair and skin can be a clue to damaging, invisible bone changes inside.

Before you get expensive medical evaluations, supplements, medications, or beauty products at least get a careful and reliable blood test of your ovarian and thyroid hormone levels, including thyroid antibodies. *Saliva hormone levels do not give you an accurate picture of actual hormone delivery to the hair follicle.*

Estrogen and Your Sinuses

Some of you may have suddenly begun having "chronic sinusitis," "sinus headaches", or "sinus infections."

The nose and sinus cavities of the face and forehead are lined with mucous membranes sensitive to the loss of estradiol. Just as the loss causes dryness of the lining of the vagina, it also causes moisture loss and diminished mucous production by the tissues lining the nose and sinuses.

Mucous helps to trap viruses, allergens, and bacteria from the air you breathe. When mucous membrane becomes drier, it can't clear out all these invaders.

Small arteries become constricted when estradiol levels fall, decreasing blood flow. Immune cells and proteins carried by the blood aren't as available to tissues to ward off or destroy the invader particles.

Taking antihistamines and decongestants daily just makes this worse, since these medicines cause more drying and constriction of the blood vessels.

Boosting your hormone levels may be more appropriate than taking decongestants and antihistamines every day.

Use natural saline nose sprays, or a steam bath for your face several times a week, as a helpful solution for sinus congestion, especially if you put a few drops of eucalyptus or peppermint oil in the hot water.

If you notice marked changes in your hair, skin, and eyes along with other hormone-related symptoms, it is time to check your hormone levels and your bone density as well.

Hormones and Your Voice

Josie is a professional opera singer. She had a hysterectomy and removal of the ovaries for endometriosis and ovarian cysts in her early 40s. Her gynecologist initially prescribed Premarin, but it caused migraines and increased blood pressure. Then he tried Estratest, a combination of estrogen and testosterone, to see if this would relieve her headaches and improve libido.

By the time I saw her, a year later, she had *completely lost her soprano voice*, and could not perform concerts. She was losing her career and livelihood.

She had also gained a great deal of weight, in spite of careful attention to diet. She still had frequent migraine headaches, and her blood pressure had skyrocketed. She had not experienced either problem prior to the initial hormone therapy.

Her hormone evaluation explains why she lost her soprano voice: estradiol was far too low at less than 30 pg/ml, and total testosterone significantly elevated at 176 ng/dl (normal for women is about 50 ng/dl). Her free testosterone level was also markedly elevated.

Sinus problems? Hormone changes play a role here too. Get your hormone levels checked.

Alert! Estratest may make your soprano an alto or bass!

Man's hormone balance, man's appetite Too much testosterone made her ravenously hungry, contributing to weight gain.

Male voice?
The excess total and free testosterone, along with very low estradiol, causes a women's voice to become very deep.

Right Rx
I prescribed a transdermal patch because it lowers blood pressure better than oral estrogen.

Hitting the high notes
Loss of estradiol also leads to loss of elasticity in the vocal cords, making it harder to hold notes, particularly high notes in the soprano range.

The fixed hormone combinations in products like Estratest make it impossible to regulate each hormone for optimal individualized amounts each woman needs. In combination with low estradiol, excess testosterone also raises blood pressure and causes headaches.

I recommended she change to an FDA-approved 17-beta estradiol and stop the Estratest. Headaches can be caused by rapid rise and fall in estradiol. The patch form gives gradual absorption and reduces the rise and fall in blood level. The steadier estradiol delivery decreased her migraines. I taught her to recognize signs the patch was wearing off. When she felt irritable, foggy, headachy, or could not sleep, she could put on a new patch. Since her testosterone was too high, I suggested she let the levels fall gradually after stopping the Estratest, which should help her voice return to normal.

Three months later, she was exuberant. She was using one Climara transdermal estradiol patch every 5 days, and occasionally added another patch when under a lot of stress and metabolizing estrogen faster.

"I feel so much better now! My voice is completely clear and back to normal. I am so grateful that my vocal cords weren't permanently damaged by all that testosterone. My headaches are much less frequent, and my blood pressure is back to normal."

Her estradiol is 120 pg/ml and testosterone is 13 ng/dl, quite a dramatic difference from Estratest levels. Six months later, she headed to Italy for a series of concerts, her voice completely restored. A year later, she says,

"We got the voice fixed and I am really pleased with that part. I haven't had a migraine headache since the change to estradiol. My energy level is great. My primary care physician was pleased that my blood pressure is staying normal, and he agrees to work with all the things I learned from you."

The title of a 1998 French medical article says it all: *"The Voice and Menopause: The Twilight of The Divas."* The larynx is a target of hormonal action. The tone of our voice depends on the balance of estrogen and androgens.

With hysterectomy and surgical menopause, or the decrease in estradiol from natural menopause, the balance changes toward androgen dominance. Excess treatment with androgenic hormones can cause changes in vocal fold structure and voice quality that may be irreversible for some. For example, Danazol, an androgen-like treatment for endometriosis, has the potential to cause significant voice deepening.

French researchers found that a significant percentage of menopausal women had a *"menopausal voice syndrome,"* manifested by *lack of power and intensity, voice fatigue* and *a narrower range of notes.*

Their conclusion is similar to observations from my practice. I find that with optimal hormonal replacement, the singing, and speaking voice recover.

I was saddened to read in the news what happened to Julie Andrews following vocal cord surgery attempting to correct her menopausal voice problems. I often wonder whether surgery could have been avoided if anyone had checked her hormone levels and tried estradiol first. None of the news articles even mentioned a possible hormone connection.

Due to hormone imbalance
Voice changes are not just a problem at menopause. Women with PCOS, endometriosis, and thyroid problems can also have adverse voice effects

Ovaries and Your Gut: A Panoply of Problems

Irritable Bowel Syndrome (IBS)

IBS causes chronic, recurrent, crampy, colicky abdominal pain, and bouts of severe diarrhea, alternating with constipation.

In spite of intensive research efforts, no one has found a single structural or biochemical "lesion" to define IBS. A variety of factors trigger these painful symptoms, including interactions between the gut and the brain, and between the gut and hormone fluctuations.

Women with IBS typically say their symptoms get significantly worse around menstruation, suggesting ovarian hormones play a role in the gut.

Progesterone slows down the smooth muscle action in the walls of the intestine, leading to slower transit time of food through the intestine. Women typically describe feeling an abdominal fullness, bloating, and mild constipation during the ten days or so in the cycle when progesterone is high, even if they don't have IBS.

If you are experiencing decline in estradiol and you still have normal levels of progesterone in this cycle phase, constipation can be a major problem, especially if you do not get enough magnesium.

IBS and Women
"Irritable" Bowel Syndrome affects far more women than men, but no one seems to know what causes it.

Hormone help

Women notice bowel movements are easier, and looser, during menstrual days than the week before menstruation when progesterone is high.

Estradiol improves the muscular contractions of the intestinal smooth muscle, and prevents constipation when levels are in balance. This is usually the week after your period when estradiol rises and progesterone is not produced.

When estradiol levels fall sharply, either with ovulation or just prior to bleeding, the falling estrogen triggers firing of the brain's alarm center, causing a burst of "fight-or-flight" chemicals that in turn cause spasm and hyperactivity in the gut wall muscles that can lead to diarrhea.

Imagine how a decrease in estradiol and the surge of "fight-or-flight" hormones, plus a loss of ovulation that produces progesterone to slow the gut, can cause significant problems for women who do have IBS!

The *vagus* nerve helps regulate normal gut function and motility. Vagal tone has to be normal for food and wastes to move properly through the intestinal tract. The neurotransmitter serotonin also plays a critical role in normal gut function.

Women with the constipation-dominate form of IBS appear to have abnormal stimulation from the vagus nerve to the intestine.

Effects

Low estradiol levels decrease serotonin production, another way that low estradiol aggravates IBS.

Women with diarrhea dominant IBS often improve when they take a serotonin "booster" such as Prozac, Paxil, Luvox, Zoloft. We know also that excess serotonin activity from these same medicines can also cause diarrhea, so the right balance of serotonin and other chemical messengers is crucial.

Estradiol has direct effects on the intestinal muscle and nerves to maintain gut motility and function, and also enhances serotonin levels. If estradiol is restored to healthy levels, many women with IBS improve enough that they do not need the serotonin-booster medicines.

Women with IBS also tend to have backaches, headaches, painful menses (*dysmenorrhea*), painful sex (*dyspareunia*), fibromyalgia, and sleep disturbances (multiple awakenings, fragmented sleep). Many of these other problems are influenced by abnormal serotonin activity as women lose optimal estradiol, and some are triggered by release of other chemical messengers called *prostaglandins*.

We know that a rise in progesterone increases the production of several prostaglandins, increases the breakdown of serotonin, and blocks estradiol binding at a number of different estrogen receptors.

All of these patterns lead me to focus on the estradiol-progesterone *balance* in young women with these problems, in addition to the actual *levels* of these critical hormones, and incorporate estradiol into my treatment approaches.

Chronic Constipation

There are many causes for chronic constipation. Some are simple and straightforward, such as lack of dietary fiber and too much fat. Some are due to treatable medical disorders like hypothyroidism or diabetes. Some are due to more serious medical conditions, such as toxic megacolon.

Estradiol and progesterone affect the smooth gut muscle and motility of the intestinal tract: too little estradiol with too much progesterone causes constipation.

Calcium and magnesium must be in the right balance for the bowels to work smoothly and not get "stuck" in slow gear. When your estradiol is too low, it leads to decreased stomach acid production, which means you don't absorb calcium, magnesium and other minerals from food or supplements as well as you should.

Estradiol also enhances magnesium use by our muscles and bone. If you don't have sufficient estradiol, you won't absorb magnesium as well *and* magnesium won't be taken up into the smooth gut muscles for normal bowel movements. Constipation gets worse.

Magnesium is depleted in many ways: high coffee consumption, stimulant medications (decongestants used in cold and allergy products, some antidepressants, many asthma medicines, over-the-counter diet pills, the herb ephedra, to name a few), cortisone medications used to treat asthma and arthritis, and the ever-present stress in our lives.

Women consume large amounts of soft drinks that contain phosphates (sometimes called phosphoric acid), that attach to magnesium and calcium from foods and supplements diminishing absorption. At the same time, glutamate (MSG) and aspartate (Nutrasweet) in soft drinks *increase* the body's need for magnesium.

Add all these hormone effects to the typical American diet, about ¼ the fiber and twice the fat we need, along with low magnesium—you can see why the bowels rebel, become sluggish or stop working properly.

Workings
Estradiol improves intestinal function and motility in another way: it aids calcium and magnesium absorption in the gut.

Less is not good
Women today have much lower magnesium intake than women of earlier generations.

Ovaries and Your Heart: Hormone Effects on Palpitations, Flutters, and Arrhythmias

Type A problems
Type A women leading a high stress life, and drinking lots of soft drinks deplete magnesium stores rapidly.

Remember the young woman who had three serious heart attacks, each with falling estradiol at the beginning of her bleeding days? She had severe PCOS causing low estradiol and excess androgens, that triggered spasms of the coronary arteries leading to heart attacks.

You may have experienced mild versions of some: all of a sudden you have horrendous palpitations, flutters, and pounding sensations. You feel anxious; your stomach is upset; your skin cool and clammy.

What's going on? You're healthy, and never had these problems before. Is it a panic attack? A heart attack?

You see your family doctor, who checks you over, says you're too young for heart problems, you're fine. He tells you to relax more and reduce your stress. With a deep sigh of relief, you go on about your daily routine.

Then a few weeks later, it happens again. *What is this?*

Kerry was 34 and worked as a respiratory therapist at a large urban hospital. She had been diagnosed with *ventricular tachycardia* (VT), an abnormal heart rhythm manifested by extremely rapid heartbeat that causes dizziness, lightheadedness, and fainting.

Caution
Hormone imbalances can cause other heart-related problems as well.

These symptoms happen when the heart is beating too fast and the ventricles don't have time to fill with enough blood to pump with each beat. As a result, the brain doesn't get enough blood flow, causing fainting episodes (*syncope*). It is quite frightening, but the primary danger of VT occurs if it degenerates into more serious arrhythmias, such as ventricular fibrillation (or *V-fib*, as you have probably heard many times on *ER*) that can lead to death.

She had been in the ICU on three separate occasions for particularly bad attacks. Her doctors were puzzled. The cardiologist did not find an underlying disease. She did not have plaque build-up in the arteries of the heart causing a blockage.

She was diagnosed as "anxious and stressed" and her doctors prescribed Xanax. But with her medical background, Kerry was trained to think about patterns and connections. Her observations about the timing of VT episodes led her to the consult with me.

This is her story, in her own words, from her first appointment:

"I have had a miserable year with 3 hospitalizations for arrhythmias. First time, it was hot and I was taking care of my horse, and I got so dizzy I couldn't stand up. It passed and I didn't think much about it.

"Then it happened again while I was at work at the hospital. I had a run of V-tach (ventricular tachycardia); they called a code (medical term for emergency treatment of cardiac arrest), did all kinds of tests, and found nothing wrong.

"I was put on Tenormin (a beta-blocker), and that really affected me badly. Now I know what low blood pressure feels like. I could hardly get off the couch! I was tapered off it, but I still had very low BP, and then I had another episode of those horrible arrhythmias. They checked me out and sent me home, but this time with meds for anxiety. My doctor just told me I was stressed and anxious. I took Buspar, but it kept me up all night, so I weaned myself off. Then they recommended Xanax to take as I needed it and that seemed to at least help some."

"The next time it happened, I was having palpitations really bad, so I put myself on the monitor, and found I had an irregular heart beat. I showed the cardiologist, and they put me back in the hospital, but then another physician said there was nothing wrong, I was just anxious.

"It was getting so that it happened like clockwork every month right before my period. (Do you see a major clue here?) Right before my period starts, I have these feelings like I am going to pass out. This is a miserable way to live; I only have two weeks of feeling good.

"I am an outdoors person, I love riding, and I want to be active, but I can't do what I want to do when I feel so lousy. I do everything right, I have very moderate alcohol, I don't drink caffeine, I don't smoke, I eat well, and my stress is no different than it has ever been. I need something to help this."

All her episodes happened with the onset of menstrual bleeding, an important clue to a potential hormone change setting off a heart rhythm change. I sometimes find it hard to understand why this isn't more obvious to health professionals, particularly when an educated, medically trained patient gives such a descriptive history of the association.

She was carefully checked for all the "usual" causes of heart problems and nothing abnormal was found. When your period starts, the drop in blood levels of estradiol affects the brain's cen-

Coincidence

"I remember it was right before my period was supposed to start, and it struck me as odd, because that's when it happened the last two times."

"I suffered a lot of humiliation and I was really upset; they should have known I was an intelligent woman and a medically-trained person."

ter that regulates heart rate and blood pressure, in several ways. I show this sequence of events in the chart that follows. It occurs whenever estradiol falls abruptly, whether during your monthly cycle, or after a baby is born, or leading up to menopause.

So there is a cascade of responses affecting heart rate and rhythm from a hormone-triggered release of the brain's alarm chemicals.

Then, when we don't understand what is happening, our *psychological* fear response intensifies the body's *physical* responses from the drop in estradiol.

This is such a common occurrence, many women don't notice it until the hormone drops are so marked that the body's responses are more intense. If your estradiol declines for any reason, then the fall in estradiol before menses triggers a much more pronounced physical response and suddenly, you are aware of it and perhaps even frightened.

Remember

Hormones can trigger these disruptions in heart rhythm.

Most doctors don't ask you *when* in the menstrual cycle you have palpitations, panicky episodes, heart flutters, racing or pounding, feeling queasy or nauseous, sweating, or feeling anxious for no apparent reason.

That's because physicians are *not* taught to think that women's unique hormone shifts are that important, even though we know that estradiol, testosterone and progesterone have diverse effects throughout the brain and body. They don't realize that women's observations of menstrual cycle timing are clues to *physical* changes *triggering symptoms*.

Doctors forget

Hormone changes affect the heart in many ways.

Other than reproduction, I wasn't taught about ovarian hormone connections in medical school or during my formal specialty training. When I first started as a physician, it didn't occur to me to ask *when* in the menstrual cycle a symptom appeared.

It was not until I had been in practice for a few years, listening carefully to women's vivid descriptions, that I realized I was hearing the same patterns and connections from many different patients.

I started asking *why* these similarities? Women say they know "its a physical, chemical kind of thing." They describe it well, but are told that "it can't be" or "it's caused by stress," so their body knowledge is written off and lost, connections between the dots aren't made, and women suffer.

Dr. Vliet's Guide to Hormone Heart Effects

Decreased estradiol from the ovary

Decreased estradiol at brain centers

Decreased brain endorphins and serotonin

Burst of epinephrine and norepinephrine (epi, NE—the "fight or flight" hormones) in the brain's "alarm center" (locus ceruleus)

Epi and NE set off multiple responses in cardiovascular system

Results in:

- *Increased heart rate,*
- *Disrupted heart rhythm (palpitations, flutters, pounding)*
- *Blood pressure rises*
- *Dilation of blood vessels to critical organs (causes lightheadedness because heart beats too rapidly and doesn't fill with enough blood for each beat)*
- *Fear of symptoms intensifies the "alarm reaction" which in turn increases all of the above responses*

© 2001–2007 Elizabeth Lee Vliet, M.D.

In Kerry's situation, her doctors had ruled out more serious causes of the arrhythmias, but had not considered the known *heart effects* from the physical hormone changes of menses. *Her treatment with Xanax or beta-blockers did not correct the underlying cause.*

When working with patients like Kerry, I want to know why a *recurring* pattern happens. I research the medical literature to see what I can find to explain it. The more I do this, the more information I find that has been in the peer-reviewed, published menopause and endocrine literature, sometimes for decades.

It is sad, and costly, such information is overlooked and not incorporated into treatment plans to help prevent overuse of other medications and needless expensive testing.

We know us best Women's descriptions are "on target" more times than not. Doctors need to listen to what *women* say, and value their input.

Falling estradiol was the likely cause of Kerry's problems, so it made sense to try an estradiol patch applied two days before her next period to keep her estradiol steadier. I could test this theory easily. If Kerry didn't like how she felt, she could simply take the patch off, and the added estradiol would metabalize quickly and be gone in about 24 hours.

She was thrilled, and quick to understand the concept of stabilizing estradiol because of her training in cardiac function. She used the estradiol patch during bleeding days for her next several cycles and did not have any cardiac episodes. It worked so well we began a trial on a combined estrogen-progestin low dose birth control pill.

A constant daily dose of estrogen and progestin effectively suppressed the ovarian cycles so she didn't experience the normal ups and downs of a menstrual cycle. I recommended she take the active hormone pills daily without stopping to have a period each month. This prevented the "destabilization" of the brain centers regulating heart rate and rhythm, stopping the fall in estradiol from triggering arrhythmias.

Six months later, she said,

"I am doing wonderfully, absolutely fine! I sleep better, my skin and hair are better, I am not having any palpitations. I am not on any other medications—I was on a ton of stuff before to control arrhythmias. I was able to wean off everything else. I don't have any runs of PVCs the way I did before. I am feeling really well now."

Cardiovascular Symptoms or Disease? How Do You Tell the Difference

Symptoms are changes and sensations you experience, such as headaches, racing heart, clammy skin, pain, flushing, and tingling, among many others. These changes can indicate a normal body response to environmental stimulus or even to your own thoughts. These sensations can also be a potential warning of *disease*.

Hypertension and osteoporosis are classic examples of diseases that do not produce symptoms until the damage is done.

As a physician, my role is to help patients sort out symptoms, links to possible diseases, and what disease could explain the entire cluster of symptoms, as well as what disease could be present but silent and symptomless.

Dr. Vliet's Guide to Summary of Key Estradiol (E2) Benefits on Our Heart and Blood Vessels

- E2 lowers blood pressure by dilating blood vessels
- E2 increases HDL ("good") cholesterol
- E2 decreases total cholesterol and ("bad") LDL
- E2 improves carbohydrate metabolism, decreasing risk of diabetes, a risk factor for heart disease
- E2 reduces platelet stickiness and clumping that causes clots, artery-   clogging plaque, strokes
- E2 reduces risk of blood clots by several mechanisms
- E2 has antioxidant effects on artery walls, helps reduce plaque
- E2 reverses the impaired blood vessel response to the chemical messenger acetylcholine in plaque-filled coronary arteries. A gender specific effect.
- E2 increases release of endothelium-derived NO (nitric oxide), a potent vaso-dilator, that helps to open up blood vessels, increase blood flow
- E2 acts as a calcium-channel blocker which also helps blood vessels dilate, improving blood flow, and also lowering blood pressure
- E2 alters synthesis, release and response to peptides (e.g. endothelin-I and angiotensin-II) that constrict blood vessels, raise blood pressure, and reduce blood flow to tissues
- E2 increases transport of oxygen in the blood across the cells (endothelium) lining arteries so more oxygen is delivered

©Elizabeth Lee Vliet, MD 1995, revised 2001–2007

Palpitations, fluttering or pounding sensations in the chest, can be disturbing. They can occur when we are frightened as part of the normal "fight-or-flight" response, a normal response to a fearful situation. They can occur in certain types of *benign* heart disease such as mitral valve prolapse; or in potentially serious heart disease such as *atrial fibrillation*. They can occur from something as simple as falling blood glucose.

Most doctors evaluate possible *heart disease* causes thoroughly; they often just forget to explore other *metabolic* causes, such as the heart's response to brain effects from declining estradiol, as we saw with Kerry.

Finally In the 21st century, physicians are beginning to pay "official" attention to these issues.

Palpitations become more frequent, and more intense, as women move into the perimenopause hormonal declines. But *palpitations can occur at any age* if dieting, illness, surgery or stress has pushed estradiol too low. In numerous studies, palpitations occur in 40 to

60 percent of women during the menstrual cycle when estradiol levels drop (bleeding days and around ovulation).

Diverse diseases such as anemia and hyperthyroidism can also produce palpitations through other mechanisms. Palpitations can be a side effect of many medications, herbs, allergy and cold products. (See Chapter 8.) Panic disorder is a biological condition of excess, and erratic, production of adrenaline-type compounds in the brain that can produce palpitations. You need a careful, comprehensive evaluation *that should include a test of your hormones.*

Balance
It also makes sense to use treatment approaches that better correct and stabilize hormone levels.

Ovaries and Your Lungs: Asthma and Your Menstrual Cycle

Asthma is another illness that hits men and women, and doctors have traditionally thought treatment is the same for either sex. But the more we study differences in body chemistry and disease patterns in women and men, the more we find that women's unique hormonal make up governs body chemistry, response to medicines, and also affects *when* asthma flare-ups are likely.

In ancient Greece, Hippocrates, the father of modern medicine, observed that the wheezing and difficulty breathing (now called asthma) became worse in women around their menses.

Hippocrates astute observations about women's health, like his observations about muscle and joint pain and it's relationship to menses and menopause, lay gathering dust in libraries for the last 2500 years.

Fact
About one-third of women with asthma experience more intense asthma attacks in the few days before, and during, menses.

In the early 20th century, other observant physicians published a classic paper describing asthma in the premenstrual and menstrual phases of women's cycles. Again, these observations were overlooked until the last two decades of the 20th century when several other studies documented the association between menstrual cycle phase and increased asthma attacks.

Interesting data from Finland show that hospital admission rates for treatment of asthma were about the same for young girls and boys, but rates for were much higher for women age 25–55 (the reproductive and perimenopausal years) than for men the same age.

Finnish researchers also looked at occupational asthma rates, and found alarming trends in the gender differences. From 1986 to 1993, the annual incidence of persistent asthma among people age 15 to 64 years was *stable in men,* but *increased* 43% in women. During that same period *occupational* asthma *increased* 70% in women.

That's a significant percent of patients with obvious evidence of hormone changes triggers. Ovarian hormones *must* play a role, yet most physicians still overlook this connection.

Another interesting finding is that women with these menstrual asthma flare-ups do not respond as well to corticosteroid treatment. Women with increased asthma attacks in the days just prior to and during bleeding report significantly *greater* use of their inhalers and other medicines, yet still have a much *lower* peak expiratory flow rate (PEFR), longer asthma episodes, and more severe attacks than those without menstrual exacerbation. These are times of the cycle when estradiol and progesterone fall to their lowest levels. This means that women whose asthma is worse with falling hormones do not respond as well to the usual medications for asthma treatment. This observation shouldn't be surprising.

> **Rx**
> When I work with women with asthma that is worse around their periods, I prescribe daily birth control pills with no break for menses.

If the trigger is a fall in the hormones causing the reaction of constricted airways and changes in the immune system, it makes intuitive sense that standard asthma medications might not work as well as at other times.

One hormone-based theory explains the link between asthma and menses based on the changes in airways that occur with the drop in progesterone the 2–3 days before menses. Progesterone relaxes smooth muscle tissue. In the gut, this action causes constipation, but in the lung, smooth muscle relaxation acts to dilate the bronchioles increasing air flow, which is a good thing.

But progesterone also acts as an immunosuppressant hormone as well, so when levels fall, the immune system is *more* reactive, making asthmatics more sensitive to environmental allergens.

The drop in both progesterone and estradiol before menses can also destabilize the walls of tiny capillaries, leading to fluid leakage from these tiny vessels in the airways which causes edema of the mucosa lining the airways, making it harder to breathe.

I typically use pills with a higher estrogen to progestin ratio.

Other physicians who have tried birth control pills to prevent asthma flares describe mixed results. This happens, in part, because most physicians still tell women to *stop the pills* for a period each month. Other doctors use pills too high in progestin relative to the estrogen. This can cause more constriction of airways because of progestins' effects that are different from our body's natural progesterone.

Vital role
Ovarian hormones play crucial roles in regulating immune function.

Intramuscular injections of progesterone are sometimes used to prevent severe menstrual asthma attacks, but some women have more depressed mood and fluid retention with this approach. This happens because their estradiol balance isn't addressed at the same time. If progesterone is injected to prevent asthma without following the usual menstrual cycle, it changes your cycle and actually contributes to heavier, more irregular bleeding.

In some severe cases of menstrual asthma attacks, some physicians try medications such as Lupron, which suppresses ovarian cycles and reduces the menstrual asthma attacks. But women then developed *menopausal* symptoms if estradiol was not added back.

Bad cure!
Women who have Lupron treatment with no estrogen replacement often tell me the "cure" is far worse than the original problem!

For most women with asthma worse around menstrual days, episodes are still relatively mild. Some women have such a mild increase in asthma symptoms they do not recognize deterioration in their breathing during menstruation.

Then there are a few women who have such severe asthmatic attacks with menses they require hospitalization and need ventilators.

If you have asthma, speak up and ask your doctors about these connections in the hormones, if you have noticed it is worse at certain times of your cycle.

Asthma Triggers in Your Medicines and Foods

During specialty training at Johns Hopkins, I became aware of potentially serious, and bizarre, patients' reactions to things as seemingly innocuous as the coloring agents in medicines. Even vitamins and herbal products have coloring agents that cause these problems.

One patient with asthma was admitted for another problem. In treating that illness, the asthma was getting worse. I could not figure out what was happening, since asthma medications were stable and blood levels therapeutic. My mother, a research scientist at the time, was studying the role of tartrazine-based dyes in allergic reactions. After talking with her, I raised the possibility that the orange-colored tablets we used to treat the other illness affected this patient's asthma.

We changed medication to a *white* tablet, and within a short period the asthma cleared. Since the patient was curious about the orange dye, she took the pill one more time. The wheezing returned rapidly. She was convinced.

This happened over 20 years ago, and remains a lesson I share with patients and other physicians. Asthma is a complex disease, with many causes and triggers. Obviously, colorings on medicines is not a primary cause for most people, but we learn from situations like this.

Beware!
If you have asthma, watch out for any food colorings that could be a hidden trigger of attacks.

Immune System Goes Awry: Allergies, Food and Chemical Sensitivities

In my practice, I see a striking number of women with ovarian hormone imbalances who also have an increase in allergies, chemical sensitivities, intolerance to perfumes, and a variety of adverse reactions to environmental chemicals.

Progesterone, for example, is the hormone that suppresses a mother's immune system so she won't destroy the foreign tissue of a developing baby. Without progesterone to thwart her immune response, the mother's body would attack the fetus like the body attacks transplants.

Estradiol revs up the immune response, and when estradiol is too low, we are more easily "overloaded" by common chemicals, fragrances, and allergens that we tolerated just fine when hormones were in balance.

Relief
I hear so many women say that after their estradiol balance is restored to healthier levels, they also notice their allergies are less severe.

Ovaries and Your Bones: Osteoporosis Isn't Just for Older Women

Over the last 20 years, I have diagnosed many *young* women in their 20s and 30s with osteopenia or osteoporosis. And then there is the damage to ovaries from cigarette smoking, chronic dieting, or excessive exercise—all of which can stop or decrease normal menstruation and hormone production.

While the cause may vary, the result of too little estradiol is poor absorption of calcium and magnesium, poor deposition of these crucial minerals into bone, and an increase in bone breakdown compared to the rate of *building* new bone. They can't

Why?

Significant bone loss can happen to young women because of environ-mental, dietary, autoimmune and other disruptors of the ovaries' optimal production of estradiol and often testosterone.

Wrong

Her doctor told her she was too young for a bone density test, and said "Besides, you look too healthy to have any bone loss."

Shock!

Fredricka had osteoporosis at age 28!

build healthy new bone in a normal fashion. Low calcium and magnesium intake, or loss of these minerals from drinking too many soft drinks, alcohol, or coffee, rob bone. You won't reach menopause with a normal bone level, and are at even greater risk of debilitating fractures.

Fredricka's Story

Fredricka was 28, and already had many symptoms of ovarian decline and low estradiol. Her doctor would not check her actual serum hormone levels, even though she had marked insomnia, fatigue, loss of sex drive, weight gain, PMS, and a depressed mood the second half of her cycle.

I tested her hormone levels and the results indicated the need for a bone density test. She was shocked to find that, compared to a healthy peak bone mass for a woman her age, she was already 2.5 standard deviations *below* the desirable level at *both* spine and hip.

This is the cut-off used by the World Health Organization to defines osteoporosis.

Her serum estradiol level on Day 2 of her cycle was only 15 pg/ml, instead of the normal 80–90 pg/ml at this cycle phase, and her testosterone was 10 ng/dl instead of 40–50 ng/dl. For day 20, her estradiol was 74 pg/ml when it should have been in the 200–250 pg/ml range. Even with such low levels of estradiol and testosterone, her progesterone was still at the upper end of a healthy ovulatory range level at 18 ng/ml.

Her NTx, a marker of bone break-down products in the urine, was 65, much higher than the 35 or lower considered healthy for her age.

What caused this young woman's osteoporosis? She was very thin, and pushed herself with dieting to keep her weight "ideal." In reality, she was underweight.

She smoked 2 packs of cigarettes a day, and had done so since she was 15 years old. On weekends, she often had 8–10 beers as well as 1 or 2 after work each evening. She often skipped lunch, and drank 4 to 6 Cokes a day for energy. Her mother had developed severe osteoporosis about 10 years earlier than average, which further increased Fredricka's risk.

I checked her for other causes of early bone loss and did not find evidence of other underlying diseases. Fredricka was an attractive woman by society's standards, and "looked" healthy in spite of her significantly abnormal ovarian hormone levels, poor nutrition, and lifestyle habits.

Our female hormones play a critical role in bone growth. Estradiol and testosterone both facilitate calcium and magnesium deposits into bone for strength. These two hormones also regulate the rate of bone breakdown carried out by bone cells called *osteoclasts* so that breakdown doesn't occur faster than new bone is made.

Estradiol "primes" the bone cells called *osteoblasts* that stimulate new bone formation. Progesterone has a slight effect on the bone-building cells (osteoblasts) and assists in simulating new bone growth, but progesterone is only a "helper" that can carry out its job only *if* adequate estradiol is present to prime the osteoblasts.

Testosterone has a much greater bone-building effect than progesterone and it not only stimulates new bone *growth* to build bone density, it enhances bone *strength*.

You may not need to add hormones from an *outside* source for enough circulating hormones to prevent bone loss. Fredricka could help her ovaries return to producing the hormones she needs to improve her bones if she cleaned up her lifestyle.

Cutting out the soft drinks and alcohol would help her body use the calcium and magnesium from foods or supplements.

The problem is, if you are a younger woman, no one thinks you are losing bone. Until you actually measure bone density and hormone levels with reliable tests, you just can't know.

National statistics for young women's use of alcohol and cigarettes are alarming. This doesn't include the staggering numbers of women who are dieting with deficiencies of calcium and magnesium.

We are sitting on a time bomb of bone loss in young women today. It is too late to wait until menopause to check a woman's bone density.

This is tragic, since osteopenia (early, less severe bone loss) and osteoporosis are highly preventable and treatable if caught early. I check NTx, a marker of bone breakdown, on all new patients regardless of age. If it is too high, and there is low estradiol and/or testosterone levels, I definitely recommend a bone density test.

Causes

She unknowingly depleted her "bone bank account" with the soft drinks, alcohol, cigarettes, and dieting.

Rx Trap

You can't tell from the outside how healthy a woman is on the inside. Her doctor fell into that trap, and as a result, missed crucial problems.

Other Risk Factors for Bone Loss in Young Women

Essential for women
Studies on bone metabolism worldwide show women need a certain minimum level of estradiol, usually about 80–90 pg/ml, to prevent excess bone breakdown.

There are several medications that increase the risk of bone loss in younger women: corticosteroids, gonadotrophin-releasing hormone (GnRH) antagonists such as Lupron or Synarel, anticonvulsants such as Dilantin, beta-blockers, and high doses of thyroid medication.

Medical conditions such as hyperthyroidism, malabsorption, prolactinoma, hyperparathyroidism, or immobilization due to trauma are also situations that can lead to bone loss in younger women.

Corticosteroids cause more rapid bone breakdown. They also cause the bone that remains to become increasingly brittle. If you have one of these illnesses and are on corticosteroid therapy long term, you must urge your doctor to order both the NTx and DEXA tests. You can work with your physicians to prevent bone breakdown and rebuild what you lost.

Excess cortisol in all of its forms hastens bone breakdown, even in young women. Many women are advised to take adrenal glandulars as a treatment for "chronic fatigue" on the theory that they are tired because of "adrenal insufficiency" or "adrenal exhaustion."

Men, too!
Similar studies in men find that men also need a minimum level of estradiol, about 50–60 pg/ml, working with their testosterone, to prevent bone loss.

Using the "adrenal glandulars" or "adrenal support" products sold in health food, naturopath and chiropractic offices can cause excess corticosteroid effects leading to bone loss over time, even if these products are milder than the prescription forms of these hormones.

Avoid taking medicines like Cortef for "chronic fatigue" unless you have a well-documented deficiency of cortisol (adrenal insufficiency). This must be diagnosed using the standard, reliable laboratory measures (See Chapter 17), not the highly touted *inaccurate* saliva tests.

On the other hand, if you truly do have adrenal insufficiency (AI, also called Addison's Disease), adrenal glandulars sold over the counter are *not adequate* treatment. AI is a serious medical disorder and can be life threatening. It must be treated appropriately with prescription medication monitored by a endocrinologist experienced in the treatment of adrenal insufficiency.

Dr. Vliet's Guide: Techniques for Measuring Bone Density

Each of these techniques offers advantages and disadvantages in accuracy, precision, radiation exposure, cost, and information obtained

- *dual-energy x-ray absorptiometry (DEXA)* measures bones in the hip, lumbar spine, total body, or wrist; indicated for diagnosis, evaluation of fracture risk, and monitoring therapy. DEXA is the diagnostic tool of choice because it measures multiple sites with the least amount of radiation exposure, about 1/10th that from a chest x-ray according to 1998 guidelines from the National Osteoporosis Foundation. It is noninvasive, quick, and precise. Younger women need to have the BMD tests done on the hip and spine because tests of heel and wrist are not reliable in women under age 65. DEXA is the tool used to measure bone density in most of the clinical trials of osteoporosis medications. Cost ranges from $125–350. Most states now require insurance carriers to pay for this test in women with multiple risk factors for osteoporosis.

Definitions based on World Health Organization (WHO) criteria:
T-score less than or equal to –1 = normal BMD.
T-score between –1 and –2.5 is *osteopenia*, or low bone mass.
T-score greater than or equal to 2.5 is *osteoporosis*

- *quantitative computerized tomography (QCT)* measure bones in the hip, lumbar spine, or total body (but most common site is the spine); indicated for diagnosis, evaluation of fracture risk, and monitoring therapy. This is much more expensive, often costing around $1000, and it exposes you to much more radiation than DEXA. It is not the preferred test.
- *single- energy x-ray absorptiometry (SXA)* measures bones of the forearm, finger or heel; precise but not able to detect sufficient change in bone mass required to monitor effectiveness of therapy. Especially in younger women, there are very high rates of *false negatives* that make you think you are fine, when you can actually have significant bone loss in the hip or spine.
- *quantitative ultrasound (QUS).* Measures bones of the heel, proximal tibia, wrist or finger; these are precise, but are not able to detect sufficient change in bone mass required to monitor effectiveness of therapy. Again, this test is not useful for women under age 65 due to high rates of false negatives. Heel measurements are of little value if you have had previous ankle trauma or a fracture requiring immobilization of the lower leg.

© 2001–2007 Elizabeth Lee Vliet, M.D.

Vital Test

You may have read about bone density tests using the heel or wrist scans; research shows these are not reliable for women under age 65. If you are a younger woman with risk factors for bone loss, you need to have the DEXA hip and spine test.

Warning!

Young women with asthma, Lupus or early onset arthritis syndromes taking daily cortico-steroids are at especially high risk for developing pre-menopausal osteoporosis.

Testing for Bone Loss

Until 1985, the only way to diagnose osteoporosis was to wait for fractures, rather like waiting for a stroke as the sign of high blood pressure. Bone mineral density (BMD) testing, primarily with dual-energy X-ray absorptiometry (DEXA) of the hip and spine now gives an accurate and precise diagnosis of osteopenia or osteoporosis *before* a fracture. See preceding chart.

There are several excellent medications—Actonel, Boniva, Fosamax—approved for prevention and treatment of bone loss. These medicines prevent the breakdown process, called *resorption*, and also aid development of new, strong bone. Forteo is a new medicine that stimulates the parathyroid hormone and helps prevent bone loss.

Oh My Aching Muscles: Hormone Connections in Aches and Pains

Muscle aches (*myalgias*) and joint pain (*arthralgias*) are common complaints in women with low levels of ovarian hormones. Hippocrates first described the connection 2,500 years ago in menopausal women and "women with scant menses." Modern research confirms that low estradiol levels play a role in these symptoms. But what about younger women? Is it possible for hormone changes to cause stiff, sore muscles and aching joints?

At different times in the lives of younger women, hormones can be out of balance and lead to arthralgias and myalgias when 17-beta estradiol is low or falls sharply, or when progesterone, testosterone, or DHEA are out of balance with the estradiol. Unfortunately, these potential hormonal connections are simply "off the radar screen" for most doctors, so young women usually get pain medicines rather than testing of hormone levels to identify a cause of the pain.

Mechanisms of Hormone Effects on Muscles and Joints

There are a variety of pathways by which estradiol has positive effects on the health of muscle and joints, via effects on serotonin, endorphins, pain threshold, muscle tissue, cartilage formation, and blood flow to joints and muscle, to name a few.

Loss of estradiol means decreased blood flow to muscles and joints, less elasticity of connective tissue such as the cartilage supporting joints, lower levels of serotonin to modulate pain,

Dr. Vliet's Guide to Common Hormone Changes Causing Muscle and Joint Pain Problems in Women

- Postpartum (particularly if the pregnancy is after age 35),

- Women with PCOS who have high androgens, low estradiol

- 2 to 4 years after tubal ligation

- 2 to 4 years after hysterectomy if ovaries are not removed

- 2 months to 1 year after hysterectomy if ovaries are removed and hormone therapy either is not prescribed or hormones are not optimally restored to healthy levels

- women with premature ovarian decline (POD), particularly following viral illnesses

- women with autoimmune ovarian disorders, particularly if severe enough to cause Premature Ovarian Failure (POF)

- during times of loss of menses and optimal hormone levels: dieting, prolonged stress, prolonged illness, during active alcohol and drug abuse

- perimenopause, associated with sleep changes

- after menopause, particularly if not on ERT/HRT or if hormone therapy is giving suboptimal replacement

©Elizabeth Lee Vliet, MD 1995, revised 2001–2007

and nerve endings more sensitive to pain. Loss of estradiol also makes you less sensitive to the effects of pain medicines.

Declining estradiol disrupts the brain centers that regulate sleep. Sleep disruption decreases Stage 4 deep sleep reducing Growth Hormone secretion, so muscles can't repair normally at night, and you wake up stiff and sore. There are more sleep disrupting factors: with lower estradiol nerve endings more susceptible to pain disrupt sleep; muscle and joint pain disrupts sleep; the stress to the body of continued sleep loss increases imbalance in cortisol, norepinephrine, serotonin and endorphins.

All of these lead to more pain and more sleep disruption, further decreasing your ovary hormone production. The following diagram summarizes these connections.

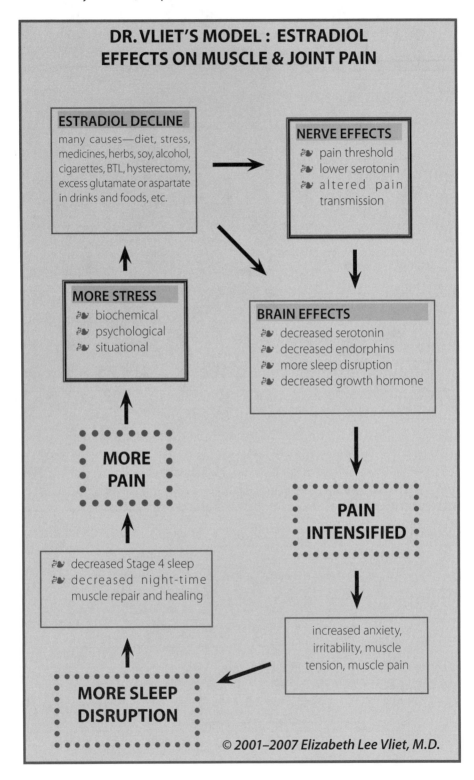

DR. VLIET'S MODEL : ESTRADIOL
EFFECTS ON MUSCLE & JOINT PAIN

ESTRADIOL DECLINE
many causes—diet, stress,
medicines, herbs, soy, alcohol,
cigarettes, BTL, hysterectomy,
excess glutamate or aspartate
in drinks and foods, etc.

NERVE EFFECTS
- pain threshold
- lower serotonin
- altered pain transmission

MORE STRESS
- biochemical
- psychological
- situational

BRAIN EFFECTS
- decreased serotonin
- decreased endorphins
- more sleep disruption
- decreased growth hormone

MORE PAIN

PAIN INTENSIFIED

- decreased Stage 4 sleep
- decreased night-time muscle repair and healing

increased anxiety, irritability, muscle tension, muscle pain

MORE SLEEP DISRUPTION

© 2001–2007 Elizabeth Lee Vliet, M.D.

Summary

There is so much confusing media coverage about the benefits of estrogen. Health writers, and physicians as well, overlook crucial and essential differences between the 17-beta estradiol our body makes and the foreign, mixed estrogens in Premarin, the product given to about 85% of women in the U.S. There is little awareness of FDA approved bio-identical hormone options that have been available for many years.

All estrogens preparations are not the same, and should not be confused. Articles in women's magazines, newspapers, and TV medical news spots don't address these points either, to help you understand what research findings really mean.

Media stories never point out that most of the studies in this country are based on use of Premarin or PremPro, estrogens significantly different from that which your body produces naturally. Few talk about 17-beta estradiol and what it does to keep you healthy and feeling well. Every system in your body uses this hormone to help the cells work properly.

For example, if a study like HERS only measures hormone effects after cardiovascular disease has already blocked the heart's arteries, it isn't surprising that they said there was no significant benefit. It's too late. The horse is already out of the barn, so to speak.

Our ovaries really are at the "hub" of a wheel symbolizing our entire body. With the many connections via the "spokes" of hormone pathways and receptors touching all the tissues and organs of our body, estradiol, progesterone, testosterone, and DHEA have profound effects.

Today most doctors practice specialties based on organ systems around the rim of the wheel, and they typically don't follow the spokes of hormone connections back to the hub. That's why they commonly miss the many effects of our ovarian hormones.

You are not imagining it.

Pay attention. You hormones affect all your body systems!

Trust your observations.

Find a physician who will be responsive to your concerns.

Have your ovarian hormones checked.

Get it RIGHT! Media sources of information for the general public consider all estrogens and progestins to be the same! No wonder you get confused reading the headlines.

Vital info You need this information to make choices will help you maintain your health, energy and vitality, as well as choices that help reduce your risk of diseases later in life.

Be alert *Nothing* is impossible when it comes to the diverse ways the body expresses imbalance.

Chapter 16
Balancing Ovarian Hormones for Optimal Health

Finding YOUR Hormone Balance

Getting anything *just right* takes a little time, patience, and work. Balancing hormones is no different. There are many hormone treatment options available to you, both in prescription form and over the counter.

ஒ What should you use?

ஒ How do you start?

ஒ What tests should you ask your physician about?

ஒ How do you interpret the results?

ஒ What are the optimal hormone levels for most women to feel their best?

ஒ What are the critical levels to prevent disease?

ஒ How do you identify risk factors?

ஒ What are the best hormone approaches?

This chapter walks you through the answers, step by step.

Step 1: Get Tested

If you scored high on the self-test at the beginning of the book or have symptoms of ovarian decline, the first step is a comprehensive hormone evaluation.

This is important; don't skip this step. Reliable hormone levels validate your suspicions about a connection between hormones and symptoms. Proper testing also indicates *which* hormones need adjusting, since symptoms are often similar.

Alert

Symptoms of low thyroid can mimic those of low estrogen and vice versa.

What is the best method of testing hormones?

I have explored many ways to test hormones but have found that serum (blood) tests are the most reliable method, and accurately correlate with the symptoms patients describe.

Saliva, hair analysis or urine tests of hormone levels are not reliable or complete and generally don't correlate with symptoms. They aren't even always less expensive.

Saliva and urine hormone tests are widely touted through newsletters, direct mail and the Internet by "experts" because they are available without a physician's order. You wind up wasting money because these tests are often wrong. Blood tests must be done before your physician can decide correct treatment.

Serum (blood) tests have been, and still are, the *gold standard* for researchers and physicians in need of reliable measurements to successfully make treatment decisions.

Serum hormone levels are the ones used by fertility specialists. If the blood tests of ovarian hormones are reliable and widely used to help women get pregnant, they should certainly be reliable for other types of hormone-related problems.

The reason serum tests better reflect hormone levels is that your ovarian hormones are transported in the blood *three* ways: **bound**—attached to sex-hormone binding globulin (SHBG), a carrier protein; **weakly bound**—attached to albumin; and **free**—*not bound* to carrier protein. The free amount is typically only 1–2% of the total circulating hormone.

The portion bound to Sex Hormone Binding Globulin (SHBG) is your reserve, like a savings account, ready for use the instant the body needs it. Measuring free, bound, and weakly-bound hormones is much like looking at all of your bank accounts to figure your total money available.

Saliva levels of ovarian and other hormones *only show the small part in the free fraction,* and the amount of the free fraction excreted into the saliva from serum.

As an analogy, a saliva test is like only counting the money in your hand, not what is in your pocket (free) or checking account (weakly bound), or savings account (bound).

Urine hormone assays only measure the metabolic break-down products of the various forms of the hormones, not the active forms.

What serum blood tests should I request?

Ovarian Hormones: Estradiol, progesterone, testosterone (free and weakly bound, and total), DHEA (conjugated and unconjugated), along with FSH and LH, drawn on day 1 to day 3 of your menstrual cycle. Measure the estradiol and progesterone levels again on day 20 if you are menstruating.

If you no longer menstruate, or had a hysterectomy, or take birth control pills, then measure all the ovarian hormones once, at any time.

Have the tests done *in the morning before any hormone medication*, or just before a new patch, or before you start a new pill pack of birth control pills.

Recheck these levels 2–3 months after you start hormone therapy, change medications, or have a surgical procedure such as a tubal ligation or hysterectomy.

Checking levels after starting Rx tells whether your therapy meets currently accepted minimum thresholds for preserving bone, brain, heart and other benefits of your hormone therapy.

Thyroid: For women, this should include TSH, free T4, free T3 and thyroid antibodies (anti-thyroglobulin and anti-microsomal). Together, these are more sensitive indicators of subtle (subclinical) thyroid disorders, long before the TSH moves out of the normal range.

Prolactin: This test measures the hormone produced by the pituitary. An elevated prolactin level can indicate a pituitary hormone-producing tumor. These are usually benign, but the hormone production from a small tumor (*microadenoma*) is enough to disrupt ovarian cycles, cause loss of menstrual periods, and contribute to headaches, depression, and weight problems.

Elevated prolactin is also a side effect of many medicines. (See Chapter 8.) Have your prolactin level checked between 7–8 AM for the most accurate results.

Important
Urine tests are less useful in measuring the circulating levels of the active forms of the ovarian hormones, the important information for treatment decisions.

High TSH
If your thyroid is failing (hypo-thyroidism), TSH is high (i.e., greater than 4 or 5 on most lab ranges).

See p. 53
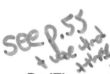

Alert!

I do not use this test to diagnose ovarian cancer, but it is the best early warning at this time. If CA 125 is elevated, you need further evaluation, such as a pelvic ultrasound.

Do IT!

Have the right tests, then know how to interpret the results correlated with your symptoms

CA 125: This is a test that can be elevated by ovarian cancer. *But benign conditions* such as endometriosis, fibroids, ovarian cysts, or even an early pregnancy can also elevate CA 125, so this can also be useful information to help decide the best treatment.

I encourage doing a CA 125 for all patients, especially if there is a family history of ovarian cancer, or if you have vague abdominal symptoms (gas, bloating, distension, change in bowel movements, or pain) that do not respond to other treatment.

What are the "optimal" hormone levels for well-being that also reduce risk of later problems, such as osteoporosis, and adverse cardiovascular changes?

When you don't feel well it is disappointing to be told "Good news, everything is normal!" It is not that you want to be sick, but the fact is you don't feel well, and want to know why.

Your physician may interpret the results based on lab "normals" rather than what your body needs to function best. Test results can fall within the lab reference range considered "normal," even though this range is too broad to be meaningful. This broad range, however, is not necessarily the "optimal" number for you to feel your best.

For **estradiol**, women generally say they feel their best when serum levels of estradiol are *above* 90–100 pg/ml. This is actually the *lower* end of the range for healthy menstrual cycle levels. Levels up to about 200 or so, are the *normal estradiol levels* of the first half of the menstrual cycle in premenopausal women.

Around ovulation, estradiol levels typically peak in the range of 300–500 pg/ml, and then in the luteal phase a healthy level of estradiol is generally in the 200-300 pg/ml range. International research finds that estradiol levels should be above 80–90 pg/ml to prevent bone loss, maintain brain function and provide cardiovascular benefits.

For **testosterone**, I find women typically feel best when serum levels of *total* testosterone are between 40 and 60 ng/dl (400–600 pg/ml), with the percent of free testosterone at about 1–2% of the total.

Levels below 30 ng/dl are generally too low to maintain your usual libido, intensity of orgasm, energy level, and bone mass.

The majority of menopausal women I evaluate, particularly those with surgical removal of the ovaries in their thirties and forties, have total testosterone levels of less than 10, and barely detectable amounts of free testosterone.

No wonder they don't have any sexual desire! This is also a significant factor in fatigue, as well as loss of muscle and bone.

Progesterone, the dominant hormone in the second half of the menstrual cycle, is measured and compared with the amount of estrogen present to decide which hormone is too low and causing symptoms. If you have ovulated, luteal phase progesterone level rises greater than 5, up to about 25 ng/dl, while follicular levels will be *less than* 1.

Thyroid Stimulating Hormone (TSH) is the hormone that stimulates the thyroid gland to produce more T3 and T4. Women can have symptoms of low thyroid when the TSH is over about 3. An optimal range of TSH for most women is generally between 0.5 to 2.0, especially if you are trying to conceive.

Follicle Stimulating Hormone (FSH) is produced by the pituitary gland, and its main function is to stimulate the ovary to produce new follicles every month. The follicles produce estradiol and progesterone. When estradiol levels drop, the FSH rises as the brain works to stimulate the ovaries to continue hormone production.

High FSH (above 20 MIU/ml) indicates estradiol is too low, and is one marker used to define menopause.

DHEA. Levels vary greatly, depending on the type of assay and reference ranges used by the lab, so I can't give specific "numbers" here. Significantly elevated DHEA is typically seen in PCOS, Syndrome X, and adrenal adenomas, and is a major cause of the adverse physical and metabolic changes.

What other tests are important in a comprehensive hormone evaluation?

The goal of a comprehensive hormone evaluation is to make sure *which* hormones are too low or too high and that you really have a hormonal imbalance causing your problems. Many disorders, such as PCOS, PMS, or premature menopause as well as other medical conditions, can cause similar symptoms.

The goal is to avoid the common mistake of misdiagnosing hormonal imbalance as psychiatric disorders—somatization, manic-depressive illness, major depressive disorder, anxiety, stress; or chronic fatigue, or chronic candidiasis.

Misery
Patients drag themselves into my office with estradiol levels of 10–30 pg/ml, yet were told it was "normal" because it fell within the reference range on the lab report. "Normal" doesn't mean what YOU need!

Low TSH
If there is excess thyroid hormone (hyperthyroidism), TSH is less than 0.3.

Reliable, objective measures identify the cause more accurately than symptoms that can be similar among many different disorders.

Vital

Insist doctors treat *you, not just your lab numbers.*

In addition to the serum hormone levels, have a mammogram and bone density test if you are 35 or over. You also need a breast and pelvic exam with a Pap smear, which can be done either by your primary care physician, gynecologist, or nurse practitioner. Physical exams provide other clues to hormone imbalance such as excess body hair (*hirsutism*), loss of body hair (alopecia), changes in skin pigmentation, enlarged or painful thyroid, patterns in body fat distribution, atrophic changes of breast and vagina, loss of height, and abnormal pulses, to name a few.

With all of the tests, it is important to integrate the "numbers" with symptoms to correlate the pattern of body changes with the fluctuations in blood levels.

The findings may lie at any point in the "normal" range, and still not be right for your body's needs. Sometimes your results may be *slightly* outside the "normal" range, but not medically significant.

Step 2: Evaluating your risks and identifying your needs

The next step is to determine how the results clarify causes of your symptoms and identify your **individual risks.** Compare your test results with the information I gave on **optimal** hormone levels.

Then you and your physician can discuss hormone options to help you make an educated decision about treatment.

1. Evaluate your lifestyle habits (diet, exercise, sleep habits, and work habits, whether or not you take the right vitamins and minerals, smoking, alcohol use, drug use, OTC and prescription medications) and work to eliminate the unhealthy ones.

2. Examine your own health risks, illness patterns, and any diseases that can be helped by hormone therapy, such as high cholesterol, high blood pressure, memory loss, depression, diabetes, osteoporosis or osteopenia, to mention a few.

3. Check your family history, especially first-degree relatives (parents, siblings) for common problems that can affect symptoms and future disease risks, such as diabetes, PCOS, elevated cholesterol, heart disease, high blood pressure,

thyroid disease, obesity, depression, cancers, osteoporosis and dementias. All can have a bearing on the importance of optimal estradiol balance as you get older.

This "risk-benefit" analysis should be based on medically sound, up-to-date information, not based on fear from an internet or "news magazine" piece or a friend's opinion.

You need to ask questions specific to YOU: "What are my health risks? Which will be *helped* by hormones? Which of my health risks can be *made worse*? Are hormones appropriate for me? Which type of hormone therapy, and route of taking hormones, is best suited to my needs? What options do I have?"

The following sections will help answer these questions.

Risk analysis
Based upon your risk assessment, weigh the potential benefits of hormone therapy against the risks.

Setting the record straight on hormones

Hormones don't *cause* cancer. There are many risk factors for cancer including genetics, exposure to environmental chemicals and radiation, obesity, diet, smoking and other lifestyle related habits.

The highest breast, endometrial and colon cancer rates occur in post-menopausal women who are obese, which means they have an excess of estrone.

Estrogen and progesterone may both facilitate the growth of an existing cancer, but there is no data that shows either hormone causes cancers.

You decide
Take your own "values inventory" to determine what quality-of-life aspects are important to you and how hormone therapy can help.

What about the studies that show taking estrogen after menopause increases your risk of breast cancer?

The studies showing increased risk are those in which women were primarily using Premarin or Prempro, the horse-derived mixture of estrogens that are chemically very different from the human 17-beta estradiol. Prempro also contains a potent synthetic progestin that has risks very different from natural progesterone. With all the extra horse-derived estrogens, this product delivers a high total load of foreign estrogens that you don't get from either the patch or the pill form of 17-beta estradiol. These are critical points that most media articles do not tell you, and many physicians overlook.

IMPORTANT! Multiple worldwide studies also show that women who do develop breast cancer while taking estrogen develop cancers that are the less aggressive types, and more responsive to treatment, and have better survival rates than do women who develop breast cancer *when not taking hormones.*

Natural!

ॐ phyto-estrogens for plants

ॐ Premarin for horses

ॐ 17-beta estradiol for humans!

Are all estrogens the same?

No. The estrogens made by your body differ from estrogenic compounds found in plants (phytoestrogens), synthetic estrogens, and the mixed, animal-derived estrogens such as Premarin. All are chemically quite different.

The non-human forms are different molecular "keys" and don't quite fit the "locks" of the estrogen receptors in your body to cause the same responses as your own 17-beta estradiol from the ovary.

Are all birth control pills the same?

No, they are definitely not. Different pills contain different ratios of estrogen and progestin, as well as different chemical types of progestins.

The lower the estrogen (E) relative to the progestin (P), the more likely you will have increased appetite, acne, weight gain, low sex drive, fatigue, headaches, and negative moods (irritability, depression), and breakthrough bleeding. The better the E:P ratio, the less likely you are to have these side effects.

The type of progestin, as well as the amount, plays a role in the kinds of side effects you may have.

If one pill causes problems, try one with a better balance of estrogen, or a different chemical class of progestin.

Do estrogen and/or progestin in birth control pills cause blood clots?

The data on this issue is based on *oral estrogen*, primarily Premarin and Prempro, or older high dose forms of birth control pills.

Newer data on the patch (transdermal) form of estradiol, our bio-identical premenopausal estrogen, shows that non-oral estradiol actually *decreases* the risk of thrombophlebitis ("blood clots"), via lowering fibrinogen and decreasing platelet "stickiness."

Older data that suggests birth control pills (BCP) caused blood clots was based on BCP use by cigarette smokers and on high-dose pills no longer available today. Cigarette smoking was determined to be the causative factor in the strokes that occurred in women taking BCP.

Does taking hormones make you fat?

No, taking the proper type hormones does not make you fat. The right hormones, in the right balance, actually improves insulin sensitivity and helps you lose excess body fat more readily provided you follow a balanced meal plan and increase physical activity.

Fat? Loss of healthy, premenopausal hormonal balance does contribute to weight gain.

I am concerned about taking birth control pills because of previous bad experiences. Have they changed?

Yes, there are many new options available today. The older pills had much higher doses of both hormones, for example 100 mcg estrogen vs. today's 20–35 mcg pills. None of the older, high dose pills are even available today.

Today's BCP formulas are also much less in the progestin content compared to when the pills first came on the market. About 1990, birth control pills were also approved by the FDA for non-smoking women over age 40 because of the many potential health benefits and reduction in rates of ovarian and uterine cancers. The FDA concluded benefits far outweighed the slight risks.

My doctor prescribed PremPro. Why are you telling me to take something different?

Everyone is different. PremPro contains a fixed dose combination of the horse-derived mixture of estrogens, Premarin, with a synthetic progestin called Provera. The fixed dose of each is not necessarily the right one for every woman, and many women have problems with weight gain, breast enlargement or tenderness with this combination.

Longevity does not equal "right" Premarin was the first oral estrogen preparation available and has been in use since the 1940s.

There are newer, FDA-approved options available, such as Activella, that give lower doses of the progestin and also has 17-beta estradiol identical to that made by the ovary.

There are FDA-approved patches and tablets of bioidentical 17-beta estradiol, as well as pills and vaginal creams with natural progesterone available. I suggest that you talk with your physician about the more natural options available today.

Many doctors still use Premarin and PremPro because of habit and the convenience of using a "one-prescription-fits-all" approach to women's hormones. It takes time and effort to fine-tune hormones on an individual basis.

There are other options! That doesn't mean it is the *best* option for everyone. Do you still drive a 1940s car?

Why the Old? Why should you take a horse estrogen produced before technology and science could duplicate the estrogen made by your body?

Go Healthy! Your body will do better with your own kind of "hormone power" rather than one Nature gave horses!

The Model T Ford was the first mass-produced automobile, but is certainly isn't the best option for use on today's high-speed Interstates.

If you have symptoms or side effects on Premarin or PremPro, demand a different option.

A recent study showed hormone replacement therapy doesn't prevent heart disease. Is this true?

The study that made the headlines in 2000 was "The **H**eart, **E**strogen-Progestin **R**eplacement **S**tudy (**HERS**) Study," and the Women's Health Initiative (**WHI**) study in 2002. In both these large studies, using Prempro, heart attacks were higher in the first years, then decreased.

The newspapers didn't tell you the serious short-comings in these studies. Here are a critical few:

- Neither one was a "prevention" study. In the HERS study, all of the women *already had* heart disease with major blockage of the coronary arteries before taking hormones; in the WHI, many were elderly, obese, and had health problems, just did not have "hot flashes."

- We really would not expect to see a *reversal of existing disease* in the short time frame of either study.

- The hormone therapy was PremPro, a combined product of horse-derived estrogens and a potent synthetic progestin (MPA) that is not the best type to improve lipids and other heart disease risk factors.

- None of the women were given natural progesterone instead of the synthetic progestin, even though we already have a number of studies showing better effects on lipids with natural progesterone.

This is another example of headlines, researchers, and many physicians missing the point about crucial differences among types of hormones.

Are hormones for everyone? Not necessarily. If you have no health risks, great bone density, and no symptoms, you may not need hormones. Just monitor your health with objective tests and evaluate hormone options later if your situation changes.

Are there non-hormonal alternatives to reduce symptoms? Yes. Many medicines, as well as other therapies, can relieve or treat *symptoms.* But many are not as effective as you may need, and most (including herbs) have side effects you must consider.

The more important issue to address with your doctor is the underlying cause of your problems. The *cause* should then be treated.

Many women take multiple medications, and still don't feel well. If this is true for you, and tests show a hormonally based problem, then it makes sense to try hormones and treat the cause.

Step 3: Choosing a hormone approach

Although many physicians think all the estrogens for ERT are essentially the same, and the manufacturers of the leading products want you to think that too, **they are not.**

There are many differences and different effects with various hormone preparations, as many studies of the past decade, and my own clinical experience prove.

But why start with hormones, and not diet, exercise and reduction of stress, as is often suggested first?

Your hormones are the metabolic fuel that power cells. It is hard to make significant lifestyle changes if you are too tired to get out of bed in the morning because your hormones are out of kilter and you aren't sleeping! I think it is crucial to address underlying hormonal imbalances first, so that you are better able to incorporate healthy lifestyle choices (see Chapters 8, 12).

This is *not* DIY

Don't just use herbal "band-aids" to treat symptoms.

Natural vs. Synthetic

A lot of women want to only take *natural* hormones. This is why many use the "wild yam" skin creams advertised as a source of progesterone, or dong quai (an herb supposedly with estrogenic compounds), or estriol (weakest of the three primary human estrogens) instead of "drugs," which are "synthetic."

The words "natural" and "synthetic" are confusing. Don't be misled by clever marketing. Actually, something *synthetic* can also be *natural*, while something *natural* be *foreign or "supernatural"* for the human body.

Premarin is a "natural" mixture of estrogens because a biological organism, a horse, makes it. *But Premarin is not natural for the human body.*

Choices

Understand the different types of hormone approaches available. Choose the best one for you.

Genistein found in soy and red clover, among others, is a "natural" substance because it comes from a biological source, the soy plant.

But genistein is *"un-natural" for our bodies.* We don't make these same compounds and don't have the enzymes to change the genistein or clover isoflavones into 17-beta estradiol, or progesterone, or testosterone.

Making "natural" hormones bioidentical to those in the human body is a process that must be done in the laboratory. We call it "synthesizing," from the Greek word meaning "a putting together, composition; to make something."

Synthetic simply means "produced by synthesis." In common usage today, "synthetic" has *come to mean "artificial,"* which is not always correct.

Unithroid and Estrace are "synthetic" in that they have been made in the laboratory, rather than within a biological organism. Yet, they are "natural" because they are the exact same molecular structure as the ones made by the thyroid and ovary, respectively. And they are FDA approved.

New start

Improving your hormone balance provides an important biochemical foundation upon which to build an integrated approach to your overall mind-body-spirit health.

"Natural," bioidentical human estrogens

The sources for the bioidentical human forms of ovarian hormones are actually building-block molecules called sterols found in plants such as soybeans and yams.

The plant sterols are purified and chemically converted in the laboratory to produce chemical molecules *identical to those made in the human body.* Our body does not have the enzymes to make this conversion.

The resulting 17-beta estradiol, progesterone, or testosterone is then compounded into standardized tablets that regulate the amount of hormone given.

The standardization of dose in each tablet allows a physician to know exactly the amount given so the prescription can be tailored to each individual woman's needs.

This method is better than using health food store mixtures from plant/herbal sources, because those don't allow you to *determine the dose of plant compounds, or their unwanted effects in your body.* Purity isn't regulated and you also get additional chemicals *native to plants* that your body does not need.

I recommend using prescription grade **17-beta estradiol,** which is what keeps your body's cellular machinery working at optimal effectiveness.

There are several FDA-approved brands of bioidentical 17 beta-estradiol commercially available in this country. All of these brands contain estradiol made from soybean or wild yam precursor molecules.

These are as follows: (as of this writing) Estrace tablets and vaginal cream (FDA approved in 1976), Gynediol tablets, transdermal patches (Climara, Vivelle, Vivelle DOT, Menostar, Estraderm), Estragel, Estrasorb lotion, combination estradiol-progestin products (Activella, Angelique, Combi-Patch), and vaginal preparations such as Estrace creams, Vagifem tablets, Femring, and Estring vaginal rings.

I do not recommend using *estriol,* the weaker placenta-derived form of estrogen, because extensive studies over the last 30 to 40 years have shown that it doesn't provide the necessary protective effects on bone, heart, brain, and nerves as does premenopausal 17-beta estradiol.

Don't believe the marketing hype that estriol is "safer." Many studies have addressed this issue and there is no reputable scientific data to support these claims.

Empty!
You may not have the *energy* to exercise and eat right if your hormone fuel tank is on empty!

Not so!
There are NO good studies that show estriol "prevents breast cancer."

Synthetic Estrogens: not native to the human body

All of these estrogens have slightly different chemical structures from the three human forms (estradiol, estrone, estriol), and are therefore more potent, as well as having somewhat different effects and side effects on the body. There are appropriate uses for each, such as contraception.

❧ **ethinyl estradiol (EE):** The most common form of estrogen found in the birth control pill. Birth control pills are widely used in perimenopausal women who need control of irregular cycles and erratic bleeding. I recommend it for this purpose. EE is not widely used in the U.S. for postmenopausal ERT because it is more potent than needed after a woman reaches menopause and contraception is no longer necessary. EE is more often used in Europe than the United States, but if used alone, it is not a contraceptive because it does not contain progestin.

Estradiol valerate

Once in the body, estradiol valerate separates into its two components and provides estradiol like your ovaries made.

FYI

Plant sterols are all chemically different molecular "keys" from our own estradiol.

Doesn't work?

You can change your mind, stop what you are doing, and start another option.

&❧ **estradiol valerate:** Estradiol valerate is a synthetic estrogen commonly used for menopause therapy in Europe and other countries, but less so in the United States. It is available for oral or intramuscular delivery, and is more potent and lasts longer than 17-beta estradiol.

Estradiol valerate is the estradiol used in the 1979 Swedish study that initially reported a higher risk of breast cancer in estrogen users. Follow-up analysis of the same data from this group in Sweden, published in 1992, shows *no increase* in breast cancer risk in users of estradiol valerate. This update, however, did not get press attention or make headlines.

Phytoestrogens

Phytoestrogens are estrogenic compounds such as isoflavones found in several hundred different plants, including soybeans, red clover, and grains. These are biologically weaker than the native human estrogens.

There is another issue to consider: concentration in the bloodstream. Isoflavone supplements can quickly give high serum concentrations of the phytoestrogens that overwhelm the miniscule amounts of estradiol and wind up competing with and inhibiting the action of your hormone. This makes your own estradiol less effective. Health articles and product ads don't tell you this part of the picture.

Although the phytoestrogens are less potent than 17-beta estradiol, herbalists often recommend them as a "natural" source of estrogen. **But they are not "natural" for a human body.**

These products are heavily marketed for PMS and menopausal remedies, with claims that they are "safer" than our own hormones. This isn't always the case. And they really provide little benefit.

Several recent double-blind, placebo-controlled, prospective studies in the international menopause literature have found that phytoestrogen products were no more effective than placebo even for controlling hot flashes, much less all the other functions of our own ovarian estradiol.

There can also be adverse effects. Ginseng, for example, can cause high blood pressure, insomnia, anxiety, and agitation if taken in the currently recommended doses, and studies clearly show it does not have measurable estrogenic effect. Black cohosh can damage the liver.

At the Fork in the Road: Deciding What to Take

Premenopausal women who are still menstruating, but experiencing ovarian decline and health risks like bone loss, or menopausal symptoms such as hot flashes or fragmented sleep, have two roads to consider:

One is *birth control pills*.

The other road is *physiologic hormonal supplementation* with estradiol, progesterone and testosterone as appropriate.

There are advantages and disadvantages to each approach. If you decide on one approach for awhile, you haven't locked yourself in for the rest of your life.

The KEY
The key is to choose the pill with the right estrogen to progestin ratio to help you feel better, calm the turbulence of your cycles, and minimize side effects.

Option I: Using Birth Control Pills As "Hormone Stabilizers"

Birth control pills (BCPs) deliver hormones constantly, putting the ovaries at rest. The steady dose of both estrogen and progestin mimics early pregnancy, and the brain does not send out the FSH and LH signals to stimulate the ovaries for a menstrual cycle.

"The pill" suppresses your cycles, and ovulation, preventing the "roller coaster ride" of monthly hormone ups and downs. As a result of the steadier hormone levels from BCP, my patients tell me their PMS symptoms are markedly diminished.

Steady is better
Monophasic E/P pills keep you on a more "even keel" than a triphasic pill.

Newer low-dose BCP provide other health benefits beyond contraception and hormonal stability. In fact, in a medical article in *ObGyn News* in 1999, Dr. Patricia J. Sulak of the Scott and White Clinic in Temple, Texas said, "*BCP are one of the most important preventive health measures in all of medicine. There's no medicine that offers reproductive-age women more benefits; there's nothing out there that even touches OCs (oral contraceptives).*"

You hear unpleasant reports of side effects with BCP, or you may have tried them and felt terrible. In my experience, this usually happens when the progestin does is too high and the estrogen too low. There are many new and more effective options available than even a decade ago. If you had a bad experience in the past, you may be pleasantly surprised with modern BCPs.

Fewer problems
Better E:P ratio pills have many fewer side effects!

Many studies show that women who don't stay on the pill have heavy periods and irregular periods, premenstrual syndrome, functional ovarian cysts, and a higher likelihood of endometriosis and fibroids.

Good News!
BCP reduce the risk of ovarian cancers by about 50–60% and endometrial cancers by 70-80% if taken for at least 5 years!

Women with PCOS can actually help preserve future fertility by starting BCP at a younger age, and stay on it except when attempting pregnancy, and when breast-feeding.

BCP work especially well for women over 30, whose ovaries often start acting up with the beginning of ovarian decline. Since about 80–90% of all women develop irregular bleeding before menopause, BCP can help reduce the amount of menstrual flow as well as the common erratic bleeding.

In addition, 1994 studies from Italy, along with others since, show a significant protective effect on maintaining bone density in women taking OCs during perimenopause. Other health benefits of birth control pills include those in the chart that follows.

In my practice, I find patients have additional benefits of BCP:

Bleeding
When you stop the active hormone pills in the birth control pill pack, it is the drop in progestin that triggers a period.

- Better preservation of bone mass
- Reducing menstrual migraine frequency by continuous pill use, with no break for periods
- Reducing excess androgen effects in PCOS
- Improving muscle and joint pain
- Improving cyclic mood swings, decreasing cyclic anxiety
- Improving energy, decreasing fatigue
- Improving vulvar and vulvodynia pain (if low progestin pills are used)
- Improving vaginal lubrication and interest in sex

So how do you choose a birth control pill?

If you are using BCP to decrease symptoms of PMS, PCOS, endometriosis, fibroids, heavy bleeding or migraines, I recommend a BCP pill formula with a low progestin content relative to the estrogen to reduce typical progestin side effects like depression, weight gain, headaches, fatigue, acne, low sex drive, vaginal dryness, and other unwanted side effects.

Other symptoms
The drop in estrogen causes headaches, muscle aches, insomnia, pain flares, or mood symptoms.

A pill that contains a steady-dose (*monophasic*) of both estrogen and progestin gives better suppression of ovarian cycling than does a tri-phasic pill that has varying hormone levels.

BCP with better estrogen content (30–35 mcg of ethinyl estradiol), such as Ovcon 35, Modicon, Ortho-Cyclen, Ortho-Cept, Yasmin or Diane 35 are important for maintaining bone mass, improving mood/sleep/hot flashes, maintaining normal libido and orgasm ability, for example. Another good option is the non-oral Nuvaring.

Pills with *high* progestin and low estrogen ratio (such as Alesse, Mircette, Loestrin) have more unwanted side effects of weight gain, bloating, constipation, acne, fatigue, depression, low sex drive, difficulty having an orgasm and vaginal dryness.

In control!
Yes, you can be in control of when you have a period!

You need a certain amount of progestin (1) to suppress ovary cycles and prevent hormone fluctuations that trigger symptoms and (2) to protect the lining of the uterus from becoming too thick ("hyperplasia") as it would if you took estrogen alone.

A low progestin pill still accomplishes both of these goals. The disadvantage is that with less progestin you can have more break-through bleeding and spotting that can be annoying. This is temporary and should resolve after about 3–6 months on the BCP.

Myth
"BCP make you gain weight." Not so!

If bleeding remains a problem, a straightforward way to manage it is to increase the progestin content for just a few months. You aren't likely to become depressed on the higher progestin if you just take it for a short time. Taking a higher progestin pill for 2–3 cycles usually stops the bleeding problems effectively. You can do this every few months if needed.

If bleeding remains heavy after increasing the progestin content, then your physician may suggest a pelvic ultrasound to measure the thickness of the uterine lining and check for polyps or fibroids.

BCP and weight gain
This is usually fluid, not fat. Eat right and exercise and you're not likely to get fat on the pill.

To keep the estrogen level steady to prevent headaches or other symptoms between BCP packs, I recommend you use an estradiol pill or estradiol patch for the days off BCP to prevent the drop in estrogen between pill packs.

If you prefer NOT having periods every month, you can take the active hormone pills every day, with no break between packs. This is safe, but this option is a well-hidden secret. You simply throw away the placebo pills and go right into your next pill pack.

You can do this for 3 to 6 packs and then stop for 3–4 days to have a period, if you wish. If you are taking the pills continuously and start to have bothersome break-through bleeding, stop them at any time to have a period, which should typically alleviate that problem.

Warning!
Do not smoke cigarettes while taking birth control pills, as smoking may increase your risk of stroke.

Follow the suggestions above, and ask your doctor about supplemental estradiol whenever you stop the active BC pills to prevent symptoms from the drop in estrogen during your period.

Common Side Effects with BCP:

Whenever you increase the female hormones, estrogen and progesterone (or the progestin in birth control pills), you can expect some breast tenderness and fullness, mild feelings of fluid retention or bloating, headaches, cramps, feelings of tiredness and possibly "queasiness" or nausea like early pregnancy.

Initial weight gain of a few pounds is typically due to *fluid* balance changes, not increased body *fat*. These are usually *temporary* side effects and commonly resolve by about the third pill pack.

Be patient
Most common side effects are temporary and resolve in 3–6 months.

Break-through bleeding and spotting are also quite common in the early months of using birth control pills, especially those with low progestin content. This usually stops by 3 to 6 months on the pill. Be patient.

Most women tell me they feel much better overall with less progestin, so it can be worth the inconvenience of some spotting for a while to achieve these other benefits.

Most studies to date show no increased risk of breast cancer in women who use the birth control pill. Check the National Cancer Institute graphs for the last forty years. You will see that over the time that BCPs exponentially increased in use, the graph for breast cancer has remained steady, and even began decreasing slightly in 1996. These graphs are available from the American Cancer Society (see Appendix II).

Menopause yet?
If your FSH is greater than 20 mIU/mL on the days off the hormone-containing birth control pills, then you have reached the endocrine stage of menopause.

Please read your pill package insert for possible serious reactions. Notify your gynecologist or primary care physician promptly if you have any of these problems.

Transitioning: BCP to Menopause HRT Options

By using an oral contraceptive in the years of hormone decline, you typically do not experience the hot flashes and other symptoms that mark the endocrine transition to actual menopause.

How do you decide when to change to *post*menopausal hormone options? This is best done with the assistance of a knowledgeable health professional, so you don't experience any unwanted effects from stopping oral contraceptives abruptly or from differences in potency of the birth control pills and the natural hormones.

I recommend that you have an annual blood test to measure FSH, beginning at age 50 or so. Do this test on the 5th to 7th days *off the active birth control pills, during the "placebo" week when you menstruate.*

If the FSH is checked at the end of the week of placebo pills, you are off hormones long enough for FSH to rise into the meno-pausal range, if you are menopausal. If you have not yet reached menopause, the FSH will still be low on these days.

If you check FSH while taking the *hormone-containing* pill, it is suppressed to a level usually less than 3 or 4 and *will not give an accurate determination of your menopausal status.*

Your physician may not yet be aware of how and when to check FSH, since it is still relatively new to use oral contra-ceptives for perimenopausal women into their early fifties. I suggest a switch to the postmenopausal hormone options when your FSH is above 20. If the FSH is still less than 20, you could possibly still become pregnant (although it is uncom-mon), and you may want to stay on the oral contraceptives until your FSH is menopausal.

Good news
You do not have to stop the oral contraceptives for several months in order to check the FSH, as many women are told.

Option II: The Other Fork in the Road

What if you are still premenopausal and need a hormone "boost" but do not want to take birth control pills? There are other op-tions. You can choose to follow your cycle and supplement with 17-beta estradiol pills, patches or creams to compensate for ovar-ian decline. This is a bit more complicated and unpredictable to manage, but it still can work well for some women.

With this approach, you would still experience the ups and downs of your cycle, but you ease the symptoms of low estradiol with the pill or patch, or lotion. You also have estradiol's other benefits.

When your own ovaries stop making progesterone, you need to add it to trigger a regular shedding of the uterine lining and prevent bleeding problems or excess build up of the uterine lining (hyperplasia). There are several FDA-approved options available, as I explain below.

Keep at it!
You and your physician must work together to adjust your dose to give you levels closer to the healthy menstrual cycle range.

For women with a normal cycle who have regular bleeding, body markers of ovulation with a rise in progesterone from the ovaries, you may ask your doctor about adding supplemental progesterone later, after regular cycles stop, or you start skip-ping periods, and can no longer feel yourself ovulating, or you have erratic bleeding. This has to be monitored closely to avoid bleeding problems or hyperplasia.

Forms of Estradiol

In my experience, FDA-approved bioidentical 17-beta estradiol options typically give better relief of symptoms than conjugated equine estrogens (Premarin and PremPro) or esterified estrogens (Estratab, Estratest, Menest, and Cenestin).

For optimal benefits on pain, mood and sleep pathways in particular, the dose may need to be higher than traditional HT doses, which are based on the *minimally* effective dose to relieve hot flashes.

FDA-approved Bioidentical Estradiol Options

Bioidentical Estradiol

Many options are available and FDA-approved! You do not have to get them from compounding pharmacies!

- Transdermal estradiol (Climara, Vivelle DOT, Menostar, and generics) patches
- Oral micronized estradiol (Estrace and Gynediol brands) or generic 17-beta estradiol ("estradiol")
- If the transdermal route is preferable, but you have rashes with patches, try the new FDA-approved estradiol gel (Estragel), or lotion (Estrasorb)
- The vaginal ring (Estring), vaginal cream (Estrace), or vaginal tablets (Vagifem) are very good options for topical vaginal and urinary urogenital effects but these doses are too low for significant systemic benefits (i.e. to relieve hot flashes, improve sleep, etc.)
- Femring is a systemic dose vaginal ring works well, but doesn't always last the full 3 months it is supposed to.
- Injectable estrogens, or pellets and implants, may be an option as well. These deliver higher levels initially, with an unpredictable fall in levels prior to next injection or implant. I use injectable forms occasionally, but they are more difficult to regulate and fine-tune, especially if your own ovaries still make any measurable estradiol.

Patch or Pill?

The brands of transdermal estrogen patches, lotions, and gels listed earlier are recent innovations. Their delivery of the human 17-beta estradiol is the most "natural" of all. The estradiol is absorbed through the skin, directly into the bloodstream, much like the ovary does before menopause, without going through the stomach and liver *first*.

BENEFICIAL EFFECTS OF ORAL CONTRACEPTIVES
Condition or Disease Decrease Compared to Non-pill Users

1. Menstrual Disorders   DECREASE:

Dysmenorrhea	63%
Menopausal symptoms	72%
Menorrhagia	48%
Irregular menstruation	35%
Inter-menstrual bleeding	28%
Premenstrual tension (PMS)	29% (I find the reduction in symptoms is better than this with low progestin, higher estrogen pill

2. Reproductive Organ Tumors DECREASE:

Breast: fibrocystic/fibroadenomas	60–75%
Breast biopsies	50%
Benign ovarian cysts	65% (if using Monophasic, steady-dose pills)
Uterine fibroids (fibroma)	59%
Ovarian cancer	40%
Endometrial cancer	50%

3. Other Reproductive Disorders DECREASE:

Endometriosis	50%–60%
Pelvic inflammatory disease	10%–70%
Toxic shock syndrome	60%
Uterine retroversion	24%

4. Other Health Problems   DECREASE:

Rheumatoid arthritis	50%
Iron deficiency anemia	45%
Duodenal ulcer	40%
Sebaceous cysts	24% (better decrease with some progestins than others)
Acne	20% (better response rate with low progestin dose, and androgen-blocking progestins)

Ref: Richard P. Dickey, MD, Ph.D. *Managing Contraceptive Pill Patients*, 11th edition, Essential Medical Information Systems, 2002. *Comments in brackets by Dr. Vliet.*

The estradiol patches all look like a clear circular, oval or rectangular "Band-Aid" that sticks to the skin and stays in place for several days as the hormones are slowly absorbed. As the hormone delivery falls, the patch is replaced. Each brand of patch lasts for a slightly different time, and because women metabolize the hormones at different rates, it can take some experimentation to find the right change schedule and dose strength for you.

First pass

The "first pass" metabolism in the liver breaks down some of the estradiol into estrone, making it less effective for estradiol's normal functions.

Patches are a very good option for estrogen therapy, with only two primary drawbacks: (1) the skin irritation from the adhesive bothers some women, and (2) if you have a low level of HDL, you may need the extra "plus" of oral estrogen stimulating the liver to make more HDL.

The patch, lotion, gel and vaginal ring give the beneficial *physiological* (normal) effect of estrogen to maintain the normal level of HDL cholesterol, but not the *pharmacologic* (greater than normal) effect of extra liver stimulation to make more HDL as seen with the oral estrogens.

If you have a normal cholesterol profile, the patch is all you need to give the physiologic benefits. If you have high total cholesterol and *low* HDL, an *oral* form of estradiol provides greater *decrease* in total cholesterol and *increase* in HDL for cardiovascular protective effects.

Transdermal has several advantages over oral delivery, as summarized in the chart on the next page.

Migraines and Estradiol and Patches

A typical example of my unifying approach happens when I see a woman who has suffered from migraines. I ask detailed questions about the relationship of the headaches to her menstrual cycle, in addition to all the usual history and workup identifying the typical triggers like foods, stress, weather changes, etc.

If a woman tells me she has a regular migraine every month when her period starts, it makes sense! There is a hormone connection here! Science shows that falling estradiol decreases serotonin, constricts blood vessels and lowers pain threshold. This sets off the migraine just as bleeding begins.

One approach I use for headache sufferers is to teach them to use an estradiol skin patch to avoid the drop in estradiol level and prevent the headache from beginning. Using estradiol patches this

Dr. Vliet's Guide to Advantages of Transdermal Estradiol Over Oral

- Non-oral forms keep blood levels of estradiol fairly steady, similar to ovarian hormone production.
- Bypassing the liver's "first-pass" metabolism can decrease triglycerides (TG). Oral estrogen in some women increases TG, which is not desirable because high TG is an independent risk factor for heart disease and diabetes in women.
- Transdermal delivery of estradiol improves glucose-insulin pathways, an important benefit for women with insulin resistance or diabetes.
- Non-oral forms provide better relief of hormonally-triggered migraines due to slower rise and fall in blood levels.
- Non-oral forms typically have better dilating effects on blood vessels and lower blood pressure more than oral estrogen does.
- Non-oral delivery decreases clotting factors like fibrinogen and factors such as rennin substrate that can raise blood pressure more than oral estrogen does.
- Non-oral forms don't increase estrone like oral forms, an advantage for overweight women whose body fat makes excess estrone, a risk factor for breast cancer.

© 2001–2007 Elizabeth Lee Vliet, M.D.

way doesn't stop the menstrual flow, which is triggered by the fall in progesterone. It seems such a logical approach for a migraine that always comes with menses. Of course, if the estradiol patch does not work, I use other approaches. Women frequently tell me that their migraine headaches are relieved, or are less frequent and or less severe when we find a way to keep the estradiol steady. I consider this a *crucial first step* with menstrual migraines. I can always go to the standard medications later, if needed.

specifies natural non-oral progesterone for PCOS on p.429

Progesterone

I use FDA-approved products for many of my patients, Prometrium or Prochieve. For many women, the natural hormone progesterone causes fewer side effects than the synthetic progestins (Provera, Cycrin, MPA, norethindrone, levonorgestrel, etc).

There are also times when the potency of the synthetics provides better control of medical problems such as heavy bleeding or endometriosis. ***There is a great deal of individual variation, so ignore sweeping generalizations that one is always better than another.***

Current accepted doses for progesterone to provide therapeutic effects on the uterine lining (endometrium) without excess buildup (hyperplasia) are as follows :

NO! I do ***not*** recommend such high doses of progesterone. It has many adverse breast AND metabolic AND mood effects.

Warning!
If you use natural progesterone for hormone therapy, stick with the FDA-approved and medically-accepted dose ranges.

Options
There are also women who just feel better on one of the synthetic progestins than they do with natural progesterone.

Do the Math!
100 mg/gm cream is roughly equivalent to about 1,000 mg oral progesterone.

1. For a **cyclic regimen,** the usual dose is 200 mg of **oral** micronized progesterone (i.e. Prometrium) for 10–14 days a month. If you are allergic to peanut oil you can't use Prometrium, but compounded prescriptions are available. **Prochieve** is a vaginal gel in sustained release form, and the 4% strength is given **every other night for 6 doses a month.**

The FDA-approved dose schedule gives 40 mg every other day, or an *average daily* dose 20 mg. If Prochieve isn't readily available, a similar preparation can be made up by a compounding pharmacist.

2. For a **continuous daily regimen** the accepted dose is 100 mg oral progesterone every day, usually best given at bedtime because of the sedative side effects for most people.

Note: progestins are more potent than natural progesterone, and are therefore used in much lower doses. For example, Provera or Aygestin 2.5 mg is usually given for a daily schedule, or 5 mg is used for 10–14 days in a cyclic regimen. Some women do fine on even the lower dose of Micronor, 0.35 mg.

Caution: Progesterone doses in excess of 300 mg a day orally (or creams containing more than 20–30 mg per day) cause blood levels of progesterone that are as high as those found in the *third trimester of pregnancy.*

I see women getting prescriptions for 100 mg per gram of progesterone creams, to be applied twice daily. Such a dose is seriously excessive, particularly since the FDA-approved dosing for transdermal vs. oral is usually for transdermal forms to be about 1/10 a typical oral dose. Two applications of such a cream each day would give you roughly the equivalent of taking 2000 mg in a pill or tablet! *No wonder women using this feel fat, bloated, and depressed!*

Higher doses of progesterone are often recommended by other doctors for PMS treatment, but can cause or aggravate many other problems: (1) marked weight gain similar to pregnancy, (2) high blood glucose and decreased glucose control in diabetics or women with insulin resistance, (3) high triglycerides, (4) high cholesterol, (5) higher than normal insulin production, (6) more backaches, due to ligaments becoming lax or "loose" from progesterone effects, (7) headaches, or intensified migraines, (8) decreased sex drive, and (9) depressed, lethargic mood.

One problem is that many health specialists who recommend such high doses of natural progesterone do not check serum levels of progesterone, do not monitor the cholesterol-triglyceride profile, and do not check for changes in fasting glucose and insulin. They then miss these developing problems.

Downer! Excess progesterone often causes lethargy, fatigue, and low libido!

Be careful about too much progesterone, especially if you are overweight, have diabetes, hypertension, elevated cholesterol or triglycerides, or a history of depression.

If you think progesterone is a "wonder" hormone and doubt the potential for serious side effects with it, simply recall two common pregnancy-related problems most women know: (1) pregnancy-induced ("gestational") diabetes, and (2) toxemia or pre-eclampsia, a severe form of high blood pressure that occurs in the latter part of pregnancy. These two problems often occur in the last stages of pregnancy when progesterone levels are at the highest levels.

If You Are Sensitive to Progestins—What Else is Available?

Nuvaring is a combined estrogen-progestin contraceptive that comes as a soft vaginal ring. It contains ethinyl estradiol (15 mcg or 0.015 mg) and a new progestin called etonogestrel (0.120 mg). I use it often for my patients as a "hormone stabilizer" for women with disruptive PMS or PCOS mood swings, or to help decrease cramps, pelvic pain, or heavy bleeding.

Nuvaring allows both hormones to be slowly released into the vaginal tissue and then absorbed directly into the bloodstream, bypassing the "first-pass" effect through the liver. This means lower doses of both hormones can be used, which in turn helps to minimize the typical side effects that women experience with oral BCP.

Nuvaring is very soft and pliable, making it easy for a woman to insert and remove on her own. If you want to have your usual menstrual period, you remove it at the end of three weeks. If you want to skip a menstrual period or prevent cramps and heavy bleeding, you may leave the ring in place for three weeks, and then immediately replace it with a new one. This keeps the hormone delivery steady and prevents the drop in progestin that triggers a period and cramps.

Nuvaring has worked very well for many of my patients who had bothersome side effects with oral birth control pills, so it may be

Progestin IUDs

Very low doses have less systemic effect and are better for the body and the breast.

Go Trans...

Sometimes oral doses are not absorbed adequately for desirable blood levels or cause adverse changes in cholesterol. Changing to a gradually absorbed transdermal cream often improves the overall response.

an option to discuss with your physician. To read more about it, check the website www.nuvaring.com.

Mirena and **Progestasert** are two *intrauterine* progestin-delivery systems approved as contraceptives rather than as progestin therapy in peri- or menopausal women, but they are options if you have side effects with oral progestins.

Both release a small amount of progestin daily directly into the lining of the uterus, and very little progestin is absorbed into the total body circulation. This reduces the likelihood of the unpleasant side effects such as headaches, depression, low libido, weight gain, and vaginal dryness often associated with progestins in hormone therapy and birth control pills.

Some women use these intrauterine delivery systems successfully if they cannot tolerate any other form. A number of studies show that these products deliver enough progestin to effectively suppress the build-up of the uterine lining.

There are some drawbacks, however, so it is important to discuss these with your health professional. Possible problems with either Mirena or Progestasert include increase in ovarian cysts, increased risk of pelvic inflammatory disease if there are multiple sexual partners, increased risk of ectopic pregnancy, erratic bleeding, and menstrual changes.

If you need a progestin and nothing else has worked, ask your doctor about these products. Pregnancy rates are less than 0.02%, and it also reduces the amount of monthly bleeding for most women after the initial 3–6 month adjustment. After a year, about 20% of women have no further bleeding, and there is much less progestin being delivered to the rest of your body, especially the breasts.

Testosterone or DHEA

Consider adding either one of the androgens if you have documented *low serum* levels, but do *not* base a treatment decision on the highly variable and unreliable saliva test for testosterone and DHEA. Serious side effects can occur with too much of either.

In addition, it is far better to restore testosterone directly than to try DHEA, since the conversion of DHEA to testosterone is fairly unpredictable, especially if your ovaries are declining or have been surgically removed.

Women's testosterone levels are obviously not the same as men. For some time the only synthetic testosterone available was *methyl* testosterone, the one associated with causing liver damage, and a few others not natural to the human body.

Until recently, doctors were not aware that women needed considerably lower doses of testosterone. This is the root of horror stories about testosterone causing moustaches and a beard, voice changes, and liver damage.

Through the miracle of the laboratory, soybeans are turned into *boy*beans, now that scientists can synthesize exact molecular replicas of women's own testosterone. Using the micronization process, we now have a form of natural testosterone that is not lost to the digestive process when taken orally, as we have for progesterone and estradiol.

Unlike OTC DHEA, prescription grade (USP) DHEA or *testosterone* is standardized so I know exactly how much of the hormone I prescribe and can fine-tune it for each individual.

Until we have a FDA-approved bioidentical testosterone, it has to be made by compounding pharmacists, as skin cream, skin gel, tablets, injections or vaginal suppositories. The method of delivery determines the amount absorbed, how it metabolizes into other forms, and the effects—desirable or undesirable.

Gels and troches are being touted as "best," but I prefer the slower absorption forms because a *rapid* rise in blood level of testosterone can cause **aggressiveness, pounding headaches, insomnia and irritability.**

We do not yet have a FDA-approved product of bioidentical testosterone for *women*, even though there are several approved by the FDA for *men*. The bioidentical testosterone patch for women was not approved by the FDA in 2004 in spite of excellent data on safety *and* effectiveness. This is a major loss for women's health, particularly for women who have loss most of their testosterone due to surgical removal of their ovaries.

Until such time as we can in the U.S. can get FDA-approved bioidentical options for women, *as men have had for years*, we have to use *compounded* testosterone. This process uses *testosterone USP*, a pharmaceutical-grade, bioidentical form

Testo is good! It isn't that testosterone is bad, it is that we haven't had the native form available, and it hasn't been used with much finesse for women!

Warning! Pain, headaches, acne, hair loss, insomnia, anxiety and irritability are worse if androgens are given *before* optimal estradiol is restored.

like the ovaries make. I don't recommend synthetic *methyl* testosterone.

Currently, commercial brands of testosterone don't have doses low enough for women on a daily basis, or the bioidentical form made by our bodies. Compounded prescriptions allow a fine-tuning of the dose. I use a sustained-release tablet or capsule, or a slow-release cream form. Oral doses generally are 1–4 mg daily.

2% Testo cream

Dose is much to high for a woman! This is a man's dose!

Transdermal cream doses need to be lower non-oral routes (transdermal, vaginal, sublingual) have more rapid and more complete absorption from bypassing the first pass metabolism in the liver, which increases breakdown.

You and your health professionals need to understand this, because *many women get excessive doses of testosterone creams or sublingual troches, which can create horrible side effects.*

For example, a 2% testosterone cream (widely recommended in a number of women's health books) contains **20 mg/gram** of cream delivering about **20 times** the dose most women need in this readily absorbed form.

By comparison, most of my testosterone prescriptions are for 0.25 mg/gram up to about 1 mg/gram (0.1%) of cream (1 gram = ¼ teaspoon of cream).

Most women need only very small amounts of testosterone to achieve desired benefits. I start patients on 1.00–1.25 mg of oral sustained-release micronized testosterone, and gradually increase based on the woman's description of symptoms and her serum levels.

Most women achieve the desirable response at a dose between 1 and 4 mg a day. Re-check the testosterone level in the morning before your next dose, to be sure it isn't too high 24 hours after you take it.

The transdermal cream form of testosterone (and DHEA, when appropriate) may be less likely to cause the negative changes in the good HDL cholesterol, since absorption into the bloodstream through the skin bypasses the liver "first-pass" metabolism. Cream forms are an option for testosterone therapy for women with high cholesterol or low HDL who need the other benefits of testosterone. But this form doesn't last as long as over the day as tablets do.

I have summarized in the following table the benefits of adding testosterone to a hormone therapy regimen. I have also given you some pointers on what to look for to know if you have too little or too much testosterone, or DHEA.

Dr. Vliet's Guide to Testosterone And DHEA Effects

TOO LITTLE	JUST RIGHT	TOO MUCH
low energy	normal energy	hyper feelings
loss of sex drive	normal libido	increased libido
slowed down	alert, interested	"scattered" thoughts similar to A.D.H.D.
depressed mood	positive mood	irritable, anxious, edgy, tense, aggressive
fewer dreams	normal dreams	intense dreaming, aggressive dreams, violent dreams, disrupted sleep
thin, fine hair	hair thicker	increased facial hair
hair loss (alopecia)	normal hair growth	hair loss (alopecia)
dry, thin skin	normal skin	acne, oily skin
loss of muscle mass and strength	healthy muscle mass	muscle spasms and tenseness, aching

© 2001–2007 Elizabeth Lee Vliet, M.D.

Step 4: Monitor Effectiveness and Adjust as Needed

The importance of checking estradiol levels to monitor progress and effectiveness of treatment was shown dramatically in a 1998 study by Drs. Vihtamaki and Tuimala. They evaluated whether women and their doctors correctly judged estrogen dose solely based on the degree of improvement in symptoms.

Interestingly, they found that as many as 45% of women, who had reported their symptoms completely relieved, but actually still had serum estradiol levels below the currently accepted thresholds for protective effects of estradiol on the brain, bone and other target tissues. These physicians concluded that we cannot tell by symptom relief alone that women are getting the right amount of estradiol. They stated definitively that *follow up blood tests are necessary for proper monitoring*, just as with other hormones like thyroid.

How often do you need to recheck levels? Generally, about every 2–3 months after the start or change of medication, or when new symptoms appear or grow worse. Make treatment decisions based on both clinical symptoms and objective laboratory results.

Summary

If you decide to use hormone approaches to correct health problems and relieve troublesome symptoms, there is a systematic way to achieve your goals, and many options to try.

Work with a knowledgeable health professional to create a hormone supplement program fine-tuned to your body needs that restores balance to your natural levels. It can be done.

If you have complex problems and many different symptoms, or are sensitive to medications, it could take six to twelve months to find exactly the right combination for your needs so your body can heal and repair for overall improvement.

There are reliable, objective measures that will help you track your progress, in addition to your observations and feelings.

Don't settle for feeling lousy every day. Don't continue what doesn't work.

There are a variety of ways to rekindle your sexual spark, energy level, and vitality.

Dr. Vliet's Guide to Tests for an Overall Health Assessment

Comprehensive metabolic profile: Includes tests for liver, kidney, adrenal function, electrolytes and complete blood counts. It helps to screen for serious metabolic disorders that may cause similar symptoms to those seen with decline in estradiol or thyroid hormones. (See *Women, Weight and Hormones* for more detail).

Fasting lipid profile: This includes cholesterol, HDL, LDL, triglycerides to help check your risk of later heart disease. Elevated triglycerides are a risk factor for both diabetes and heart disease, and are also a reason to use the patch form of estradiol instead of oral.

Fasting glucose and insulin: This checks for diabetes or insulin resistance (both are risk factors for heart disease). Fasting glucose should be between 70-100. Low blood glucose, or **hypoglycemia**, is a fasting glucose less than 60. Glucose intolerance is now considered to be a fasting glucose of 111-125, and above 126 is the new cut-off to indicate diabetes.

8 AM cortisol: The "stress" hormone produced by the adrenal glands. Levels that are too high can indicate a stress response to physical factors, benign effects on binding proteins from birth control pills, or could mean the presence of a disease like Cushing's Syndrome. 8 AM cortisol levels less than 7 can indicate chronic stress effects (sometimes called adrenal "exhaustion"), or the serious adrenal insufficiency (Addison's Disease).

Ferritin: A measure of iron stores. If too low, (more common in women who still bleed monthly), it is associated with fatigue, hair loss, "restless legs," insomnia, and muscle aches; if too high, ferritin is associated with increased risk of cardiovascular disease as well as fatigue, aching muscles or joints, and headaches.

Bone density of the hip and spine: DEXA—Dual Energy X-ray is the most reliable test. for women under age 65, heel and wrist bone density tests do not correlate well with degree of bone loss at hip and spine, which are the really critical areas. Heel or wrist tests may be cheaper, quicker and easier but may give you false reassurance. DEXA tests of hip and spine are now covered by most insurance plans. Costs vary widely; shop around for the best price.

©Elizabeth Lee Vliet, MD 2001–2007

Dr. Vliet's Guide to Tests for an Overall Health Assessment

Urine or serum test of N-telopeptide: This measures the rate of bone building vs. bone breakdown. If this number is higher than 35, it indicates that you are already beginning the process of excessive bone breakdown and are at higher risk for osteoporosis and fractures later. You should begin to take aggressive steps now to build and preserve bone.

Glucose Tolerance Test (GTT) with Insulin levels: If you have this test, you need to do the full five hour version; a three hour test misses important symptom information from *falling* glucose in the 4th and 5th hours. A GTT should be done in the luteal phase of the menstrual cycle (three to five days before the start of your period) if you have risk factors for PCOS, Syndrome X or insulin resistance risk factors (See chapter 13 and 17). This allows for early identification of women at high risk for developing diabetes and heart disease. A patient symptom log should be coordinated throughout the test.

Waist to Hip Ratio: This ratio gives an idea of your health risks based on *where* the fat is located as well as by *how much fat* you have. As women get older, the ratio of testosterone to estradiol increases, and there is more gain in fat around the waist and upper body. **Waist-to-hip ratios of more than 0.8 for women or 1.0 for men means you have become an "apple,"** and you are at increased health risk of diabetes or heart disease. To calculate waist to hip ratio, measure your waist at its narrowest point, then measure your hips at the widest point. Divide the waist measure by the hip measure. Example: A woman with a 35-inch waist and 46-inch hip has a WH ratio of 0.76 (35÷ 46).

©Elizabeth Lee Vliet, MD 2001–2007

Chapter 17

Test and Treat Strategies for Optimal Thyroid, Adrenal, and Glucose-Insulin Balance

Although this is an "ovary" book, I can't take the isolationist approach of talking about one body part or one hormone system separate from all the rest. You have seen the many ways that the ovaries interact with other body systems and how the ovarian hormones affect multiple other pathways and functions of the body beyond reproduction.

Now I want to explain how you can get checked for other common hormone imbalances, describe some pitfalls to avoid with treatment, and review techniques I use to help women restore optimal hormone balance.

Many women have the mistaken idea that if their basal body temperature is lower than 98.6 in the mornings, it automatically means they have hypothyroidism, even if other thyroid tests are in the desirable ranges.

There are many causes of lower than normal body temperature, including ovarian hormone decline. If you want a clear picture of what is out of balance, and how to fix it, you must have a careful, complete, systematic hormone evaluation that looks at all these pieces of the puzzle.

You cannot just rely on a list of symptoms for a "diagnosis."

Fact
There is a great deal of overlap in symptoms from thyroid, ovarian, adrenal, and glucose-insulin imbalance.

Thyroid Tests: What to Have Checked, How To Interpret Your Results

Thyroid disorders can be a significant cause of infertility, menstrual irregularity, and abnormal ovarian hormone production.

Young women can and do experience thyroid problems even when TSH is normal. We see a lot of women in their 40s and 50s that have had hypothyroid symptoms for years, going back to their 20s and 20s, and have been unable to have them properly diagnosed even though their quality of life was eroded away. I want you to understand some basics about thyroid testing and treatment approaches. Then find a physician who will work with you to get it done right.

Complete thyroid testing (including antibodies) is crucial if there are any of the mood or fatigue symptoms described earlier, *particularly during the post-partum period.*

You also need complete tests of thyroid function if you have developed other problems such as high blood pressure, heart arrhythmias, high cholesterol, marked weight gain, diabetes, depression, anxiety, or memory and concentration difficulties.

Most standard thyroid panels, particularly in HMO settings, only check TSH and *total* thyroid hormones because this standard profile is cheaper and saves the insurance company money.

Thyroid antibodies not checked in the standard profile may be significantly elevated causing thyroid dysfunction and infertility, even though the TSH is within the normal range. In addition, it is really the amount of thyroid hormones present in the bloodstream in the free, active form that determines how effectively your thyroid hormones are working, especially for women taking birth control pills.

Consequently, **I always check free T3 and free T4 as well as both types of thyroid antibodies in my patients.** I suggest you ask your doctor to do the same. There isn't a major difference in cost. The information is more helpful in finding the cause of problems, as well as fine-tuning any thyroid medicines.

Go for What's Optimal, Not Just What's "Normal"

If a health professional tells you that your thyroid tests are "normal," that doesn't mean you still could not have a subtle thyroid dysfunction contributing to your menstrual disturbances, or infertility or fatigue or mood or weight problems.

Dr. Vliet's Guide to Thyroid Tests
(can be done on any day of your menstrual cycle)

- ஃ Ultra-sensitive Thyroid Stimulating Hormone (TSH)
- ஃ Free T4 (levothyroxine)
- ஃ Free T3 (triiodothyronine)
- ஃ Antimicrosomal antibody (also called anti-thyroid peroxidase antibody, or anti-TPO), an antibody to the thyroid gland tissue
- ஃ Antithyroglobulin antibody, an antibody to the T4 thyroid hormone itself
- ஃ Thyroid binding globulin, a measure of the carrier protein level in the bloodstream. It can be increased or decreased by a variety of medicines and dietary factors, so checking the level may help sort out a puzzling thyroid problem.
- ஃ Thyroid Releasing Hormone (TRH) Stimulation test is also available, but I generally don't find that this is necessary if the ones above are done. Ideally, this test should be done by an endocrinologist, since it requires awareness of pitfalls and special considerations to interpret it properly.

©Elizabeth Lee Vliet, MD 2001–2007

In fact, for women, these symptoms *commonly* occur before TSH goes up into an obviously abnormal range. It's a little like waiting for the lake to go bone dry before you call it a water shortage, instead of taking steps to conserve low water supplies before they dry up.

I find that women are often told their thyroid is "normal," without having the complete thyroid tests done. When I do my more complete testing, I often find the culprit is elevated antibodies or low free fractions of T3 and T4 hormones.

Another key point is that many women, and too many physicians, don't take into account that a "normal range" on a laboratory report is just that: a range. Each one of you will feel your best at a somewhat different point along that range. Some of you will require higher or lower levels than we may think are "normal" in order for you to feel well and to function optimally. We must look at the lab results in conjunction with the symptoms described by each individual.

This is when it is very important to listen with an open mind to each woman, and her descriptions of what is wrong, and trust in what she says and knows about her body.

Warning
"Normal" for lab range does *not* mean *optimal for your body.*

A Note
After all, as a physician, I am treating *people*, not lab values.

As a general rule of thumb, I like to see women's TSH between 0.5 and about 2.0 for optimal thyroid function. I can't easily give you actual numbers for optimal levels of free T3 and free T4 because these will vary depending on what lab you use, what test they do, and what units of measure they are using, all of which affect the reference range.

The Dangers of "Wilson's Syndrome" Protocols and Relying on Basal Body Temperature Tests

Women often ask me about a condition of impaired conversion of T4 to T3 that Dr. Denis Wilson purportedly "discovered" and named for himself ("Wilson's Syndrome"). This condition has actually been in thyroid medical textbooks for many years, and was not "discovered" by Dr. Wilson. It is one of the many defects in the thyroid pathways that come under the larger heading of "thyroid resistance syndromes." Failure to adequately convert T4 to T3 can have many causes. (See Chapter 10 for a list related to diet and lifestyle.)

Difficulty making sufficient T3 clearly exists and is more common in women than men. In women with disturbed menstrual cycles, a test of free T3 is actually more critical than the standard T4 measures. The blood test for free T3 is accurate and answers the question of whether the body converts T4 to T3 or not.

Proponents of Wilson's Syndrome tell you that blood tests are not reliable and recommend checking your morning basal body temperature under your arm (axillary temperature) to see if you have low free T3. They ignore the advances in blood testing methods in the two decades.

They further direct you to increase the amount of T3 you take until your morning body temperature is back to normal at 98.6 degrees.

This can be a very dangerous thing to do, and can lead to serious thyroid overdosing. There are many causes of lower than normal body temperature, including ovarian hormone decline.

Doctors who recommend the basal body temperature method, like Wilson, Broda Barnes, and many fibromyalgia specialists, have ignored basic female biology. Women's *ovarian* hormones are *also* important body temperature regulators. Most women know this from their own experiences each month. How many of you have checked your body basal temperature to determine ovulation?

Today, with the sensitivity of current test methods, we can get a reliable answer to the T3 issue to determine a thyroid problem, along with reliable blood tests of estradiol and cortisol. Your physician needs to adjust thyroid medication carefully to avoid serious problems from too much.

Excess T3 alone can also cause high blood pressure, severe palpitations, and shortness of breath, nervousness, anxiety attacks, agitation, increased sweating, and fatigue from over-stimulation throughout the body.

All of these problems are intensified by low estradiol. (Remember, *excess* thyroid will suppress normal ovarian function, which then makes the estradiol even lower.) Even with excess T3, however, basal body temperatures typically *remain* low unless you also restore estradiol levels to optimal ranges.

And, YOU should not change your thyroid medication on your own, without specific guidance from your physician, *based on reliable blood test results.*

Warning

Low estradiol and excess T3 can cause lethal heart rhythm disturbances, dangerously high blood pressure, and sudden death.

When To Consider Starting Thyroid Medication

On many laboratory scales, hypothyroidism is diagnosed with TSH values greater than about 4 or 5. Many physicians still don't treat with thyroid medication until the TSH rises over 8.

In my opinion, such rigid adherence to TSH overlooks the point I made earlier: weight gain, menstrual irregularity, infertility, PMS, depression and memory loss in women are occurring long before the TSH goes that high.

In addition, current studies in the infertility field have found that women often have difficulty conceiving if their TSH is much above 2.0. In my view, if we wait until TSH is above 5, it allows all of these problems to get worse unnecessarily.

I prefer to begin treatment earlier, in a preventive approach. I may start thyroid medication when the TSH is only 3 or so, especially if thyroid antibodies are high, or if the free T3 or free T4 are lower than optimal or women are having a lot of symptoms of low thyroid.

Fact

Excess T3 and low estradiol can also accelerate bone loss and cause severe insomnia.

Smart
The earlier treatment is begun, the less likely you are to have other adverse effects of low thyroid such as high blood pressure, elevated cholesterol, impaired cognitive function or serious weight gain.

Note
FDA-approved commercial thyroid products for levothyroxine are *bioidentical* to your body's own T4.

It will also be easier to regain optimal health if you aren't starting from rock bottom. In the lake analogy, I used earlier, it is easier and faster to replenish the water supply if it is just *low*, not bone dry!

Thyroid Medication Options:

If you need to take thyroid medication, or are already taking it, you may be wondering if is it better to take synthetic pure bioidentical T4 (*Synthroid, Unithroid, Levoxyl* and generic levothyroxine) or a mixed, animal-derived T4–T3 blend (such as Armour thyroid).

Should you take "Natural" or "Synthetic"? And what is the difference? Remember, "natural" can mean "bioidentical" to what your body makes, or it can mean coming from a biological (natural) source, which could be chemically different from the molecule made by your body.

"Synthetic" can simply mean "made in laboratory" to be identical to what your body makes, or it can also mean "chemically new" and unlike that which your body makes. Don't get caught up in misleading marketing ploys!

Now that scientists have identified the exact molecular make-up of T4, they have been able to create ("synthesize") a carbon-copy that is identical to what the body makes. This has given us standardized commercial preparations of the T4 thyroid hormone, such as the brands *Unithroid, Synthroid, Levoxyl*, and the generic tablets of L-thyroxine (T4, or levothyroxine) made by different manufacturers.

All of these are identical to the human T4 thyroid hormone even though they are made in a laboratory. These are "natural" for your body because the body can't tell the difference between this carbon-copy molecule and the T4 molecule made by your own thyroid gland.

These commercial products have been successfully used to manage thyroid problems in millions of people over the last 4 decades. For most people, the T4 in these products will be converted by the thyroid gland and body tissues such as the liver to adequate amounts of T3.

If this conversion does not take place normally, you can take natural, bioidentical T3 using either a commercial, short-acting one called Cytomel, or a specially compounded, sustained release form of T3 (tri-iodothyronine).

It has become quite confusing to consumers because there has recently been a lot of marketing of one brand, Armour thyroid, as a "natural" thyroid that's better for you than Unithroid, Synthroid, or Levoxyl.

Armour thyroid is "natural" because it is derived from a biological source: desiccated (dried) pig thyroid tissue, and it contains both T4 and T3.

This pig blend of T3 and T4, however, is not the natural ratio of these two hormones that we have in our body. As a result, this product often provides more T3 than you need and not enough T4, so the balance isn't quite right.

Since Armour thyroid is a fixed-dose combination, it cannot be individually fine-tuned for your body as we can do if we use separate tablets of T4 and T3. I prefer to get the best balance that is natural for your body and not use a ratio natural to a pig or cow!

With the increasing concern about prion contaminants (viral-type particles) in livestock that can lead to such lethal brain diseases such as "mad cow" disease, I am concerned about the safety of taking thyroid tablets made up of ground-up animal glands.

While the meat supply in the United States is considered safe, we don't always know the true source of animal tissue used for some of these products.

This is a risk I prefer not to take when we have standardized, effective, non-animal-derived bioidentical thyroid hormone product available.

My other concern with *animal-derived hormones* is that they have the *potential to cause our bodies to form antibodies to the hormones* and to our own endocrine glands.

This was one of the early problems recognized decades ago with the animal-derived insulin given to diabetics, and also with the allergies to horse serum when this was used in the past as a base for many injections in the past.

Most of these problems have been resolved with the development of synthetic human insulin and injections no long being given in a horse serum base. Similar problems occurred with

Caution Don't be misled about their safety and effectiveness by all the marketing hoopla about "natural" products being "better" for you.

Fact Armour is "natural" for pigs… not natural for humans!

Caution I don't recommend thyroid products made of ground-up animal glands! It's a risk you don't need.

Evidence

I have seen too many women develop high levels of both types of thyroid antibodies when taking animal-derived thyroid products.

animal derived thyroid products when they were all we had and therefore used more widely.

Unithroid, Synthroid, Levoxyl, and the generic brands of levothyroxine (T4) are not animal-derived, so they don't have animal residue to stimulate our antibody production. This is a good example that "natural" sources are not always natural or better for humans.

If you need T3 in addition to T4, there are better options than Armour thyroid. Cytomel is a commercial, FDA-approved T3 product that has been in use in the United States for several decades. It can be effective, but it has a very short duration of effect. That means people often experience too much T3 stimulation soon after taking it, and then feel a "crash" when it wears off.

I have prescribed Cytomel over the years, but my patients often don't like the "rise" and "fall" feeling they have with it. That led me to try and find a longer-lasting preparation of T3.

Wisdom

Separate tablets for T4 and T3 allow individualized dosing for each person.

About 1986, I asked a pharmacist if he could compound a sustained release T3. He was able to make a very successful, long-acting T3 tablet. He uses a hypoallergenic base to help reduce the possibility of allergic reactions, which is very good for chemically-sensitive people with a lot of allergies.

Since that time, I have primarily prescribed this sustained-release compounded T3 whenever I have patients who need T3 added to a commercial T4 product.

Doses can be made up to be as low or as high as needed, rather than being limited to the few commercial strengths available. Your doctor will be able to order sustained-release T3 prescriptions if it is appropriate for you.

To Be Safe: Start Low, Go Slow

Remember

Symptoms of too much thyroid are the same ones that occur if your estradiol is too low.

Too much thyroid, too fast, will commonly cause rapid heartbeat, palpitations, headaches, anxiousness, irritability, or insomnia. If thyroid is added too quickly before estradiol is optimal, it is a like someone pouring gasoline on a fire! Your heart races, your mind races, you are not sleeping, and your head pounds. Not much fun.

So don't over do the thyroid thinking you can feel better faster. Start with a low dose, and increase slowly, using laboratory results and your doctor's advice, as well as your body response, to guide the dose changes.

When I prescribe one of the T4 products, especially for women who have other hormone imbalances, I usually start at half of the lowest commercial dose, for about two weeks.

I then work to increase the dosage gradually based how my patient tells me she feels, and on how the TSH is responding. I'd like to see the TSH in the range of about 0.5 to 2.0.

Then, if there are remaining symptoms of low thyroid function and the free T3 is low, I may add T3 starting with a very low dose, such as 5 mcg. Again, I increase very slowly.

If 5 mcg feels like too much at once, I suggest splitting the tablet, taking half in the morning and half at lunchtime.

It can become complicated when working with the ovarian and thyroid hormones at the same time, since they affect each other in a variety of ways and the symptoms of both too high and too low often mimic each other. Therefore, I prefer to stabilize the ovarian hormones with whatever approach a woman prefers, and **then** work with the thyroid balancing—*unless* the TSH is so high that the hypothyroidism simply must be treated right away.

It can be quite a juggling act, and I often find I have to combine our "science" (lab tests) along with a lot of "art" (clinical judgment and listening to the woman) in order to decide what to do at any given time.

Thyroid hormone replacement is a clearly a complex topic. These are the highlights of some crucial issues I think are important for you to address in working with your physicians.

I do not advocate using thyroid hormone supplements just because you feel tired all the time, or just based on low body temperature, or solely for weight loss if all of the laboratory studies are completely normal, including thyroid antibodies.

Too much thyroid can actually cause fatigue, and also causes weight gain in the early stages, by stimulating appetite to fuel the excess thyroid-induced metabolic demands.

Excess thyroid can also cause significant wasting of skeletal muscles throughout the body, leading to more weakness and more fatigue that makes you incorrectly think you need thyroid. If you also have low estradiol and testosterone, this is another cause of muscle and bone loss. It is critical to check both ovarian and thyroid hormones carefully before making treatment decisions.

Oops!
If you take T3 later than lunchtime, it may cause restless sleep.

Warning
Serious health consequences can occur if you are given thyroid hormones when you don't really have a thyroid problem.

News reports from Florida and Georgia describe the deaths of several women due to complications of excess thyroid. Don't be tempted to take a "quick fix" approach to fatigue, low energy or weight problems by increasing thyroid medication. Especially do not increase your medicine on your own. It is dangerous and you may get more problems than you bargained for.

Caution

Myths abound about "adrenal fatigue" or "adrenal exhaustion" based on unreliable saliva tests.

Cortisol: What to Have Checked, How To Interpret Your Results

You're tired, your muscles feel weak, or you're gaining weight. Is it an *adrenal* problem?

A serum cortisol at 8 AM or 4 PM is the most reliable *first* step in checking for low or high cortisol; sometimes endocrinologists also do a 24-hour urine for free cortisol. Saliva tests are not reliable measures of cortisol to diagnose Cushing's or Addison's disease.

High cortisol: An 8:00 AM *serum* cortisol level *higher* than about 20–25 µg/dl is considered abnormal and suggests the need for additional tests to clarify the cause. The typical ones that are done include serum *free* cortisol, corticotropin binding globulin (CBG), ACTH, 24-hour urine for urinary free cortisol, and Dexamethasone Suppression Test (DST).

Warning

True adrenal insufficiency causes weight *loss* in virtually *all* people who have it. If you are *gaining* weight, it is highly unlikely that you have adrenal insufficiency.

If the DST shows morning or afternoon cortisol higher than 5 µg/dl the day after you take 1 mg of dexamethasone, then I recommend you have a thorough evaluation for possible Cushing's disease. This will involve further tests, such as serum ACTH, 24-hour urine for urinary fee cortisol. A Corticotrophin Releasing Hormone (CRH) Stimulation Test may be appropriate, and this is usually done by endocrinologists.

If these follow up tests are abnormal, imaging studies (MRI, CAT scans, etc.) are usually ordered to check the adrenal glands and pituitary to check for possible tumors causing the excess cortisol production.

Low cortisol: An 8:00 AM cortisol lower than about 5 to 7 µg/dl is suggestive of AI if your electrolytes are also abnormal. If the 8:00 AM cortisol is greater than 10 µg/dl, and your serum electrolytes (sodium, potassium) are normal, this makes it *very unlikely* that you have adrenal insufficiency, or "adrenal exhaustion," the current buzzword.

If your cortisol is low and you have a low sodium and high potassium, and you are losing weight, I urge you to see an endocrinologist who has experience with these disorders.

AI, or Addison's disease, is a serious metabolic illness that can cause death if not evaluated and treated properly. It should *not* be self-treated with over-the-counter adrenal supplements.

There are additional tests that normally should be done to confirm the diagnosis, and identify any possible causes. A serum ACTH, and ACTH (Cortrosyn) stimulation tests are generally done next to evaluate the cause of adrenal insufficiency (for example, adrenal destruction or pituitary dysfunction).

Caution
It can be dangerous to take over-the-counter "adrenal support" supplements, or "adrenal glandulars."

If you are having fatigue, weakness and low energy level and your cortisol is above 10 and below 20, you should have tests of your other hormone systems tested as I have discussed, since these symptoms have many causes in addition to adrenal problems.

Make sure you see a physician experienced with the various medicines used to replace inadequate adrenal production of cortisol, and who are knowledgeable about side effects and problems that can occur.

I have seen many women over the years who have been told that they have "adrenal exhaustion" based on unreliable tests such as saliva or kinesiology ("muscle testing"). When serum cortisol assays were done at the proper times of day, they actually had *high* cortisol reflecting the stress response from other hormone imbalances and/or the excess corticosteroid medicine.

Warning
Taking glandulars may actually suppress your own adrenal hormones further, or could cause menstrual irregularities.

Adrenal glandulars and "herbal adrenal support" products sold in health food stores are animal-derived, with the same potential problems I described for animal-derived thyroid products—*allergic reactions, stimulation of antibody formation, or prion contamination.*

Getting Tested for Insulin and Glucose

Chapter 13 describes the multiple health problems that occur when glucose and insulin get out of kilter. Here's how to get properly tested.

Fasting Tests:

First, have a blood test for fasting glucose and insulin, measured first thing in the morning, at least 12 hours after your last meal.

Normal fasting insulin is usually 6 to 25 micro-international units per milliliter (mIU/ml), depending on which assay the lab uses.

Fact
A healthy fasting glucose should be in the 65–100 mg/dl range.

Some labs still show that a "normal" fasting glucose goes up to 115 mg/dl, but the latest guidelines are that fasting glucose should be less than 100 mg/dl. Fasting glucose above 100 mg/dl suggests the beginning of glucose intolerance, which can lead to insulin resistance, and later diabetes.

These are the new diagnostic criteria for Diabetes from the American Diabetes Association:

- fasting glucose greater than 126 mg/dl,
- a casual (random) glucose greater than 200 mg/dl along with symptoms

Warning
A 2-hour post-prandial glucose of 140 mg/dl but less than 200 mg/dl indicates you have impaired glucose tolerance.

- or, a two-hour post-prandial glucose greater than 200 mg/dl.

Post-prandial (after meals) Tests:

Measuring glucose and insulin at two or three hours after a typical meal is another way to check for early stages of glucose intolerance, insulin resistance or diabetes.

This test is called a *2- or 3-hour post-prandial glucose and insulin*, and tracks how high your glucose and insulin rise in response to eating. The results are more helpful if you eat a meal that is usual for you, rather than "loading up" on protein, as some lab staff tell women. If your 2-hour post-prandial glucose is over 200, you likely have diabetes and need a thorough evaluation by your physician.

There are different insulin assays used in laboratories throughout the country with different reference ranges so the numbers may be different at your lab. Insulin values are not as standardized as are glucose values, so interpretation is a more difficult.

Fact
A typical two-hour post-prandial insulin range is 6–35 mIU/ml.

If your 2-hour post-prandial insulin is at the high end or over the lab's normal range, you are likely insulin resistant. High fasting and post-prandial insulin levels are common in young women with significant weight gain, in women with PCOS, and in perimenopausal women losing the beneficial effects of their estradiol.

Other Tests:

Hemoglobin A1C measures the amount of glucose incorporated into hemoglobin, the oxygen-carrying molecule in red blood cells. If you develop inability to handle glucose, this test is a sensitive marker that detects problems earlier and gives a picture of blood glucose levels over the past three months.

If you already have diabetes, Hemoglobin A1C is used to monitor the impact of diet and medications on your glucose control. The desirable goal is a Hemoglobin A1C less than 6, which indicates good glucose control.

Insulin Resistance: More Complete Testing

One way to detect insulin resistance is the *"Insulin Response to Glucose Test."* You drink a measured amount of glucose, then test glucose and insulin at regular intervals over six hours to see the pattern in rise and fall of both, correlated with any symptoms as the levels change. Women are often told this longer test is not necessary.

I disagree. So does the World Health Organization, which now recommends using the oral glucose tolerance test to identify early insulin resistance and those at higher risk for diabetes.

Your doctors may say "We don't do those to diagnose diabetes," or "A three hour test is fine, you don't need the full six hours," or "It doesn't matter when in your cycle you do a glucose tolerance test, it's all the same."

I disagree on all points.

We are not simply looking for diabetes; we are looking for the early change of insulin resistance, and for objective laboratory data that explains your descriptions of uncontrollable food cravings, difficulty losing weight, mood swings, and other physical symptoms.

If you only have a three-hour measure of glucose-insulin response, you miss the last 2 hours when additional abnormal changes often occur, such as a reactive hypoglycemia or a persistently elevated insulin value.

The luteal stage rise in progesterone, and the relative balance with estradiol, affects both your symptoms and your body's insulin-glucose response.

At mid-life, insulin resistance often gets worse, especially if you have ovulatory levels of progesterone with decreasing estradiol and androgens "unmasked" by the decline in estradiol. These

Caution
High insulin levels can cause weight gain, heart disease, diabetes, and even increase women's risk of breast cancer.

Vital
Brain symptoms such as memory loss, concentration difficulties and mood swings are especially likely to get worse in the last two hours of the 5-hour test.

Important
In menstruating women, the glucose/ insulin testing should be done about days 20–23, the "food craving" days.

Vital
Log any symptoms you have during glucose– insulin testing and note the time they occur.

Caution
The balance and timing of *foods* you eat each day is critical.

combined hormonal shifts cause more glucose changes that trigger physical and emotional symptoms.

I often do these tests in the office whenever possible, for several reasons. Labs often mess up the tests and don't do what I ask. Most physicians have the patient go to a lab, then only look at the numbers for each hour of the test. If the numbers fall into the "normal" range, the patient is told "everything is normal," without being asked how you felt during the test.

This overlooks the most crucial information of all: what you have to say about your symptoms as the glucose and insulin levels rose and fell.

This integrated information allows you to correlate symptoms with "the numbers" and determine a course of treatment, such as the balance of carbohydrate, fat, and protein, the spacing and number of meals, and what medications your doctor may think are needed.

Effective Treatment Strategies to Get Your Glucose and Insulin in Balance:

Step 1: Nutrition is your first line of defense to regulating insulin—and there is no way around it. Medication alone will not do it.

Eating smaller, balanced meals throughout the day provides the cornerstone of your insulin-balancing program. You also need adequate protein and the right balance of healthy fats—all are the most important steps you can take to keep excess insulin from destroying your health. Skipping meals and eating large amounts in the evening leads to more insulin and more fat storage. High carbohydrate foods increase insulin production.

Detailed meal plans to improve glucose-insulin balance are described in *Women, Weight and Hormones*. (See Appendix II).

Step 2: Exercise acts like an "invisible insulin" to improve muscle use of glucose from the bloodstream so it can be used for energy instead of floating around in the bloodstream doing damage.

Lower blood glucose then decreases the insulin pouring out of your pancreas in response to all that glucose hanging around.

Less insulin in the bloodstream means you burn fat for fuel more effectively, and also build more muscle, which then increases your metabolic rate.

Step 3: Restore Ovarian Hormone Balance to get your estradiol, progesterone, testosterone, and DHEA back into healthy ranges. They all work together improving your insulin response, increasing your metabolic rate, and helping you build healthy muscle.

If you are overweight, have glucose intolerance, insulin resistance, or actual diabetes, and need contraception: avoid the higher progestin pills such as Loestrin, Alesse, Mircette, and others.

Contraceptives with less progestin and better estrogen ratios work better to improve insulin sensitivity and do not over-stimulate your appetite: Ovcon 35, Modicon (and their generics), Yasmin, Orthocyclen, Orthocept, and Nuvaring.

If you do not need contraception, or have had a hysterectomy, then focus on using FDA-approved bioidentical hormone preparations. If you have a uterus and are not producing your own progesterone adequately, *non-oral* natural progesterone such as Prochieve typically causes fewer adverse effects on blood sugar swings and insulin production than with oral forms.

Don't use over-the-counter progesterone ("wild yam") creams, since many of these contain enough added progesterone to seriously throw your insulin-glucose pathways out of whack, and are not reliable in preventing excess build-up of the lining of the uterus.

In my experience, the following hormone preparations are *more likely to aggravate insulin resistance and glucose intolerance* since they do not give optimal levels of estradiol and/or contain higher doses of progestins: mixed estrogens (Premarin, Estratab/Estratest, Cenestin), synthetic progestins (Provera, MPA).

Step 4: Decrease your stress to lower cortisol. Remember, cortisol helps make more body fat for storage. The higher your stress, the higher your cortisol, and the more problems with insulin resistance. Take stress-busting steps now. (See Chapter 7 for more information)

Step 5: Insulin "Sensitizer" Medications. If balancing your ovarian hormones doesn't improve insulin resistance, you may want to talk with your doctor about other medications, such as Glucophage (metformin), Actos (pioglitazone), and Avandia (rosiglitazone). All of these improve insulin sensitivity.

I use these quite successfully for many women of all ages, especially those suffering from PCOS. Lifestyle strategies are the first course

Tip

Walking for 5–10 minutes a few times a day is one of the simplest, quickest, and least costly things you can do to reduce the deadly consequences of insulin resistance.

Smart

The patch form of estradiol, compared to oral, gives better results for insulin sensitivity

Warning

Progestin-dominant combination products such as PremPro, Prem Phase, Combi-patch, Femhrt can make it harder to control insulin resistance and cause weight gain.

of treatment, but many women need additional medicines to get the insulin resistance under control and facilitate healthy weight loss.

Once normalized, many women are able to taper down or stop the medication and maintain the improvements with healthy eating, regular exercise, and good hormone balance.

With these medicines I prescribe a lower than usual dose, and increase very gradually. This way, side effects are minimized. The American Diabetes Association and Joslin Diabetes programs recommend combination therapies of two or more of the above medications, even in younger women, to control insulin resistance early and prevent full-blown diabetes and all its complications later. The specific combination must be tailored to your body responses by your physician, looking at all the variables described.

Summary

It is becoming increasingly common to see younger women struggling with the early stages of hormonal imbalance. There are effective medication options to help you achieve improved thyroid, cortisol, and insulin balance. Addressing these hormonal imbalances when you are *young* can help prevent many of the chronic weight and health problems as you get older.

Don't depend on saliva tests. If you are not satisfied with your physician's evaluation, don't hesitate to get a second opinion. Look for FDA-approved bioidentical human hormone formulations when possible. Try to avoid animal-derived products.

Remember to individualize your treatment by starting with low dosages and work with your physician to gradually increase the dose depending upon your response to the medication and the results of appropriate lab tests. Keep symptom logs to help you focus on how you are feeling with each change in medication.

If these issues are addressed properly, you may not need so many antidepressant or anti-anxiety medicines to improve mood, decrease anxiety and improve your energy and sleep. This will help reduce both side effects and lower medication costs.

Careful monitoring and communication with your physician is key. There is no need to wait to address the situation "later." You deserve to feel better!

Chapter 18
Starting Your "Clean-Up Campaign": Get Rid of Ovarian Disruptors You Can Control

Now that you have read about the many ways that your ovaries can be damaged by the environment and your lifestyle, let's explore ways to "clean up" and improve your overall health.

Eliminating Hormone-disrupting Habits

Cigarette Smoking

When you smoke, you don't even *look* healthy. I can easily spot a smoker just by her skin and her voice, regardless of age.

Cigarette smoking damages more than just appearance, however: *your ovaries, your unborn children, your brain,* and *body.* Don't forget secondary smoke has many adverse effects of on children and others around you.

Tobacco is a highly addictive drug that seduces you, only to then steal your health.

To stop smoking is easier said than done, I know. There are excellent smoking cessation strategies available to help you clean up the habit.

One highly effective way is the nicotine patch, in gradually decreasing doses, to help you taper off the nicotine addiction and reduce withdrawal symptoms. You must avoid smoking cigarettes while using the patch, however, or the excess nicotine can cause a serious heart rhythm disturbance from nicotine toxicity. There are also other medications, such as Zyban and some antidepressants, that diminish nicotine withdrawal, and help you get over the hump.

First! If you smoke and have hormone problems, your first clean-up prescription is **stop smoking!**

Yes! You *can* do it. Your life and health depend on it.

Alcohol

Alcohol has an ancient history in cultures around the world. Studies show that people who drink small amounts of alcohol regularly gain some health benefits that lower heart disease risk. Moderate use means a *glass* of wine or beer, not a whole bottle of wine in one evening.

Warning

If you have symptoms of declining hormonal levels, alcohol further suppresses poorly functioning ovaries.

For women, however, even moderate use may increase risk of menstrual disturbances, changes in fertility, and later increased risk of breast cancer.

Women react differently to alcohol than men. We have fewer gastric enzymes to metabolize alcohol, so we absorb approximately 30 percent more alcohol into our bloodstream, even if we drink the same amount.

If you take birth control pills or prescription hormone therapy, alcohol increases liver production of estrone, the unwanted type of estrogen, and can interfere with the positive effects of hormone therapy.

Daily use of alcohol, even in moderate amounts, suppresses immune response and can aggravate allergies and chemical sensitivities. Alcohol adds significantly to daily calories, doesn't add any nutritional value, and makes you get fatter around your middle.

Enjoying wine or beer or other alcoholic beverages on special occasions may be fine, but *don't drink alcohol every day*, even in small amounts. It saps your brainpower and your energy, and increases later risk of breast cancer.

Pinkies Up!

Tea (more so than coffee) contains modest amounts of antioxidants that are potentially beneficial.

Excess Caffeine

I certainly enjoy a good cup of coffee in the morning —I love the aroma as it fills my kitchen, and I enjoy the taste. Go ahead and enjoy yours too. Two or three cups of coffee or tea a day has never been shown to have any adverse health effects.

Recent studies have found that regular, moderate coffee intake is associated with lower risk of Type II Diabetes. There aren't any serious health problems in either coffee or tea, as long as you keep total caffeine intake to less than about 200–250 mg a day (the equivalent of 3–4 cups of coffee, depending on size of the cup).

Recent studies have shown that "caffeine" in soft drinks leads to high blood pressure in women, though this effect was not shown in either coffee or tea. My theory is the sodium and other additives in soft drinks are the culprit, *not caffeine.*

Like many things, caffeine becomes a problem when you overdo it. If you are chronically tired, and use caffeine as a "pick-up" to get through the day, it can actually make fatigue worse.

Caffeine acts as a diuretic, so it dehydrates your body, makes you lose water-soluble vitamins, and depletes calcium and magnesium needed for healthy muscle function and mood regulation, to name a few of its energy-sapping effects.

Caffeine also disrupts the healthy balance of serotonin and norepinephrine in the brain and nerve tissues. This means excess caffeine also increases pain sensations, makes you irritable, anxious, intensifies PMS, and also causes rebound headaches when it wears off.

If you drink beverages with caffeine late in the day, it disrupts your sleep cycles. Deep stage 4 sleep is the time your muscles repair themselves, so if you have caffeine or alcohol at night, you'll wake up tired with sore, aching muscles the next morning. Then you use more caffeine to pick you up, and the cycle continues.

> **Wisdom**
> Limit yourself to 2 cups of your favorite caffeinated beverage in the morning and switch to water for the rest of the day.

Many women don't realize that "fatigue" is also a symptom of dehydration from too little water intake.

If possible, purchase "organically-grown" coffee and teas to avoid residual pesticides often present on the leaves of tea and coffee plants. If you can't find it locally, check the Internet for on-line and mail order services.

Stimulant "Diet" Pills

Using stimulant diet pills on a regular basis causes some of the same problems as excess caffeine: disruption of the brain's endocrine regulating pathways, alteration of weight-regulating pathways, mood crashes when they wear off, anxiety, insomnia, and chronic fatigue from revving your body engines too fast and depleting its energy reserves. If you take stimulants every day, talk with your physician. You may need medication to get off them safely and avoid withdrawal problems.

Stop using these drugs! Proper hormone balance, diet and exercise are still the best way to lose weight. Sorry, there is no quick fix!

Cocaine

Even though this drug is illegal and there are stiff consequences for its use, it is still widely abused in this country. Young women are especially vulnerable to its endocrine and mood effects.

Cocaine is one of the most powerful stimulant drugs of all, blasting neuro-transmitters out of their nerve cell storage sites with a vengeance. Because of its potency, even one "hit" can permanently alter the brain, leading to addiction. The high that follows release of this flood of chemical messengers is fleeting, which is why it triggers such intense cravings for more. The "rush" cans stimulate the heart so intensely that it leads to sudden death.

Cleaning Up Your Diet, Getting Rid of Excitotoxins

The typical American diet of "fast foods," lots of soft drinks, high salt, high fat processed foods contain significant amounts of additives and flavor enhancers, such as MSG or *monosodium glutamate* and hydrolyzed vegetable protein (HVP). This compound imparts an "excited," intensified taste to foods. Unfortunately, it also is an *excitatory amino acid* (like aspartate in sweeteners found in soft drinks) that over-stimulates brain cells, including pathways regulating the menstrual cycle.

MSG is ubiquitous today in frozen, canned and processed convenience foods and difficult to avoid unless you carefully read labels. Manufacturers are clever at disguising it under other names, such as "natural flavorings" and *hydrolyzed vegetable protein* (HVP).

HVP is a product high in three different excitotoxins —glutamate, aspartate, and cystoic acid. The amino acid glutamate is even sold in supplements at the health food store, supposedly for memory enhancement. Start looking for ways to eliminate these chemicals—you may even find you have better "brain power" when you cut the excitotoxins from your diet.

Families, especially when both parents work outside the home and time is at a premium, have difficulties preparing healthy meals. Despite your best efforts, fast food restaurant meals seems to increase steadily with the number of children family activities on a given day. Sales pitches aimed at kids for "fun foods" make it doubly difficult for parents to set limits and serve wholesome foods.

Hidden Sources of MSG and Excitotoxins

I.   Food Additives Always Containing MSG

- Monosodium glutamate, MSG
- Hydrolyzed vegetable protein - HVP (contains 3 different excitotoxins, aspartate, glutamate, and cystoic acid that is converted to cysteine).
- Hydrolyzed plant protein, or hydrolyzed protein
- Textured protein
- Plant protein extract
- Hydrolyzed oat flour
- Yeast extract, autolyzed yeast
- Sodium or calcium caseinate

II.   Food Additives Frequently Containing MSG

- Malt flavorings or extract
- Bouillon cubes, dry soup powders, canned chicken or beef stock
- "Flavoring" or "natural flavoring"
- "Natural spices"
- "Seasoning," or "natural seasoning"

III.   Food Additives That May Contain MSG

- Carrageenan
- Soy Protein Concentrate
- Soy Protein Isolate
- Whey Protein Concentrate (depends on manufacturer)
- "Enzymes" (protease enzymes break food proteins into their component amino acids, some of which are excitatory amino acids like glutamate)

IV.   Other Excitotoxin Sources

- Foods containing aspartate, aspartame, aspartic acid
- Nutrasweet
- Glutamate (glutamic acid) amino acid supplements
- Cysteine (cystoic acid) amino acid supplements

Reference: *Excitotoxins: The Taste That Kills*, by Russell L. Blaylock M.D., 1994, Health Press, Santa Fe, NM

The quick and easy convenience foods available everywhere just add to the problem. If you ever wonder why it's difficult to resist these delights, just remember there are a lot of talented, experienced marketing experts working for savvy food manufacturers whose sole goal is to make you desire these foods—most of which are high in fat, sugar and salt.

It takes detective work to identify all these damaging additives, and the results are worth the effort.

For more on how these chemicals can adversely affect your health, read the book I used as a reference for this chart, *Excitotoxins: The Taste That Kills*, by Russell L. Blaylock M.D. (1994, Health Press, Santa Fe, NM).

Take a look at the chart to the left to see just how many different food additives contain these compounds, and start being aware of how much aspartate, glutamate, HVP or MSG are actually in what you are eating. Work to eliminate as many as possible.

Cleaning Up the PVCs

Common everyday plastic cling wrap is another source of unwanted chemicals in your food. If it is made of clear polyvinyl chloride (PVC), an inherently brittle plastic, it will contain a plasticizer, DEHA, to make it more flexible.

DEHA leaches into the food it surrounds. The molecules migrate from the packaging into the food until the wrapping is depleted of the chemical.

DEHA is not the same chemical as the hormone DHEA.

A Consumers Union test showed that DEHA reached levels of 153 parts per million (ppm) in cheddar cheese samples wrapped in packaging containing DEHA.

The Commission of the European Communities sets a limit of 18 ppm, quite a difference. PVC packaging includes plastic trays in boxed cookies or chocolates, and may also be in plastic bottles, and the lining of cans. Meat and poultry is often packaged in PVC.

Bottles with PVC can often be identified by the #3 recycling label on the bottom. Be sure your cling wrap is *polyethylene* based, *not polyvinyl*. Check the label. Only buy products that clearly state the contents.

Cleaning Up Your Bedroom Habits

Good sleep is absolutely critical to our health. Women with hormone problems can't sleep, yet sleep is the crucial time our body replenishes and recharges itself for the next day's activities. Excess androgens, excess thyroid, low estradiol—all can cause disrupted sleep.

To sleep well, we need quality mattresses and bedding. We often spend less money on a mattress than most other furniture we own. Some types of mattresses contain synthetic chemicals that "outgas" or emit vapors that can interfere with sleep and aggravate allergies. Check both foam and inner spring mattresses for content. Synthetic materials such as polyfoams, styrene, butadiene rubber, and toxic glues are an unsuspected problem for many people.

In addition, bedding fabrics are often made of synthetic fibers that don't "breathe," so they trap moisture that attracts dust mites and promotes growth of various microorganisms such as mold.

To help eliminate these problems, dry your bedding outside in the sunshine. If that's not possible, then use your clothes dryer, but AVOID perfumed fabric softener strips that add more noxious chemicals to the mix. Sunlight helps kill troublesome microorganisms and dust mites, and the fresh air gives a fresh, natural smell that is much better than the chemicals in fragranced products.

Avoid *fragranced candles, air fresheners and other sources of petroleum-based chemicals in your bedroom* especially if you have allergies or are sensitive to chemicals. These produce combustion by-products and volatile organic compounds. Use pure, unscented candles of 100% bees wax or vegetable wax.

Your bedroom should be an oasis, as free of chemical contaminants as possible, an environment that promotes a restful night's sleep. Your body needs this time to recoup each day.

In the table that follows, you'll find more tips to improve sleep. If these approaches don't work, and you've restored hormones to optimal levels, talk with your doctor about formal sleep studies.

Fact

The average human body releases up to a *pint* of moisture each night. Women with "night sweats" from hormone imbalance may lose even more.

Warning

Don't use fragranced products at all, especially if you have hormone problems.

Don't...

It is all too easy to get caught in the vicious cycle of perfectionistic workaholism, endlessly trying to do everything.

Cleaning Up Your Workaholism

Take Heed
Workaholism will eventually force *you* to stop and listen to your body's cries for a rest.

You're the "Type E woman"—being *everything* to *everybody everyday*. *"Just one more hour, and then I'll be finished. Just one load of wash, then I'll stop. Just one more report and then I'll take a break. Just one more room and then I'll be finished."*

Take an inventory of your daily time sheet:

- ❧ How many hours do you work outside your home?
- ❧ How many hours do you work *inside* your home?
- ❧ How many hours do you spend on the needs of others?
- ❧ How many hours do you spend on your needs?

Warning
All of these chemicals affect your health in ways you never dreamed, including causing daily headaches.

Maybe you don't define yourself as a workaholic, but take a close and honest look at the hours you just totaled up—do you see a destructive pattern here?

Workaholism can rob you of your health and vitality. (Remember Harriet in Chapter 7). You can ignore the signals for a while, but they catch up with you.

I have personally been dealt that lesson in spades many different times in my adult working life. I think my body will go on and on and on. I think I am immune. And guess what? If I push too hard at work, have too many stresses from patient load, business or family issues, and too much to accomplish in too short a time, eventually it catches up with me. Although I generally know at some level what I am doing at some level, if I ignore early warning clues that I'm on overload, I get slapped down every time.

Fact
These compounds are *neurotoxins*, chemicals that damage nerve cells and disrupt major pathways in the limbic system.

No one is immune to the destructive effects of over work, and lack of rest and recovery. Heed your body. Spend some time on you. Relax more.

Clean Up Endocrine-Disrupting Chemicals Around You

The National Institute of Environmental Health Sciences (NIEHS) oversees a variety of studies that suggest many of the women's health problems, including autoimmune diseases, breast cancer and reproductive cancers and reproductive dysfunctions including infertility, premature menstruation and premature menopause, are connected to chemical exposure from everyday products at home and work. (See Chapter 5 for more detail). So, how do you reduce exposure and health risks?

Let's start with things you use every day...cosmetics, lotions, conditioner, shampoo, gel, hair spray, nail polish and remover, perfume, deodorant, toothpaste, mouthwash, among others.

All of these are heavily fragranced, and most people's noses are now numb to the smells. But your brain isn't; it gets the full impact because the smells are carried along the olfactory nerve directly to the limbic system areas that regulate mood, sleep, memory, and other vital functions. That's one way that strong chemicals can disrupt memory and cause you to feel suddenly irritable.

Except for *very few, very expensive* perfumes that use only plant-based compounds, over 95% of the chemicals in today's scented products are derived from *petroleum-based* compounds. Even the potent synthetic "musk," in many popular perfumes, colognes and after-shave products, falls into this group of chemicals.

Studies show that these chemical fragrances can cause central nervous system disorders, immune disorders, headaches, allergic reactions, birth defects and even cancer.

This is really not new. It was reported to the U.S. House of Representatives in 1986 by the Committee on Science and Technology, based on extensive scientific evidence. These reports have been overlooked and ignored in terms of their potential to cause such varied health problems. Most of the research focus is on the cancer-causing potential of these chemicals rather than the subtle types of brain and immune system effects.

The dyes, dry cleaning solutions, laundry products, fragrances from perfumes and household products, mothballs, and a host of other products in your home environment—all have the potential to further disrupt neuroendocrine pathways.

Most of you use scented products and do not notice problem right away. Over time, and with hormone imbalances, you may develop traditional allergies, or what is known as *multiple chemical sensitivities* (MCS).

I encourage my patients to eliminate as many of these scented products as possible, particularly if they have hormone and allergy problems. Many hypoallergenic home and personal care products now help relieve allergies and sensitivities. (See Appendix II for helpful sources).

Watch out! Mothballs, Lysol spray, and Pine-sol— all have harsh chemicals that release noxious vapors and are severe irritants for women with hormone problems who are chemically sensitive.

It works I have used these approaches for the last thirty years, since I first began having problems with sensitivity to a lot of perfumes and chemicals. They are inexpensive and they work.

There are other sources of chemical vapors in our homes. It is important to minimize these, as well as eliminate mold and mildew that release toxic vapors.

Have you ever noticed the strong plastic smell when you open a new shower curtain liner? New sheets, pillowcases, carpets, and permanent press clothes are usually treated with formaldehyde, another chemical smell that causes problems for many women.

Advertisements bombard us with a different cleaning product for every purpose, all containing these strong chemicals.

Options

There are many less toxic options for getting rid of pests, inside and outside your home.

But how do you suppose our grandmothers got along? They used simple nontoxic remedies to handle most cleaning problems. We can reduce our household chemical overload, and save money at the same time, by following their example.

I use simple white cider vinegar and tap water for cleaning just about everything from shower tiles to glass table tops to windows to kitchen counters and floors. It works better than many commercial products, and doesn't contaminant your living and working environment with chemicals. If I need an abrasive for various tasks, I add simple baking soda.

My grandmother used a concoction of vinegar, water, and a small amount of olive oil on a cloth, an excellent solution that trapped dust effectively.

Lemon juice makes a fine brass polish. Instead of the strong-smelling silver polish, use Spic and Span in an aluminum-foil lined pan full of hot water. It whisks the tarnish away without the harsh chemicals and odors of the usual silver cleaners.

There are additional excellent ideas in the series of healthy cleaning books by Anne Berthold-Bond, or in *Less Toxic Living,* by Carolyn P. Gorman.

Clean Up Pesticides: They May Kill Pests, but What Do They Do to You and Your Children?

You now realize the dangers of most commercial pesticides used inside the home and outside on the yard and garden. If you must use them, be sure to follow directions and take necessary precautions.

Many pesticide chemicals, as well as medicines, fragrances, solvents, and cleaners, are absorbed through the skin. If you spill any on yourself, wash the area thoroughly.

Pesticides also release vapors that can adversely affect your brain if inhaled. This is a serious problem for older folks, but children (and your pets) are also vulnerable to residues from the sprays, and should not be outdoors when they are being used.

Glue traps work wonders on ants, spiders, scorpions, roaches, and other indoor pests. Boric acid solution is another non-toxic pest killer. (See Appendix for other non-toxic ideas for outdoor pest control).

Be Safe

Minimize exposure to potentially toxic chemicals for you and your family.

Inventory your home for products such as pesticides, cleaning products, paint and paint thinners that contain potentially dangerous ingredients. Isolate them in storage areas such as a locked garage or outside shed, rather than the basement.

Vapors from these chemicals can be as harmful as the product itself. If there is a warning label that the product is not safe for humans or pets, or is toxic, or if the label says that "special care" needs to be taken in the handling and application of the product, stop and ask yourself, "Is this product safe to have around?" Look for safer alternatives.

You may feel that not all of the following suggestions are feasible, but do what you can. Even small changes can add up over time.

Remember that all of these are *potentially harmful endocrine disruptors*. Patients say daily that they have no idea these products could cause *hormone* problems! Consumers simply are not told about potential damage. Better, safer options exist.

Check the chart that follows and begin your clean-up campaign.

Summary

We may not yet know *all* of the adverse effects these endocrine disruptors have on our bodies, yet what we do know is quite alarming. Don't take these warnings lightly. Eliminate as many of these substances as you can.

Every little bit helps. Accumulation of these endocrine disruptors, not necessarily just one or two, wreaks havoc on the health of our ovaries and the rest of our bodies.

Use common sense and caution. Scrutinize what you put in your mouth, on your body, in your home, work environment, and around your children.

Dr. Vliet's Guide to Ways to Minimize Toxic Chemicals at Home

🐦 PCBs and pesticides DDT, kepone, chlordane, lindane and benzene hexachlorane and benzene hexachloride (BCH) are banned in the U.S. but are still produced here and exported to other countries. Residential areas near these plants, workers in these plants, travel to other countries, and possibly imported produce may be sources of exposure. Check your local EPA office to see what chemical producers are near your home.

🐦 Minimize pesticide use in your home and look for alternative non-toxic products.

🐦 Avoid using pesticides such as endosulfan, methoxychlor, and triazine herbicides altogether, even though they are still made here.

🐦 Avoid traditional pesticides contained in pet collars and dips to control fleas and ticks. This minimizes children's risk of exposure to toxic chemicals when they play with their pets.

🐦 Avoid golf courses the day of, and the day after, spraying of pesticides. Call and ask when they spray, and plan your golf dates accordingly.

🐦 Keep your kids off pesticide or chemically fertilized lawns/gardens.

🐦 Ask your grocer if produce is sprayed with pesticides. If yes, let the manager know you plan to shop elsewhere unless they offer pesticide-free produce options.

🐦 Be aware of any local fish warnings to avoid fish contaminated with PCB, dioxin, and mercury.

🐦 Call your local water company and find out what is in the water and how it is treated. If you are on a well, be particularly careful when farmers spray their crops, and periodically test your water for contamination.

🐦 Install a reverse osmosis water filter with carbon system that will remove chemicals and particles (regular charcoal filters generally only remove odors and chlorine and bad tastes but not all toxic chemicals). If possible, use a shower filter or whole house carbon filter to eliminate chlorine and chlorine gas from the water and air.

🐦 Look for fresh fruits and vegetables, dairy products, poultry and meats that have not been treated with products that contain pesticides or growth hormones and chemicals. For chicken, try to buy those labeled "Free range," "no antibiotics," and "fed organic feed."

🐦 Avoid "basted" or "self-basting" turkeys that have added fat, water, broth and flavor enhancers containing MSG. Choose "fresh," or "fresh-frozen" birds instead.

🐦 If there are no local resources for organic foods in your area, check the Internet for sources of healthy, antibiotic-free and hormone free foods.

©Elizabeth Lee Vliet, MD 2001–2007

Dr. Vliet's Guide to Ways to Minimize Toxic Chemicals at Home

- Avoid plastics, particularly PVC (#3).
- Don't store or heat foods in plastic containers, styrofoam, or PVC cling wraps. Don't use plastic in microwave ovens. Instead, heat foods in porcelain or glass.
- Avoid boxed cookies and chocolates with plastic trays, which are usually PVC plastic. Check plastic bottles to see if they are marked PVC #3. Be especially careful of plastic-wrapped cheeses.
- It is best to cook with stainless steel, cast iron and glass. Teflon, aluminum, and copper are generally considered safe.
- Avoid alkyl phenol ethoxylates (APEs) found in detergents, hair coloring products, spermicides, and some plastics. Studies show these have estrogenic effects in mammals.
- Babies should not be given toys made of plastic. Use unpainted, unvarnished toys made of wood.
- Avoid lead-based paints in toys, dishes, or on walls. Lead accumulates to toxic levels that adversely affect the brain, especially children.
- Remove and dispose of plastic covers on dry-cleaning, and then air out dry-cleaned clothes outside before bringing them into your closets.
- Know where local hazardous waste sites are. People living near hazardous waste sites have higher rates of medical problems.
- Your workplace and home office should be well ventilated to prevent accumulation of fumes from toners, solvents and cleaners.
- Try new "micro fiber" cleaning cloths using only water to clean, so you can remove stains and dirt without added chemicals.
- Don't use room or bathroom fresheners. Don't use those noxious deodorizers often used in municipal public toilets. Most of these contain formaldehyde as well as synthetic fragrances that are toxic.
- Avoid the inexpensive particleboard or plywood furniture that is popular for offices and children's rooms. These need extensive airing to outgas the formaldehyde isocyanerates, and other chemicals used in the manufacturing process. They may also contain pesticides.
- The same formaldehyde problem is true for much of the carpeting sold today. Tile or wood flooring is better than wall-to-wall artificial fiber carpeting. Even wool carpeting is made with pesticides in the fibers, which can break off and become inhaled, particularly dangerous for small children and animals.
- Avoid permanent press products treated with formaldehyde, which can be irritating to eyes, skin, and cause headaches.
- Wash your hands often. Encourage your children to do the same.

©Elizabeth Lee Vliet, MD 2001–2007

Dr. Vliet's Guide to Ways to Minimize Your Body Exposure to Endocrine Disrupters

- Don't smoke.
- Limit alcohol to special occasions in small amounts.
- Increase your fiber intake to help eliminate environmental chemicals from your intestinal tract.
- Reduce your fat intake. Fats are where these chemicals concentrate.
- Work to maintain optimal percent body fat (20 - 25% for women under 50). Toxic chemicals are stored in body fat for up to 30 years.
- Exercise regularly to maintain optimal body fat and decrease your risk for breast cancer, heart disease and osteoporosis.
- Use caution with soy and phytoestrogens that mimic and interfere with your own natural estrogen
- Make sure any hormones you take are *bioidentical* to your body's own natural hormones, unless there are medical reasons (contraception, endometriosis or fibroid suppression, among others) for which the synthetic hormones work better.
- Minimize use of processed foods containing artificial sweeteners, monosodium glutamate (MSG), hydrolyzed vegetable protein, and other excitatory amino acids.
- Take anti-oxidant vitamins and minerals, magnesium, zinc to neutralize some of the cell-damaging effects of excitotoxins.
- Read your labels. Don't always assume sports supplements, diet foods, energy boosters, and products from health food stores are "safe."
- Soymilk often has glutamate in the form of hydrolyzed vegetable protein added as a flavor enhancer. Sports drinks and diet foods often contain aspartame, another excitotoxin to avoid.
- Although hormone-disruptor chemicals and environmental chemical pollutants can be transferred from mother to baby via breast milk, most experts still feel that the positive benefits of breast-feeding outweigh potential risks.

©Elizabeth Lee Vliet, MD 2001–2007

Chapter 19
Create Your Path to Optimal Energy and Health

Knowledge is power. I have often said this is crucial when it comes to your health and your life decisions.

You must first have a *reliable* information base.

As I have discussed throughout this book, there is so much information available these days, both accurate and inaccurate, it can be overwhelming and confusing. I am dismayed that even articles from reputable sources only scratch the surface of important issues and play it safe to avoid offending advertisers.

We see this especially with the issue of estrogen. Most information on estrogen never differentiates between the different types of estrogens or the brand used in the studies being headlined.

Rarely does anyone talk about how we are constantly being exposed to estrogenic chemicals from outside our body—in our foods, homes, water and air—that are far more dangerous to our health than anything that has ever been found with our own body estrogens.

In my view, this is a tragic oversight, and it leaves out an enormous, and perhaps even central, piece of the total hormone picture. I hope that with the science-based information I have provided in this book, you will be better equipped to ask probing questions, to evaluate media stories, and to make decisions about your health.

I encourage you to constantly question the information you receive. Ask what is the source, and what may be the underlying agendas. Are the studies cited funded by the industry that will profit from favorable findings?

Look for solutions and treatments that address the underlying cause and be wary of prescriptions, medications, and products that just treat the symptoms. If you do not, you may not only

Accurate knowledge is power. Power is freedom. Freedom to accomplish what is important to you for your health and your life.

put your health at risk but you may also wind up spending a lot of money on multiple medications and over the counter products that may have side effects for which you will need additional medications, products or treatments.

Wisdom
Be proactive about your health. Follow my tips for taking action.

Stop and ask, "Am I on the right path?" If you suspect you are not, do not be afraid to act quickly.

Kate's Successful Journey

I'd like to share with you is the story of a young woman I have known on both a professional and personal basis. I have seen her struggle with hormonal problems even before she realized that she had these problems. I have seen her turn disappointments into triumphs and throughout the years gain the knowledge and confidence to work with her own physicians to positively deal with her hormonal challenges. I hope her story will inspire you and give you the courage to keep reaching for your own goals.

When I first met Kate, she was 30 years old and just recovering from her second exploratory laparoscopic surgery for possible uterine fibroids and unexplained infertility. She had been trying to conceive for five years and had already had several rounds of diagnostic tests and attempts at artificial insemination with accompanying fertility drugs, without success.

Caution
Be careful about taking too many herbs and supplements.

Kate has always been a very fit and health conscious person. She exercised on a regular basis, ate well and maintained her body fat within optimal levels. The only health complaint she had, other than not being able to conceive, was severe PMS. She also experienced overwhelming light-headedness, sweats and chills, cramps and nausea prior to her period. These episodes were usually controlled by ibuprofen. What she didn't know, however, was that these were early clues of premature decline in her ovarian hormones.

Over the next few years, discouraged from unsuccessful infertility treatments and tired of the hormonal roller coaster infertility drugs can cause, she and her husband decided to explore other options for starting a family.

Adoption seemed the next logical step. They looked at working with an adoption agency or adopting a child from another country, but she quickly found out this was not an easy process either. They decided to become foster-adoptive parents with their state's child protective services. This would fulfill their desires for a family, and also give a new chance for a child in need. This process took nearly a full year to complete.

An incredible part of this story is that one month prior to their final licensing from the state, Kate was laid off from her 8-year-long administrative position with a health care organization due to downsizing.

Initially devastated, she realized this was been a blessing in disguise when she got a call from her caseworker at Child Protective Services asking if they could take an immediate placement. Three children, ages 11 months, 3 and 4 years old, seriously abused, were in *immediate* need of a foster home.

This is what Kate and her husband had been waiting for—and even more! Because of the severe abuse, neglect and parental unfitness of the biological parents, Kate and her husband officially adopted all three siblings nine months after the initial placement. This was a fast adoption.

Kate likes to call this was a "God deal." The initial timing was just right, coming after her lay-off when she could be home with the children. She felt it was just meant to be. Even more amazing, all three children looked just like her husband. Comparing baby pictures and snap shots of her husband at age 4 and 5, you could barely see a difference.

For a while though, Kate still hoped every month that she would be surprised and find herself pregnant, but this never happened. She has now accepted this, because her life is full and she is still amazed how fortunate they are and how much happiness the children have brought them.

And now the rest of the story. Throughout the years, Kate has been interested in my work and shared with me her own "hormonal" stories. She had a complete hormonal evaluation when she was 30, which showed some early hormone decline, but nothing so out of normal that she wanted to address it at the time.

Over the years, the more she learned, researched and we discussed, the more she saw in herself the hormone connections I have been writing about, and the work I have been doing with patients for the last 20 years.

She worked with her own physician to implement many of the treatments I have outlined in this book. Her PMS, and later cyclic acne, and menstrual headaches are improved. She would often tell me, "*My friends' doctors are putting them on Prozac and*

Note
Even mild symptoms can be clues to hormone decline.

Wisdom
Make sure you have a reliable hormone evaluation. Don't ignore early problems.

"I am so grateful to have this knowledge. I would have just struggled through these symptoms, felt miserable, and probably wound up paying through the nose for expensive medications that I didn't like taking."

Sarafem, or prescribing lots of other medications, or just telling them to tough it out and simplify their lives. What people don't seem to understand is that if your hormones are out of whack, you don't have a healthy foundation. Without hormones in balance its tough to make the positive lifestyle changes that in the long run will help make a difference. You just don't feel up to it." Well, obviously Kate "got" the message and was able to proactively take charge of her life and health.

Recently she had an unexpected "opportunity" to once again apply what she had learned. She had an unrecognized ruptured appendix, severe infection and adhesions that ultimately caused a total hysterectomy, with removal of the uterus, both ovaries and tubes.

This time Kate was prepared. She sought a second opinion with us prior to her surgery and we were able to guide her through the hormone options for post surgery. Immediately after the surgery, she asked her surgeon to start estrogen replacement therapy right away. She was given an injection of estradiol. She also had a prescription for estradiol patches and applied these as the injection began to wear off.

Kate is now stabilized on a regimen of low dose Estrace AM and PM with an estradiol patch to provide continuous stable estrogen levels. Recent blood work showed good estradiol levels, low testosterone levels, and borderline thyroid levels. Since we have successfully stabilized her estradiol levels, the next step will be to address the thyroid and restore her testosterone to optimal levels. Recently, she said,

"I continue to be amazed how really basic all this is when you stop and think about it. Yet no one is making these hormone connections. Even when I bring it up to friends, or other doctors, it is just dismissed. I think everybody is afraid of 'hormones.'"

"Except for the recovery from the surgeries, I feel like my transition has been very smooth. I have not experienced any symptoms from the estrogen drop, except when I forget to take my pills on time! I am so glad that I was able to get on top of this from the beginning. My body may be hormonally the equivalent of a 61-year-old lady, but I certainly do not feel like one. I am confident that if I can keep my hormones at optimal levels, continue to exercise and eat right, I will continue to feel like my old self, maybe even better! Thanks for being there for me."

No one ever found a cause for Kate's infertility, though we have often wondered if all the exposure to pesticides in the farming area in which they lived may have been a factor. She clearly had many of these warning signs that have been reported in animals and in the few human studies that have looked at this issue: unusually early decline in her ovarian hormone levels, headaches, early onset of fibroids when she didn't have any of the usual risk factors for developing these, and mild endometriosis, again without the more common risk factors or family history.

We will likely never know whether or not she was one of the silently injured ones from the widespread endocrine disruptors in her environment.

Going forward on your journey

I encourage you to do as she has done in being proactive to get her health needs met, knowledgeable about her options, and in being psychologically resilient enough to flow with the challenges and setbacks that came her way.

When we are out in a sailboat, we cannot control the direction of the wind, but we can learn to adjust the sails to get where we want to go.

That's what I hope this book has given you—the knowledge to "trim your sails" and make the adjustments in your health strategies as your conditions and needs change.

Getting older is a fact of life. It may not be as much fun as some other times in your life, but it sure beats the alternative. What is hard to accept is the feeling that our body is betraying us, letting us down, getting old before its time. This is not how it is supposed to be.

While these are natural feelings, don't let yourself get stuck in the negativity and blame. Try to understand what is going on and work to positively improve your health and fitness. Your body is telling you that you simply can no longer get away with all the 'things' you used to get away with.

You must carefully scrutinize every aspect of your lifestyle; eating habits, environment, medications, supplements, activity levels and start using many of the tools we have discussed throughout this book. Cumulatively, they will make a difference.

Get rid of as many sources of these chemicals as possible. You do not need this contamination in your home and your bodies. Do your research carefully. Check before you try something new you heard about on the evening news. The very fact that we do not yet know all the ramifications and consequences of these persistent organic pollutants is itself the very reason you need to take seriously the concerns that have been raised.

If new medicines or supplements or herbs are suggested, ask yourself:

- ❧ *What am I taking, and why am I taking this?*
- ❧ *Are there sound reasons for me to take this?*

"This is not what I thought I would be dealing with at age 35. This was not a 'club' I wanted to join. But since I am now a full-fledged menopausal woman, (although surgically induced), I am grateful that I had a knowledgeable hormone specialist to guide me through it."

Attention
Pay close attention to the early warnings I have described throughout this book.

Wisdom

Take charge of your own health. Know what your own hormone levels are, using reliable blood tests.

≥► *What is in it?*

≥► *Where does it come from?*

≥► *Do I really need it?*

≥► *What reputable scientific information backs up the claims.*

≥► *Who will profit from my buying this product?*

≥► *Who is funding the research?*

Don't let others fool you into thinking you can't be experiencing hormone decline because you are not the textbook menopausal age of 51. The sooner you get on top of your health problems the better.

As you identify potential problem areas and work toward making positive changes, be gentle with yourself. Be understanding of your body, and give it time to respond, to recover, to heal, to rejuvenate.

Do it!

Ask questions and don't be satisfied until you have confidence in the answers you receive.

Hormone imbalance doesn't turn around after one doctor visit. Your body needs time to recover, restore, repair and readjust itself. Make yourself and your health your top priority—and don't feel guilty! If you don't take care of yourself, who will? You need to take care of yourself so you can be healthy enough to give to the other people in your life.

Balance is the key. The body is an exquisitely sensitive, precious instrument and it needs the proper balance in order to function optimally.

Balance will be achieved in *different* ways, with *different* techniques and medications, for *different* individuals, using the tools of modern medicine coupled with the options and wisdom of complementary medicine when appropriate.

Each one of us is an individual with *different* needs. The key is to find a blend of therapeutic approaches that is right for you: healthy food, optimal hormonal balance, exercise, optimal vitamin and mineral supplementation, body therapies, other medications as appropriate, positive mental attitudes, meditation and prayer. All are important. Slow down and take time to do these for you.

Warning

Don't take your symptoms lightly. Don't fall into the trap of denial.

All of these approaches combine to help you regain and sustain your health, energy and vitality, and find the "old self" you know and miss. Remember to like yourself during this process. Use positive self-talk. This may sound corny, but is so important. Accept where you are and what you are experiencing, while you look at ways to move forward.

Summary

It has been an inspirational journey for me as I have worked with the women who cross my doorstep in search of answers, in search of ways to feel better, restore balance, and have the energy to lead fuller lives. I don't take these responsibilities lightly. I have seen the devastation in women's lives, as well as the lives of those who love them, when there is misinformation and mistreatment. I want to help them get better, using sound approaches.

I find myself at times overcome with anger and frustration, and immense sadness, at what women have been told, at the gross misinformation in the press and books by those who only seek to be a "guru" to sell the most books, or tapes, or vitamins, or wild yam creams, or herbs, or saliva tests or "designer" formulations... or whatever the latest gimmick may be.

The appalling morass of myth, hype, misinformation and distortion, along with the fear tactics frequently used in marketing and advertising, creates untold damage and suffering for the women who are seeking help.

Damage is also done by those who fear to venture out of the narrow tunnel vision of their specialty, who make rigid pronouncements based on their medical training from 25 years ago, and do not take the time to look, to think, to learn, or even question old theories.

I don't have an easy answer for you, but I do encourage you to rely on your own wisdom and common sense, and on medical professionals who care about you; those whose knowledge you can trust because you have done your homework, and who work with you to find approaches that help.

Hormones are your body's metabolic "power" fuel. Don't let your body run on empty. Get checked and regain your energy and vitality! I think the solution lies in these words:

*Pursuing knowledge is not
So much to get caught up in
PROOF...
as to discover
What works...
and then
Make it WORK!*   —*Rolling Thunder*

GO FOR IT!

Dr. Vliet's Tips: Your Path to Health:

- **Become proactive about getting information**, explore your options, read about pros and cons of various choices, make notes, and lists of your questions before you take action.
- **Research your family health history**, write it down, and take copies with you to your medical visits.
- **Know your health risks**, write them down, and give a copy to your physician.
- **Take an inventory of EVERY supplement you are taking**, list all the ingredients and doses and take a copy of this to every medical visit. Insist that all of your doctors keep this information in your chart. We ask our patients for this information at every visit, but I continue to be surprised at the women who say, "I don't know what I am taking," or "I don't know what's in it."
- **Keep a single list of all of your prescription medications** and the doses of each one. Share this list with each doctor. *Take a copy to every medical visit.*
- **Keep track of your past and present "health data"** (we call this your "medical records"). Get copies and keep a set to take with you if you have an emergency or see a new physician.
- **Pay attention to your "numbers"** (medical test results); ask for copies of your lab reports and key test results and keep for your records and to show other physicians you may consult.
- **Do your homework** investigating resources for health professionals who will best suit your needs for your health "team."
- **Keep track of your symptoms** (charted with your menstrual cycle, or phase of hormone therapy); take this log to your medical appointments. Write down, before each appointment, "What's better since last time? What's not better?"
- **Write a list of questions** you want answered before each appointment with your health professionals. This will focus your thoughts so that important items are not overlooked in the discussion.
- **Speak up and ask questions** if you don't understand an explanation or directions.
- **Be actively involved.** It will help reduce risk of medical errors, and will result in your receiving better care.

©Elizabeth Lee Vliet, MD 2001–2007

Appendix I

Glossary Of Medical Terms

This is a list of the medical abbreviations and a glossary of medical terms I have used throughout this book. If you are going to take charge of your health, it will help for you to become informed about what these terms mean, so you will understand terms used by your physician to explain what is happening to your body.

I. List of Medical Acronyms Used in This Book

Hormones

E1	estrone
E 2	estradiol
E3	estriol
CEE	conjugated equine estrogens (Premarin, Prempro)
T4	thyroxine (thyroid)
T3	triiodothyronine (thyroid)
FSH	follicle stimulating hormone
LH	luteinizing hormone
SHBG	Sex Hormone Binding Globulin
TSH	Thyroid Stimulating Hormone
GH	Growth Hormone

Other Terms

BCP	birth control pill (see also "OC" for oral contraceptive)
BMI	body mass index
BMR	basal metabolic rate
BTL	Bilateral Tubal Ligation
CHOL	cholesterol
CVD	cardiovascular disease
DEXA	Dual Energy X-Ray absorptiometry
DA	dopamine

EPI	epinephrine
EFA	essential fatty acids
FFA	free fatty acids
GABA	Gamma Aminobutyric Acid
GLA	Gamma Linolenic Acid
HDL	high density lipoprotein ("good" cholesterol)
HRT	Hormone Replacement Therapy
IUD	Intra-Uterine Device
LDL	low density lipoprotein ("bad" cholesterol)
NE	norepinephrine
NTx	N-telopeptide (bone breakdown product)
OC, or OCP	oral contraceptive pill
PCOS	Polycystic Ovary Syndrome (also abbreviated just PCO)
PMS	Premenstrual Syndrome, also called
PMDD	Premenstrual Dysphoric Disorder
POD	Premature Ovarian Decline
POF	Premature Ovarian Failure
POPs	Persistent Organic Pollutants
SERMS	Selective Estrogen Receptor Modulators.
ST	serotonin, also called 5-HT (5-hydroxytryptophan)
TG	Triglycerides

Measurements

cc	cubic centimeter (1 cc = 1 ml)
dl	deciliter
mcg	microgram
mg	milligram
ml	milliliter (1 ml = 1 cc)
ng	nanogram
pg	picogram

Appendix II
References

It is not possible to list the hundreds of medical and scientific peer-reviewed articles from reputable medical journals that I have read and studied for my clinical work and book writing.

This is a list of selected historical and current articles that may be of interest for those of you who want a reference for your physician, or for your own reading of the medical literature. Many times I have included the older articles to illustrate how long this information has been available and how our current understandings have evolved from this historical foundation. The historical articles will be of particular interest to women who have known intuitively for many years that something "hormonal" is wrong. Many of the concepts I describe in this book have been described in the medical literature, but ignored, for decades.

The current research articles help you see the depth and breadth of our existing science explaining these important hormone connections to the healthy function of our entire body. Each article provides additional references if you wish to pursue a topic in more depth. I have focused on medical research articles published in the major, peer- reviewed national and international medical journals.

Introduction to Revised Edition
Genazzani AR, Gambacciani M. A personal initiative for women's health: to challenge the Women's Health Initiative, *Gynecol Endocrinol* 16: 255–257, August 2002.

Schneider, HPG. The view of the International Menopause Society on the Women's Health Initiative (WHI). *Climacteric* 5: 211–216, September 2002.

Writing Group for the Women's Health Initiative Investigators. Risks and benefits of estrogen plus progestin in healthy postmenopausal women. *JAM Med Assoc* 288: 321–333, 2002.

Chapter 1: When Ovaries Go Awry: Women's Lives, Women's Stories
Abramowitz ES, Bakerk AH, Fleisher SF. Onset of depressive psychiatric crises and the menstrual cycle. *Am J Psych* 139: 475–478, 1982

Backstrom CT, Boyle H, Baird DT. Persistence of symptoms of premenstrual tension in hysterectomized women. *Br J Obs Gyn* 88: 530–536, 1981.

Coulam CB. Premature gonadal failure. Fertility and Sterility 38: 645–650,1982.

Davis SR. Premature ovarian failure. *Maturitas* 23(1): 108, 1996.

Fourestie V, DeLignieres B, Roudot-Thoraval F, et al. Suicide attempts in hypooestrogenic phases of the menstrual cycle. *Lancet*, 1357–1360, Dec. 1986.

Sarrel P. Ovarian steroids and the capacity to function at home and in the workplace. Oral presentation, North American Menopause Society, New York, September 21–23, 1989.

Vliet EL, Davis VL. New perspectives on the relationship of hormonal changes to affective disorders in the perimenopause. In *Clinical Issues in Women's Health*, vol. 2(4): Midlife Women's Health, Oct.–Dec. Philadelphia: Lippincott, 1991, pp. 453–472.

Chapter 2: Your Ovaries: An Owner's Manual

Bhatia SK, Moore D, and Kalkhoff RK. Progesterone suppression of the Plasma Growth Hormone Response. *Clin Endocrinol Metab* 35: 364–369, 1972.

Kalkoff R. Metabolic effects of progesterone. *J Obstet Gynecol* 142–6: 735–738, 1982.

Nieschlag E, Behre HM, ed. *Testosterone: Action, Deficiency, Substitution*, 2nd ed. Berlin: Springer–Verlag, 1998.

Stott CA. Steroid hormones: metabolism and mechanism of action. In *Reproductive Endocrinology: Physiology, Pathophysiology, and Clinical Management*, 4 ed., S.S., eds. Yen, R.B. Jaffe, and R.L. Barbieri. Philadelphia: WB. Saunders, 1999, p. 124.

Chapter 3: Your Ovaries and Their Life Cycle

Aoki Y. Polychlorinated biphenyls, polychlorinated dibenw-p-dioxins, and polychlorinated Dibenzofurans as endocrine disruptors—what have we learned from Yusho disease. *Environ Res (United States)*, 86(1): 2–11, 2001.

Chang KJ, Hsieh KH, Tang SY, Tung TC, Lee TP. Immunologic evaluation of patients with polychlorinated biphenyl poisoning: evaluation of delayed-type skin hypersensitive response and its relation to clinical studies. *J Toxicol Environ Health* 9(2): 217–223,1982.

Christiansen C, Christiansen M. Climacteric symptoms, fat mass and plasma concentrations of LH, FSH, PRL, estradiol 17–beta, and androstenedione in the early postmenopausal period. *Acta Endo* 10 1: 87–92, 1982.

Cooke DJ. A psychological study of the climacteric. In *Psychology and Gynaecological Problems*, eds. A. Broome and L. Wallace. London: Tavistock Publ, 1984, pp. 243–265.

Crawford S, Casey V, Avis N, et al. A longitudinal study of weight and the menopause transition: Results from the Massachusetts Women's Health Study. *Menopause: J N Am Meno Soc* 7(2): 96–105, 2000.

Giesy JP, Verbrugge DA, Othout RA, Bowerman WW, et al. Contaminants in fishes from Great Lakes-influenced sections and above dams of three Michigan rivers. I: Concentrations of organo chlorine insecticides, polychlorinated biphenyls, dioxin equivalents, and mercury. *Arch Environ Contam Toxicol* 27(2): 202–212, 1994.

Gladen B, Rogan W, Hardy P, et al. Development after exposure to polycholorinated biphenyls and dichlorodiphenyl dichloroethene transplacentally and through human milk. *J Pediatrics* 113: 991–995,1988.

Hagstad A, Janson P. The epidemiology of climacteric symptoms. *Acta Obst Gynaecol Scand Suppl* 134: 59–65, 1986.

Ho S, Chan S, Yip Y, et al. Menopausal symptoms and symptom clustering in Chinese women. *Maturitas* 33(3): 219–227,1999.

Krstevska-Konstantinova M, Charlier C, Craen M, et al. Sexual precocity after immigration from developing countries to Belgium: evidence of previous exposure to organochlorine pesticides. Presented at the International Workshop on Hormones and Endocrine Disrupters in Food and Water, May 2000; published in *Human Reproduction* 16(5): 1020–1026, May 2001.

Lu YC, Wu yc. Clinical findings and immunological abnormalities in Yu-Cheng patients. *Environ Health Perspect* 59: 17–29,1985.

Niessen, KH, Ramolla J, Binder M, et al. Chlorinated hydrocarbons in adipose tissue of infants and toddlers: inventory and studies on their association with intake of mother's milk, *Eur J Pediatr* 142(4): 238–244,1984.

Olea N, Olea-Serrano F, Lardelli-Claret P, Rivas A, Barba-Navarro A. Inadvertent exposure to xenoestrogens in children. *Toxicol Ind Health* 15(1–2): 151–158, 1999.

Rogan W, Gladen B, Mckinney J, et al. Neonatal effects of transplacental exposure to PCBs and DDE. *J Pediatrics*. 109: 335–341, 1986.

Rogan WI, Ragan NB. Chemical contaminants, pharmacokinetics, and the lactating mother. *Environ Health Perspect* 102(Suppl 11): 89–95, Dec. 1994. Review.

Sowers MR, LaPietra MT. Menopause: its epidemiology and potential association with chronic disease. *Epidemiology* Rev 17: 287,1987.

Vliet EL. Menopause and perimenopause: The role of ovarian hormones in common neuroendocrine syndromes in primary care. *Primary Care Clinics in Office Practice* 29: 43–67, 2002.

Wing R. Obesity and weight gain during adulthood: A health problem for United States women. *WHI* 2(2): 114–122, 1992.

Young CM, Blondin J, Tensuan R, et al. Body composition studies of "older" women, thirty to seventy years of age. *Ann N Y Acad Sci* 110: 589–607, 1963.

Chapter 4: Ovaries at Risk: Surprising Toxins in Your Diet

Allred J. Too much of a good thing? An overemphasis on eating low fat foods may be contributing to the alarming increase in overweight among U.S. adults. *J Am Dietetic Assoc* 95(4): 417–418, 19 95.

Ames B. Paleolithic diet, evolution and carcinogens. *Science* 258: 1633–1634,1997.

Cassidy A, Bingham S, Setchell K. Biological effects of isoflavones in young women: Importance of the chemical composition of soybean products. *Brit Nutrition* 74: 587–601, 1995.

Cassidy A, Milligan S. How significant are environmental estrogens to women? *Climacteric* 1: 229–242, 1998.

Coyle JT, Puttfarcken P. Oxidative Stress, glutamate, and neurodegenerative disorders. *Science* 262 (5134): 689–695, 1993.

Fort P, Moses N, Fasano M, et al. Breast and soy-formula feedings in early infancy and the prevalence of autoimmune thyroid disease in children (from Dept. of Pediatrics, North Shore University Hospital–Cornell University Medical College). *J Am Coli Nutr* 9(2): 164–167, 1990.

Fotsis T, Zhang Y, Pepper M, et al. The endogenous oestrogen metabolite 2–methoxytoestradiol inhibits angiogenesis and suppresses tumour growth. *Nature* 368: 237–239, 1994.

Halliwell B. Reactive oxygen species and the central nervous system. *J Neurochem* 59(5): 1609–1623, Nov. 1992.

Hunt J, et al. High versus low meat diets: Effects on zinc absorption, iron status, and calcium, copper, iron, magnesium, nitrogen, phosphorous, and zinc balance in postmenopausal women. *Am J Clin Nutr* 62: 621–632, 1995.

Hunter B. Some food additives as neuroexcitors and neurotoxins. *Clinical Ecology* 2(2): 83–89, 1984.

Knight, DC and JA Eden. A review of the clinical effects of phytoestrogens. *Obstet Gynecol* 87(5 Part 2): 897–904,1996.

Kronenberg F and Hughes C. Exogenous and endogenous estrogens: An appreciation of biological complexity (editorial). Menopause: *The Journal of the North American Menopause Society* 6(1): 4–6,1999.

Nagata C, Kabuto M, Kurisu Y, Shimizu H. Decreased serum estradiol concentration associated with high dietary intake of soy products in premenopausal Japanese women. *Nutrition and Cancer* 29(3): 228–233,1997.

Pirke K, Schweiger U, Laessle R, et al. Dieting influences the menstrual cycle: Vegetarian versus nonvegetarian diet. *Fertility and Sterility* 46(6): 1083–1088, 1968.

Simonian NA, Coyle JT. Oxidative stress in neurodegenerative disorders. *Anna Rev Pharmacol*

Toxicol 36: 83–106,1996.

Yon Borstel R Metabolic and physiologic effects of sweeteners. *Clin Nutr* 4(6): 215–220, 1985.

Whitten PL, Lewis C, Russell E, Naftolin F. Potential adverse effects of phytoestrogens. *Journal of Nutrition* 125(Suppl): S 776,1995.

Chapter 5: Ovaries at Risk: "Gender Benders" and Endocrine Disruptors Around You

Abou-Donia MB, et al. Neurotoxicity resulting from coexposure to pyridostigmine bromide, DEET, and permitrin: Implications of Gulf War chemical exposures. *J Tox & Environ Health* 48: 35–56, 1996.

Allen RH, Gottlieb M, Clute E, et al. Breast cancer and pesticides in Hawaii: The need for further study. *Environ Health Perspect* 105(Suppl 3): 679–683,1997.

Arnold SF, et al. Synergistic activation of estrogen receptor with combinations of environmental chemicals. *Science* 272: 1489–1492, 1996.

Barsano CPo Environmental factors altering thyroid function and their assessment. *Environ Health Perspect* 38: 71–82, 1981.

Birnbaum LS. Developmental effects of dioxins and other endocrine disrupting chemicals. *Neurotoxicology* 16(4): 748, Winter 1995.

Carpenter DO. Human health effects of environmental pollutants: New insights. *Environ Monit Assess* 53(1): 245–258, Oct. 1998.

Chester AC, Levine PH. Concurrent sick building syndrome and chronic fatigue syndrome: Epidemic neuromyasthenia revised. *Clinical Infectious Diseases* 18 (Suppl 1): S43–S48, 1996.

Colborn T, Smolen MJ. Epidemiological analysis of persistent organochlorine contaminants in cetaceans. *Rev Environ Contam Toxicol* 146: 91–172,1996.

Colborn T, vom Saal FS, Soto AM. Developmental effects of endocrine-disrupting chemicals in wildlife and humans. *Environ Health Perspect* 102 (Suppl 2): 126, 1993.

Cooper RL, Kavlock RJ. Endocrine disruptors and reproductive development: A weight of evidence overview. *J Endocrinol* 152: 159, 1997.

Dello Iacovo R, Celentano E, Strollo AM, et al. Organochlorines and breast cancer. A study on Neapolitan women. *Adv Exp Med Biol* 472: 57–66, 1999.

Exon JH, Kerkvliet NI, Talcott PA. Immunotoxicity of carcinogenic pesticides and related chemicals. *Journal of Environmental Science and Health*, Part C: *Environmen- tal Carcinogenesis Reviews* C5: 73–120, 1987.

Feeley M, Brouwer A. Health risks to infants from exposure to PCBs, PCDDs and PCDFs. *Food Addit Contam* 17(4): 325–333, 2000.

Hoffmann W. Organochlorine compounds: Risk of non- Hodgkin's lymphoma and breast cancer? *Arch Environ Health* 51(3): 189–192, 1996.

Holladay SD. Prenatal immunotoxicant exposure and postnatal autoimmune disease. *Environ Health Perspect* 107 (Suppl 5): 687–691,1999.

Kannan K, Tanabe S, Giesy JP, Tatsukawa R. Organochlorine pesticides and polychlori- nated biphenyls in foodstuffs from Asian and oceanic countries (review). *Rev Environ Contam Toxicol* 152: 1–55, 1997.

Kimbrough RD. Human health effects of polychlorinated biphenyls (PCBs) and poly- brominated biphenyls (PBBs). *Annual Review of Pharmacology and Toxicology* 27: 87–111, 1987.

Lindstrom G, Hooper K, Petreas M, Stephens R, Gilman A. Workshop on perinatal expo- sure to dioxin-like compounds. I. Summary. *Environ Health Perspect* 103(Suppl 2): 135–142,1995.

MacIntosh DL, Spengler JD, Ozkaynak H, Tsai L, Ryan PB. Dietary exposures to selected metals and pesticides. *Environ Health Perspect* 104(2): 202–209,1996.

MacMonegle Jr, CW, Steffey KL, Bruce WN. Dieldrin, heptachlor, and chlordane residues in soybeans in Illinois 1974, 1980. *J Environ Sci Health* B. 19(1): 39–48, 1984.

Mattison DR, Plowchalk BS, Meadows MJ, et al. Reproductive toxicity: male and female repro- ductive systems as targets for chemical injury. *Med Clin North Am* 74: 391, 1990.

Mattison DR, Shiromizu K, Nightingale MS. Oocyte destruction by polycyclic aromatic hydro-carbons. *Am J Ind Med* 4: 191, 1983.

Mattison DR, Takizawa K, Silbergeld EK, et al. Genetics of ovarian benzo(a)pyrene metabolism, oocyte destruction, and impaired fertility. In *Extrahepatic Drug Metabolism and Chemical Carcinogenesis*, eds. J Sydstrom, et al. Elsevier 1983, p. 337.

Miller GW, Kirby ML, Levey AI, Bloomquist JR. Heptachlor alters expression and function of dopamine transporters. *Neurotoxicology* 20(4): 631–637, 1999.

National Research Council. *Pesticides in Diets of Infants and Children*. Washington, D.C., 1993, pp. 123–157.

Oduma JA, Wango EO, Oduor-Okelo D, et al. In vivo and in vitro effects of graded doses of the pesticide heptachlor on female sex steroid hormone production in rats. *Comp Biochem Physiol C Pharmacol Toxicol Endocrinol* 111(2): 191–196,1995.

Paumgartten FJ, Cruz CM, Chahoud I, et al. PCDDs, PCDFs, PCBs, and other organochlorine compounds in human milk from Rio de Janeiro. *Brazil Environ Res.* 83(3): 293–297, 2000.

Pittman KA, Benitz K-F, Silkworth JB, Mueller W, Coulston F. Environmental chemical-induced immune dysfunction. *Ecotoxicology and Environmental Safety* 2(2): 173–198,1978.

Porter WP, Hinsdill R, Fairbrother A, Olson LJ, Jaeger J, Yuill T, Bisgaard S, Hunter WG, Nolan K. Toxicant-disease-environment interactions associated with suppression of immune system, growth, and reproduction. *Science* 224 (ISS 4652): 1014–1027, 1984.

Porterfield S. Vulnerability of the developing brain to thyroid abnormalities: environmental insults to the thyroid system. *Environ Health Perspect* 102: 125–130, 1994.

Rao PS, Lakshmy R. Role of goitrogens in iodine deficiency disorders and brain development. *Indian J Med Res* 102: 223–226, 1995.

Smith EM, Hammonds-Ehlers M, Clark MK, et al. Occupational exposures and risk of female infertility. *J Occup Environ Med* 39: 138, 1997.

Swain, Wayland R. Human health consequences of consumption of fish contaminated with organochlorine compounds. *Aquatic Toxicology* 11: 357–377, 1988.

Tryphonas H. The impact of PCBs and dioxins on children's health: immunological considerations. *Can J Public Health* 89(Suppl 1): S49–52, S54–57, 1998.

Ward EM, Schulte P, Grajewski B, et al. Serum organochlorine levels and breast cancer: A nested case-control study of Norwegian women. *Cancer Epidemiol Biomarkers Prev.* 9(12): 1357–1367, 2000.

Weisglas-Kuperus N. Neurodevelopmental, immunological and endocrinological indices of peri-natal human exposure to PCBs and dioxins. *Neurotoxicology* 17(3–4): 945–946, 1996.

Weisglas-Kuperus N, Sas TC, Koopman-Esseboom C, et al. Immunologic effects of background prenatal and postnatal exposure to dioxins and polychlorinated biphenyls in Dutch infants. *Pediatr Res* 38(3): 404–410,1995.

Wolff M, Toniolo P, Lee E, Rivera M, Dubin N. Blood levels of organochlorine residues and risk of breast cancer. *J Natl Cancer Inst* 85(8): 648–642, 1993.

Yu ML, Hsin JW, Hsu CC, Chan WC, Guo YL. The immunologic evaluation of the Yucheng children. *Chemosphere* 37(9–12): 1855–1865,1998.

Chapter 6: Ovaries at Risk: Toxic Effects of Cigarettes, Alcohol, Marijuana, and Other Drugs

Babor TF, Grant M. From clinical research to secondary prevention: international collaboration in the development of the Alcohol Use Disorders Identification Test (AUDIT). *Alcohol Health Res World* 13: 371–374, 1989.

Baird DD, Wilcox AJ. Cigarette smoking associated with delayed conception. *JAMA* 253: 2979,1985.

Becker U, Tonnesen H, Kaas-Claesson N, and Gluud C. Menstrual disturbances and fertility in chronic alcoholic women. *Drug and Alcohol Dependence* 24: 75–82, 1989. Elsevier Scientific Publishers, Ireland.

Cooper GS, Baird DD, Hulka BS, et al. Follicle-stimulating hormone concentrations in relation to active and passive smoking. *Obstet Gynecol* 85: 407, 1995

Everson RB, Sandler DR, Wilcox AJ, et al. Effect of passive exposure to smoking on age at natural menopause. *Br Med J* 293: 272, 1986

Ferraroni M, Decarli A, Franceschi S, La Vecchia C. Alcohol consumption and risk of breast cancer: a multicenter Italian case-control study. *European J of Cancer* 34: 1403–1409, 1998.

Hommer DW et al. Evidence for a gender-related effect of alcoholism on brain volumes. *Am J Psychiatry* 158: 198–204, 2001.

Jick H, Porter J, Morrison AS. Relations between smoking and age of natural menopause. *Lancet* 1: 1354, 1977.

Kaufman DW, Slone D, Rosenberg L, et al. Cigarette smoking and age at natural menopause. *Am J Public Health* 70: 420, 1980.

Mattison DR, Plowchalk BS, Meadows MJ, et al. The effect of smoking on oogenesis, fertilization, and implantation. *Semin Reprod Endocrinol* 7: 219, 1989.

Mello N, Mendelson J, Teoh S. Neuroendocrine consequences of alcohol abuse in women. *Ann NY Acad Sci* 562: 211–240, 1981.

Mendelson JH, Lukas SE, Mello NK, et al. Acute alcohol effects on plasma estradiol levels in women. *Psychopharmacology* 94: 464–467,1988.

Modugno F, et al. Cigarette smoking and the risk of mucinous and nonmucinous epithelial ovarian cancer. *Epidemiology* 13: 467–471, 2002.

Muti P, Trevisan M, Micheli A, et al. Alcohol consumption and total estradiol in premenopausal women. *Cancer Epidemiol Biomarkers and Prev* 7: 189–193, March 1998.

Nystrom M, Perasalo J, Salaspuro M. Screening for heavy drinking and alcohol-related problems in young university students: the CAGE, the Mm-MAST and the trauma score questionnaires. *J Stud Alcohol* 54: 528–533, 1993.

Pettersson P, Ellsinger B-M, Sjoberg C, Bjorntorp P. Fat distribution and steroid hormones in women with alcohol abuse. *J Internal Med* 228(4): 311–316, Oct. 1990.

Pokorny AD, Miller BA, Kaplan HB. The brief MAST: A shortened version of the Michigan Alcoholism Screening Test. *Am J Psychiatry* 129: 342–345, 1972.

Roman P. Biological features of women's alcohol use: A review. *Public Health Rep* 103(6): 628–637, Nov–Dec. 1988.

Russell M, Martier SS, Sokol RJ, et al. Screening for pregnancy risk drinking. *Alcohol Clin Exp Res* 18: 1156–1161, 1994.

Valimaki N, Harkonen M, and Ylikahri R. Acute effects of alcohol on female sex hormones. *Alcohol Clin Exp Res* 7: 289–293, 1983.

Van Voorhis BJ, Syrop CH, Hammit DG, et al. Effects of smoking on ovulation induction for assisted reproductive techniques. *Fertil Steril* 58: 981,1992.

Wilsnack S, Klassen A, Wilsnack R. Drinking and reproductive dysfunction among women in a 1981 National Survey. *Alcoholism: Clinical and Experimental Research* 8(5):451–458,1984.

Yeh J, Barbierei RL. Effects of smoking on steroid production, metabolism, and estrogen-related diseases, *Semin Reprod Endocrinol* 7: 326, 1989.

Chapter 7: Ovary Shutdown: The Toxic Role of Stress Overload and Sleep Deprivation

Birketvedt G, Florholmen J, Sundsfjord J, et al. Behavioral and neuroendocrine characteristics of the night-eating syndrome. *JAMA* 282(7): 657–663, 1999.

Blackman MR. (editorial) Age-related alterations in sleep quality and neuroendocrine function: Interrelationships and implications. *JAMA* 284: 879–881, 2000.

Borbely AA. Processes underlying sleep regulation. *Horm Res* 49: 114–117, 1998.

Dijk DJ, Duffy JE Circadian regulation of human sleep and age-related changes in its timing, consolidation and EEG characteristics. *Ann Med* 31: 130–140, 1999.

Ho KY, Evans WS, Blizzard RM, et al. Effects of sex and age on the 24-hour profile of growth hormone secretion in man: Importance of endogenous estradiol concentrations. *J Clin Endocrinol Metab* 64: 51–58, 1987.

Howard AD, Feighner SD, Cully DF, et al. A receptor in pituitary and hypothalamus that functions in growth hormone release. *Science* 273: 974–977, 1996.

Kramer R, Cook Carlisle C, et al. Role of the primary care physician in recognizing obstructive sleep apnea. *Arch Intern Med* 159: 965–968, 1999.

Leong GM, Mercado-Asis LB, Reynolds JC, et al. The effect of Cushing's disease on bone mineral density, body composition, growth, and puberty. *J Clin Endocrinol Metab* 81: 1905–1911,1996.

McEwen BS. Stress, adaptation, and disease. *Ann NY Acad Sci.* 840: 33–44,1998.

McEwen BS, Sapolsky RM. Stress and cognitive function. *Curr Opin Neurobiol* 5: 205–216,1995.

Peeke P, Chrousos G. Hypercortisolism and obesity. Ann NY *Acad Sci* 771: 665–676, 1995.

Plat L, LeProult R, L'Hermite-Baleriaux M, et al. Metabolic effects of short-term elevations of plasma cortisol are more pronounced in the evening than in the morning. *J Clin Endocrinol Metab* 84: 3082–3092, 1999.

Post R. Transduction of psychosocial stress into the neurobiology of recurrent affective disorder. *Am J Psychiatry* 149(8): 999–1010,1992.

Van Cauter E, Leproult R, Kupfer DJ. Effects of gender and age on the levels and circadian rhythmicity of plasma cortisol. *J Clin Endocrinol Metab* 81: 2468–2473, 1996.

Van Cauter E, Plat L, Leproult R, et al. Alterations of circadian rhythmicity and sleep in aging: Endocrine consequences. *Horm Res* 49: 147–152,1998.

Van Cauter E, Plat L, Copinschi G. Interrelations between sleep and the somatotropic axis. *Sleep* 21: 553–566, 1998.

Weinstock M. Does prenatal stress impair coping and regulation of hypothalamicpituitary-adrenal axis? *Neuroscience and Biobehavioral Reviews* 21(1): 1–10, Jan. 1997.

Yager J. Nocturnal eating syndromes (editorial). JAMA 282(7): 689–690, 1999.

Chapter 8: Lifestyle Habits and Cultural Issues, Unexpected Stress for Our Ovaries

Aloia, JF, McGowan DM, Vaswani AN, Ross P, and Cohn SH. Relationship of menopause to skeletal and muscle mass. *Am J Clin Nutr* 53: 1378–1383, 1991.

Bale P, Doust J, Dawson D. Gymnasts, distance runners, anorexics' body composition and menstrual status. *J Sports Med Phys Fitness* 36(1): 49–53,1996.

Berga SL. Stress and ovarian function. Am J Sports Med 24(6 Suppl): S36–37, 1996.

Berkman S. Body image: Larger than life? *Women's Health and Fitness News* 4(8): 1–6, 1990.

Bullen B, Skrinar G, Beitins I, et al. Endurance training effects on plasma hormonal responsiveness and sex hormone excretion. *J Appl Phys: Respirat Environ Exercise Physio* 156(6): 1453–1463, 1984.

Chen EC, Brzyski RG. Exercise and reproductive dysfunction. *Fertil Steril.* 71(1): 1–6, 1999.

Dionyssiou-Asteriou A, Drakakis P, Vatalas IA, Michalas S. Variations of serum hormone levels in young exercising women. *Clin Endocrinol* 51(2): 258–260,1999. (Oxford.)

Duncan JJ, Gordon NF, Scott CB. Women walking for health and fitness: How much is enough? *JAMA* 266: 3295–3299, 1991.

Hakkinen K, Pakarinen A. Acute hormonal changes to heavy resistance exercise in men and women at different ages. *Int J Sports Med*, 16(8): 507, 1995.

Harrison RL, Read GF. Ovarian impairments of female recreational distance runners during a season of training. *Annals of Human Biology* 25(4): 345–357, 1998.

Keizer H, Janssen GME, Menheere P, and Kranenburg G. Changes in basal plasma testosterone, cortisol, and dehydroepiandrosterone in previously untrained males and females preparing for marathon. *Int J Sports Med* 10: S139, 1989.

Kyllonen ES, Vaananen HK, Heikkinen JE, et al. Comparison of muscle strength and bone mineral density in healthy postmenopausal women: A cross-sectional population study. *Scand J Rehab Med* 23: 153–157, 1991.

Lebenstedt M., Platte P, Pirke KM. Reduced resting metabolic rate in athletes with menstrual disorders. *Med Sci Sports Exerc* 31(9): 1250–1256,1999.

Locke RJ, Warren MP. Exercise and primary dysmenorrhoea. *Br J Sports Med* 33(4): 227, Aug. 1999.

Norsigian, J. Dieting is dangerous to your health. *The Network News* 1986; May–June: 4–6.

Notelovitz, M. Estrogen therapy and variable-resistance weight training increase bone mineral in surgically menopausal women. *J Bone Mineral Research* 6(6): 583–590, 1991.

Phillips SK, Gopinathan J, Meehan K, Bruce S, and Woledge R. Muscle strength changes during the menstrual cycle in human adductor pollicis. *J Physiol* 473: 125P, 1993.

Phillips SK, Rook K, Siddle N, Bruce S, and Woledge R. Muscle weakness in women occurs at an earlier age than in men, but strength is preserved by hormone replacement therapy. *Clin Sci* 84: 95,1993.

Pirke K, Schweiger U, Laessle R, et al. Dieting influences the menstrual cycle: Vegetarian versus nonvegetarian diet. *Fertility and Sterility* 46(6): 1083–1088, 1968.

Pirke KM, Schweiger U, Lemmel W, et al. The influence of dieting on the menstrual cycle of healthy young women. *J Clin Endocrinol Metab* 60(6): 1174–1179, 1985.

Sarwar R, Beltran-Niclos B, and Rutherford O. Changes in muscle strength, relaxation rate, and fatiguability during the human menstrual cycle. *J Physiol* 493: 267, 1996.

Selby GB, Eichner ER. Endurance swimming, intravascular hemolysis, anemia, and iron depletion. New perspective on athlete's anemia. *Am J Med* 81(5): 791–794, 1986.

Shangold M. Exercise and the adult female: Hormonal and endocrine effects. *Exer & Sport Sci Rev* 12: 53–79,1984.

Williams NI, Bullen BA, McArthur JW, et al. Effects of short-term strenuous exercise upon corpus luteum function. *Med Sci Sports Exerc* 31(7): 949–958, 1999.

Yen SS. Effects of lifestyle and body composition on the ovary (review). *Endocrinol Metab Clin North Am* 27(4): 915–926,1998.

Chapter 9: Ovaries At Risk: Unusual Effects of Viruses and Medical Illnesses

Anaasti, IN. Premature ovarian failure: An update. *Fertility and Sterility* 70(1): 1–15, 1998.

Arafah BM. Increased need for thyroxine in women with hypothyroidism during estrogen therapy. *N Engl J Med* 344: 1743–1748, 2001; commentary 1784–1785.

Cann SA, van Netten JP, van Netten C. Hypothesis: Iodine, selenium and the development of breast cancer. *Cancer Causes Control* 11(2): 121–127, 2000.

Des Moraes Ruesen M. Autoimmunity and ovarian failure. *Amer J Obstet and Gynecol* 112: 5–8, 1972.

Eskin BA. Iodine and mammary cancer. *Adv Exp Med Biol* 91: 293–304, 1977.

Fackelmann K. Early menopause for diabetic women. *Science News* 152: 15,1997.

Gloor HJ. Autoimmune oophoritis. *Amer J Clin Path* 81: 105–109, 1984.

Gold MS, et al. Depression and "symptomless" autoimmune thyroiditis. *Psychiatr Ann* 17: 750–757,1987.

Gregoire AJP, Kumar R, Everett B, Henderson A, Studd JWW. Transdermal oestrogen for treatment of severe postnatal depression. *Lancet* 347: 930–933, 1996.

Hagmar L, Rylander L, Dyremark E, et al. Plasma concentrations of persistent organochlorines in relation to thyrotropin and thyroid hormone levels in women. *Int Arch Occup Environ Health* 74(3): 184–188, 2001.

Hall RCW, et al. Psychiatric manifestations of Hashimoto's thyroiditis. *Psychosomatics* 23:337–342,1982.

Hall RCW. Psychiatric manifestations of thyroid hormone disturbance. *Psychosomatics* 24: 7–18, 1983.

Henry CH, Hudson AP, Gerard HC, et al. Identification of chlamydia trachomatis in the human temporomandibular joint. *J Oral Maxillofac Surg* 57: 683–688, 1999.

Hetzel BS, Chavadej J, Potter BJ. The brain in iodine deficiency. *Neuropathol Appl Neurobiol* 14(2): 93–104,1988.

Hoek A, Schoemaker J, Drexhage HA. Premature ovarian failure and ovarian autoimmunity. *Endocrinology Review* 18(1): 107–134, 1997.

Kim JG, Moon SY, Chang YS, Lee JY. Autoimmune ovarian failure. Brit J Obstetrics and Gynaecology 21: 59–66, 1995

Krassas GE. Thyroid disease and reproduction. *Fertil Steril* 74(6): 1063–1070, 2000.

Leer M, Patel B, Innes M, et al. Secondary amenorrhea due to autoimmune ovarian failure. *Australian and New Zealand J Obstet and Gynecol* 158: 1–5, 1988.

Longcope C. The male and female reproductive systems in hypothyroidism. In *Werner and Ingbar's the Thyroid*, 7th ed, eds. LE Braverman and RD Utiger. Philadelphia: Lippincott–Raven, 1996.

Massoudi M, Meilahn E, Orchard T, et al. Thyroid function and perimenopausallipid and weight changes: The thyroid study in healthy women (TSH–W). *J Women's Health* 6(5): 553–558, 1997.

Meisler, Jodi Godfrey, M.S., R.D. Toward optimal health: The experts discuss thyroid disease. *Journal of Women's Health and Gender-Based Medicine* 9: 345–350, May 2000.

Muechler EK, Huang KE and Schenk E. Autoimmunity in premature ovarian failure. *International J Fertility* 36(2): 99–103,1991.

Nakano T, Konishi T, Futagami Y, Takezawa H. Myocardial infarction in Graves' disease without coronary artery disease. *Japan Heart J* 28(3): 451–456, May 1987.

Nemeroff CB, Simon JS, Haggerty JJ, et al. Antithyroid antibodies in depressed patients. *Am J Psychiatry* 142: 84Q–842, 1985.

Prange AJ. L-triiodothyronine (T3): Its place in the treatment of TCA-resistant depressed patients. In *Treating Resistant Depression*, eds. Joseph Zohar, Robert H. Belmaker. New York: PMA Publishing Corp., 1987, 269–278.

Premawardhana LDKE, Parkes AB, Ammari F, et al. Postpartum thyroiditis and long-term thyroid status: Prognostic influence of thyroid peroxidase antibodies and ultrasound echogenicity. *J Clin Endocrinol Metab* 85: 71–75, 2000.

Reus, VI. Behavioral aspects of thyroid disease in women. In *The Psychiatric Clinics of North America: Women's Disorders* 12(1): 153–166, March, 1989. Philadelphia: W. B. Saunders Co.

Ridgeway EC. Hypothyroidism: The hidden challenge. Clinical Management conference proceedings, University of Colorado School of Medicine, Dec. 1996.

Seo BW, Li MH, Hansen LG, Moore RW, Peterson RE, Schantz S1. Effects of gestational and lactational exposure to PCB 77, PCB 126 or TCDD on thyroid hormones in weanling Sprague-Dawley rats. *Toxicologist* 15(1): 65–70,1995.

Smythe PP. Thyroid disease and breast cancer. *J Endocrinol Invest* 16(5): 396–401,1993.

Smythe PP. The thyroid and breast cancer: a significant association? (editorial). *Ann Med* 29: 189–191,1997.

Thomas R and Reid RL. Thyroid disease and reproductive function: a review. *Obstet Gynecol* 70:789–798, 1987.

Thyroid Disorders and Women's Health. National Women's Health Report. 22–56, 2000.

Vermuelen A. Environment, human reproduction, menopause and andropause. *Environ Health Perspect* 101 (Suppl 2): 91–100, 1993.

Viskin S, Long QT. Syndromes and torsade de pointes. *Lancet* 354: 1625–1633, 1999.

Wheatcroft NJ, Rogers CA, Metcalfe RA, et al. Is subclinical ovarian failure an autoimmune disease? *Human Reproduction* 12: 244–249, 1997.

Williams DJ, Connor P, Ironside JW Premenopausal cytomegalvirus oophoritis. *Histopathology* 16: 405–407, 1990.

Chapter 10: Ovaries at Risk: Unrecognized Problems from Surgery, Medications, and Herbs

Backstrom CT, Boyle H, Baird DT. Persistence of symptoms of premenstrual tension in hysterectomized women. *Br J Obstet Gynaecol* 88: 530–536, 1981.

Casper R, Hearn M. The effects of hysterectomy and bilateral oophorectomy in women with severe premenstrual syndrome. *Am J Obstet Gynecol* 162: 105–109, 1990.

Casson P, Hahn PM, Van Vugt DA, et al. Lasting response to ovariectomy in severe intractable premenstrual syndrome. *Am J Obstet Gynecol* 162: 99–105, 1990.

Challen J. The problem with herbs. Nat Health Jan.–Feb. 1999: 56–60.

Divi RL, Chang HC, Doerge DR. Anti-thyroid isoflavones from soybean: isolation, characterization, and mechanisms of action. National Center for Toxicological Research, Jefferson, AR 72079, USA. *Biochem Pharmacol* 54(1): 1087–1096, Nov. 15, 1997.

Hirata JD, Swiersz LM, Zell B, Small R, Ettinger B. Does dong quai have estrogenic effects in postmenopausal women? A double-blind, placebo-controlled trial. *Fertil Steril* 68: 981–986, 1997.

Jellin JM, Batz F, Hitchens K. *Natural Medicines Comprehensive Database*. Therapeutic Research Faculty, Stockton, Calif., 1999.

Khastgir G, Studd JWW. Hysterectomy, ovarian failure and depression. *Menopause* 5: 113–122, 1998.

Knight DC, Howes\JB, Eden JA. The effect of Promensil, an isoflavone extract, on menopausal symptoms. *Climacteric: The Journal of the International Menopause Society* 2: 79–84, 1999.

Masand P Chr. Symposium: Weight gain associated with use of psychotropic drugs. *Therapeutic Advances in Psychoses*, July 4, 1999.

Peterson HB, et al. The risk of menstrual abnormalities after tubal sterilization. *N Engl J Med* 343: 1681–1687, Dec. 7, 2000.

Sarrel P. Effects of hysterectomy without oophorectomy on menopausal symptoms. Oral presentation, North American Menopause Society, New York, Sept. 21–23, 1989.

Spector TD, Brown GC, Silman AJ. Increased rates of previous hysterectomy and gynecological operations in women with osteoarthritis. *Br Med J* 297: 899–900, 1988.

Studd JWW, Domoney C, Khastgir G. The place of hysterectomy in the treatment of menstrual disorders. *Disorders of the Menstrual Cycle* 29: 313–323, 2000. RCOG Press.

Watson NR, Studd JWW, Garnett T, et al. Bone loss after hysterectomy with ovarian conservation. *Ostet Gynecol* 86(l): 72–77, 1995.

Chapter 11: Ovaries out of Balance: Patterns in Women's Lives

Ballweg ML. Fibromyalgia/endometriosis link? Endometriosis Association Newsletter 12: 3,1991.

Barfield RJ, Glasser JH, Rubin BS, et al. Behavioral effects of progestin in the brain. *Psychoneuroendocrinology* 9: 217–231, 1984.

Brush MG. Increased incidence of thyroid autoimmune problems in women with endometriosis. Endometriosis: A Collection of Papers Written by GPs, Researchers, Specialists and Sufferers about Endometriosis. Compiled by the Coventry Branch of the Endometriosis Society, March 1987.

Campbell J. Is Reproductive Wastage and Failure Related to Environmental Pollution? Considerations of Human Data and Findings from a Rhesus Model. Presented at the Toxicological Pathology Symposium, Ottawa, Canada, September 1988.

Campbell JS, Wong J, Tryphonas L, et al. Is Simian Endometriosis an Effect ofImmunotoxicity? Presented at the Ontario Association of Pathologists Forty-Eighth Annual Meeting, October 1985, London, Ontario, Canada.

Cronje WH, Studd JWW. Premenstrual syndrome and premenstrual dysphoric disorder. *Primary Care Clinics in Office Practice* 29: 1–12, March 2002.

Donnez J, Nisolle M, et al. Peritoneal endometriosis and "endometriotic" nodules of the rectovaginal septum are two different entities. *Fertil Steril.* 66(3): 362–368, Sept. 1996.

Donnez J, Nisolle M, et al. Rectovaginal septum adenomyotic nodules: a series of 500 cases. *Br J*

Obstet Gynaecol, 104(9): 1014–1018, Sept. 1997.

Fanton JW, Hubbard GB, Wood DH. Endometriosis: Clinical and pathological findings in 70 rhesus monkeys. *Am J Veterinary Research* 47: 1537–1541,1986.

Grimes DA, Lebolt SA, Grimes KRT, Wingo PA. Two-fold risk of endometriosis in hospitalized patients with lupus. *Amer J Obstet Gyneco* 153: 179–183, 1985.

Magos AL, Brewster E, Singh R, et al. The effects of norethisterone in postmenopausal women on oestrogen replacement therapy: A model for the premenstrual syndrome. *Br J Obstet Gynaecol* 93: 1290–1296,1986.

Mayani A, Barel S, Soback S, et al. Dioxin concentrations in women with endometriosis. *Human Reproduction* 12: 373–375,1997.

Muse KN, Cetel NS, Futterman LA, Yen Sc. The premenstrual syndrome. Effects of "medical ovariectomy:' *N Engl J Med* 311: 1345–1349,1984.

Querleu D. Treatment of rectovaginal endometriosis. *Presse Med* 26(16): 774–777, May 1997.

Rier SE, Martin DC, Bowman RE, Dmowski WP, Becker J1. Endometriosis in rhesus monkeys (Macaca mulatta) following chronic exposure to 2, 3, 7, 8– Tetrachlorodibenzo-p-dioxin. *Fundamental and Applied Toxicology* 21: 433–441,1993.

Rier SE, Wayman ET, Martin DC, et al. Serum levels of TCDD and dioxin-like chemicals in rhesus monkeys chronically exposed to dioxin: Correlation of increased serum PCB levels with endometriosis. *Toxicological Sciences* 59: 147–159, 2001.

Smith RNJ, Studd JWW, Zamblera D, et al. A randomized comparison over 8 months of 100 mcgs and 200 mcgs twice weekly doses of transdermal oestradiol in the treatment of severe premenstrual syndrome. *Br J Obstet Gynaecol* 102: 475–484, 1995.

Watson NR, Studd JWW, Savvas M, et al. Treatment of severe premenstrual syndrome with oestradiol patches and cyclical oral norethisterone. *Lancet* 2: 730–734, 1989.

Chapter 12: Ovarian Hormones and the Brain: It's Not Just Stress or Your Imagination!

Abramowitz ES, Bakerk AH, Fleisher SF. Onset of depressive psychiatric crises and the menstrual cycle. *Am J Psychiatry* 139: 475–478,1982.

Ahokas A, Aito M, Rimon R. Positive treatment effect of estradiol in postpartum psychosis: A pilot study. *J Clin Psychiatry* (United States) 61(3): 166–169, 2000.

Ahokas A, Kaukoranta J, Aito M. Effect of oestradiol on postpartum depression. *Psychopharmacology* (Berlin, Germany) 146(1): 108–110, 1999.

Ahokas AJ, Turtiainen S, Aito M. Sublingual oestrogen treatment of postnatal depression. *Lancet* 351(9096): 109–112, 1998.

Akamatsu T, Akiyama T, Kimura T, Saito H, Yanaihara T. Menopausal Insomnia and Hormone Replacement Therapy. Third International Symposium, Women's Health and Menopause, June 1998.

Backstrom, T. Epileptic seizures in women related to plasma estrogen and progesterone during the menstrual cycle. *Acta Neurol Scand* 54: 321–347, 1976.

Ball DE, Morrison P. Oestrogen transdermal patches for post partum depression in lactating mothers—a case report. *Cent Afr J Med* (Zimbabwe) 45(3): 68–70, March 1999.

Bancroft J, Sanders D, Warner P, Loudon N. The effects of oral contraceptives on mood and sexuality: Comparison of triphasic and combined preparations. *J Psychosom. Obstet Gynaecol* 7: 1–8, 1987.

Barfield R, Glaser J, Rubin B, et al. Behavioral effects of progestin in the brain. *Psychoneuroendocrinology* 9(3): 217–231,1984.

Becker D, Creutzfeldt OD, Schwibbe M, Wuttke W. Changes in physiological, EEG and psychological parameters in women during the spontaneous menstrual cycle and following oral contraceptives. *Psychoneuroendocrinology* 7: 75–90, 1982.

Bennett RM, Clark SC, Walczyk J. A randomized, double-blind placebo-controlled study of growth hormone in the treatment of fibromyalgia. *Am J Med* 104(3): 227–231, March 1998.

Bereiter DA, Barker DJ. Hormone-induced enlargement of receptive fields in trigeminal: mechanoreceptive neurons. I. Time course hormones, sex and modality specificity. *Brain Res* 184: 395–410,1980.

Bernardi F, Bertolino S, Luisi S, Spinetti A, Monteleone P, Giardina L, Petraglia F, Luisi M, Genazzani AR. Effects of Hormonal Replacement Therapy on Circulating Allopregnanolone Levels in Postmenopausal Women. Third International Symposium Women's Health and Menopause. June 1998.

Bhatia SK, Moore D, Kalkhoff RK. Progesterone suppression of the plasma growth hormone Response. *J Clin Endocrinol Metab* 35: 364–369, 1972.

Bloch M, Schmidt PJ, Danaceau M, et al. Effects of gonadal steroids in women with a history of postpartum depression. *Am J Psychiatry* 157(6): 924–930, 2000.

Bromm B, Desmedt JE, eds. *Pain and the Brain: From Nociception to Cognition*. Advances in Pain Research and Therapy, vol. 22. New York: Raven Press Ltd, 1995.

Brovermann DM, Klaiber EL, Kobayashi Y, et al. Roles of activation and inhibition in sex differences in cognitive abilities. *Pychol Rev* 75: 23–50, 1968.

Buterbaugh GG Postictal events in mygdala-kindled female rats with and without estradiol replacement. *Exp Neurol* 95: 697–913, 1987.

Cauley JA, Pertini AM, LaPorte RE, Sandler RB, Baylers CM, Robertson RJ, Slemenda CWo The decline of grip strength in the menopause relationship to physical activity, estrogen use and anthropometric factors. *J Chronic Dis* 40: 115–120, 1982.

Christiansen C, Christiansen MS. Climacteric symptoms, fat mass and plasma concentrations of LH, FSH, PRL, estradiol 17-beta, and androstenedione in the early postmenopausal period. *Acta Endocrinol* l0l: 87–92, 1982.

Cullberg J. Mood changes and menstrual symptoms with different gestagen/estrogen combinations. *Acta Psychiatr Scand* (suppl) 236: 1, 1972.

Dawson-Basoa MB, Gintzler AR. 17-beta estradiol and progesterone modulate an intrinsic opiod analgesic system. *Brain Res* 601: 1–2, 241–245, Jan. 22,1993.

Ditkoff EC, Crary WG, Cristo M, Lobo RA. Estrogen improves psychological function in asymptomatic postmenopausal women. *Obstet Gynecol* 78: 991–995,1991.

Duncan A, Lyall H, Roberts R, Perera M, Petrie J, Connell J, Lumsden M. The Effect of 17 Beta Estradiol and Norethisterone on Insulin Sensitivity in Postmenopausal Women. Third International Symposium Women's Health and Menopause, June 1998.

Erlik Y, Tataryn IV, Meldrum DR, et al. Association of waking episodes with menopausal hot flushes. *JAMA* 245: 1741–1744, 1981.

Fillit H, Weinreb H, Cholst I, et al. Observations in a preliminary open trial of estradiol therapy for senile dementia-Alzheimer's type. *Psychoneuroendocrinology* 11: 337–345, 1986.

Fink G, et al. Estrogen control of central neurotransmission: Effect on mood, mental state, and memory. *Cell Mol Neurobiol* June 1996.

Finn DA, Gee KW. The significance of steroid action at the GABA receptor complex. In *The Modern Management of the Menopause: A Perspective for the 21st Century*, eds. G. Berg, M. Hammar. Carnforth, UK: Parthenon Publishing, 1994, pp. 301–314.

Fonseca E, Ochoa R, Galvan R, Hernandez M, Mercado M, Zarate A. Increased serum levels of growth hormone and insulin-like growth factor-I associated with simultaneous decrease of circulating insulin in postmenopausal women receiving hormone replacement therapy. *Menopause* 6: 56–60, Spring 1999.

Genazzani AR, Bernardi F, Spinetti A, Stomati M, Luisi S, Tonetti A, Petraglia F, Luisi M. The Brain as Target and Source for Sex Steroid Hormones. Third International Symposium Women's Health and Menopause. June 1998.

Gitlin MJ, Pasnau RO. Psychiatric syndromes linked to reproductive function in women: A review of current knowledge. *Am J Psychiatry* 146: 7–15, 1989.

Govoni, S. Estrogens as Neuroprotectants: Hypotheses on the Mechanism of Action. Third International Symposium Women's Health and Menopause, June 1998.

Gregoire AJP' Kumar R, Everett B, Henderson A, Studd JWW. Transdermal oestrogen for treatment of severe postnatal depression. *Lancet* 347: 930–933,1996.

Harnmarback S, Backstrom T, Holst J, von Schoultz B, Lyrenas S. Cyclical mood changes as in the premenstrual tension syndrome during sequential estrogen-progestagen postmenopausal replacement therapy. *Acta Obstet Gynecol Scand* 64: 515–518, 1985.

Henderson AF, Gregoire AJP, Kumar R, Studd JWW. The treatment of severe postnatal depression with oestradiol skin patches. *Lancet* 338: 816,1991.

Hermann WM, Beach RC. The psychotropic properties of estrogen. *Pharmakopsychiat* 11: 164–178, 1978.

Herzog AG. Polycystic ovarian syndrome in women with epilepsy: Epileptic or iatrogenic? *Ann Neurol* 39: 559–560,1996.

Herzog AG, Seibel MM, Schomer D, et al. Temporal lobe epilepsy: An extrahypothalamic pathogenesis for polycystic ovarian syndrome? *Neurology* 34(10): 1389–1393, 1984.

Honjo H, Ogino Y, Urabe M, et al. In vivo effects by estrone sulfate on the central nervous system-senile dementia (Alzheimer's type). *J Steroid Biochem* 34: 521–525, 1989.

Isojarvi JIT, Laatikainen TJ, Pakarinen AJ, Juntunen KTS, Myllyla VV. Polycystic ovaries and hyperandrogenism in women taking valproate for epilepsy. *N Engl J Med* 329: 1383–1388, 1993.

Jaussi R, Watson G, Paigen K. Modulation of androgen-responsive gene expression by estrogen. *Mol Cell Bndocrinol* 86: 187, 1992.

Jensen J, Christensen C, Rodbro P. Estrogen–progesterone replacement therapy changes body composition in early postmenopausal women. *Maturitas* 8: 209–216,1986.

Kaye SA, Folsom AR, Soler JT, Prineas RJ, Potter JD. Association of body mass and fat distribution with sex hormone concentrations in postmenopausal women. *Int J Epidemiol* 20: 151–156.

Keefe DL, Watson F, Naftolin F. Hormone replacement therapy may alleviate sleep apnea in menopausal women: A pilot study. *Menopause* 6: 196–200,1999.

Klaiber EL, Broverman DM, Vogel W, Kobayashi T. Estrogen therapy for severe persistent depressions in women. *Arch Gen Psychiat* 36: 550–554, 1979.

Klaiber EL, Broverman DM, Vogel W, et al. Individual differences in changes in mood and platelet monoamine oxidase (MAO) activity during hormonal replacement therapy in menopausal women. *Psychoneuroendocrinology* 21: 575–592,1996.

Kyllonen ES, Vaananen HK, Heikkinen JE, Kurttila-Matero E, Martikkala V, Vanharanta JH. Comparison of muscle strength and bone mineral density in healthy postmenopausal women: A cross-sectional population study. *Scand J Rehab Med* 23: 153–157,1991.

Logothetis J, Harner R, Morrell F, Torres F. The role of oestrogen and catamenial exacerbations of epilepsy. *Neurology* 9: 352–360, 1959.

Magos AL, Brewster E, Singh R, O'Dowd T, Brincat M, Studd JWW. The effects of norethisterone in postmenopausal women on oestrogen replacement therapy: A model for the premenstrual syndrome. *Br J Obstet Gynaecol* 93: 1290–1296, 1986.

Magos AL, Brincat M, Studd JWW. Treatment of the premenstrual syndrome by subcutaneous oestradiol implants and cyclical oral norethisterone: A placebo controlled study. *Br Med J* 1: 1629–1631, 1986.

Majewska MD, Harrison N, Schwartz R, Barker J, Paul S. Steroid hormone metabolites are barbiturate-like modulators of the GABA receptor. *Science* 232: 1004–1007, 1986. McEwen BS. Ovarian hormone action in the brain: Implications for the menopause. In *The Climacteric in Perspective*, eds. M. Notelovitz, P.A. Van Keep. Lancaster, UK: MTP Press, 1976, pp. 207–209.

McEwen BS, Biegon A, Davis P, et al. Steroid hormones: Humoral signals which alter brain cell properties and functions. *Recent Progress in Hormone Research* 38: 41–83, 1982. Discussion: 83–92.

McEwen BS, Rhodes Je. Gonadal hormone regulation of MAO and other enzymes in hypothalamic areas. *Neuroendocrinol* 36: 235–238, 1983.

Mizuki Y, Kajimura N, Miyoshi A, et al. Neuroendocrinological studies on patients with periodic psychosis of adolescence before and after menarche. 1990.

Montgomery JC, Brincal M, Tapp A, Appleby L, Versi E, Fenwick PBC, Studd JWW. Effects of oestrogen and testosterone implants on psychological disorders in the climacteric. *Lancet* 1: 297–299,1987.

Muse KN, Cetel NS, Futterman LA, Yen SSC. The premenstrual syndrome, effects of medical ovariectomy. *N Engl J Med* 311: 1345–1349, 1984.

Namba H, Sokoloff L. Acute administration of high doses of estrogen increases glucose utilization throughout the brain. *Brain Res* 291: 391–394,

Norberg L, Wahlstrom G, Backstrom T. The anaesthetic potency of 3x-hydroxy-5xpregnan-20-one and 3x-hydroxy-5B-pregnan-20-one determined with an intravenous EEG-threshold method in male rats. *Acta Pharmacol Toxicol Scand* 61: 42–47, 1987.

Ohkura T, Isse K, Akazawa K, et al. An open trial of estrogen therapy for dementia of the Alzheimer type in women. In *The Modern Management of the Menopause: A Perspective for the 21st Century*, eds. G. Berg and M. Hammar. Carnforth, UK: Parthenon Publishing, 1994, pp. 315–333.

Oppenheim G, Zohar J, Shapiro B, Belmaker RH. The role of estrogen in treating resistant depression. In *Treating Resistant Depression*, eds. Joseph Zohar and Robert H. Belmaker. New York: PMA Publishing Corp., 1987.

Paganini-Hill A, Henderson V. Estrogen deficiency and risk of Alzheimer's disease in women. *Am J Epidemiol* 140: 256–261,1994.

Parry BL. Reproductive factors affecting the course of affective illness in women. *Psychiatric Clinics of North America* 12(1): 207–220, 1989.

Phillip S, Sherwin BB. Effects of estrogen on neuronal function in postmenopausal women. *Psychoneuroendocrinology* 17: 485–498,1992.

Ravnikar VA, Schiff I, Regestein QR Menopause and sleep. In *The Menopause*, ed. H. Buchsbaum. New York: Springer Verlag, 1983, pp. 161–171.

Rhoades R, Pflanzer R. The Pituitary Gland. *In Human Physiology*. Philadelphia: Saunders College Publishing, 1989. Discussion of effects of progesterone on androgen receptors, p. 403.

Sampson GA. Premenstrual syndrome: A double-blind controlled trial of progesterone and placebo. *Br J Psychiatry* 135: 209–215,1979.

Sandyk R Estrogen's impact on cognitive functions in multiple sclerosis. *Int J Neurosci* 86: 23, 1996.

Shabas D, Weinreb H. Preventive health care in women with multiple sclerosis. *J Wom Health and Gender Based Medicine* 9: 389–395, 2000.

Shaywitz SE, Shaywitz BA, Pugh KR, et al. Effect of estrogen on brain activation patterns in postmenopausal women during working memory tasks. *JAMA* 281(13): 1197–1202,1999.

Sherwin BB. Hormones, mood and cognitive functioning in postmenopausal women. *Obstet Gynecol* 87: 20–26, 1996.

Sherwin BB, Tulandi T. "Add-back" estrogen reverses cognitive deficits induced by a gonadotropin-releasing hormone agonist in women with leiomyomata uteri. *J Clin Endocrinol Metab* 81: 2545–2549,1996.

Slopien R, Warenik-Szymankiewica A, Maciejewska M, Wiza M. Serum Serotonin Level in Postmenopausal Women. Third International Symposium: Women's Health and Menopause. June 1998.

Smith R, Studd JWW. A pilot study of the effect upon multiple sclerosis of menopause, hormone replacement therapy and the menstrual cycle. *J R Soc Med* 85: 612, 1992.

Stenn PG, Klaiber EL, Vogel W, et al. Testosterone effects upon photic stimulation of the EEG and mental performance of humans. *Percept and Motor Skills* 34: 371–378, 1972.

Studd JWW, Smith RNJ. Estrogens and depression in women. *Menopause* 1: 33–37, 1995.

Thompson J, Oswald I. Effect of estrogen on the sleep, mood and anxiety of menopausal women. *Br Med J* 2: 1217–1219, 1977.

Vliet, EL. An approach to perimenopausal migraine. *Menopause Management* 4(6): 25–33,1995.

Vliet EL, Davis VL. New perspectives on the relationship of hormonal changes to affective disorders in the perimenopause. In *Clinical Issues in Women's Health*. Midlife Women's Health, 2(4): 453–472, Oct–Dec. 1991. Philadelphia: JB Lippincott.

Watson NR, Studd JWW, Savvas M, et al. Treatment of severe premenstrual syndrome with oestradiol patches and cyclical oral norethisterone. *Lancet* 2: 730–732, 1989.

Yaffe K, Sawaya G, Lieberburg I, et al. Estrogen therapy in postmenopausal women: Effects on cognitive function and dementia. *JAMA* 279: 688–695,1998.

Young EA. Alteration of the hypothalamic-pituitary-ovarian axis in depressed women. *Arch Gen Psych* 57: 1157–1162, 2000

Chapter 13: The Perils of PCOS, Obesity, Syndrome X, and Diabetes

Batukan C, Baysal B. Metformin improves ovulation and pregnancy rates in patients with polycystic ovary syndrome. *Arch Gynecol Obstet* 265(3): 124–127, 2001.

Campaigne BN, Wishner KL. Gender-specific health care in diabetes mellitus. *J Genderspecific Medicine* 3: 51–58, 2000.

Chang RJ, et al. Diagnosis of polycystic ovary syndrome. *Endocrinol Metab Clin North Am* 28(2): 397–408, 1999.

Deedwania P. Hypertension and diabetes. *Arch Internal Med* 160: 1583–1594, 2000.

Escalante Pulido JM, et al. Changes in insulin sensitivity, secretion and glucose effectiveness during menstrual cycle. *Arch Med Res* 30(1): 19–22,1999.

Ferrara A, et al. Sex differences in insulin levels in older adults and the effect of body size, estrogen replacement therapy, and glucose tolerance status. The Rancho Bernardo Study, 1984–87 *Diabetes* 18(2): 220–225, 1995.

Folsom A, Kushi L, Anderson K, et al. Associations of general and abdominal obesity with multiple outcomes in older women. *Arch Intern Med* 160: 2117–2128, 2000.

Gambacciani M, Ciaponi M, Cappagli B, et al. Climacteric modifications in body weight and fat tissue distribution. *Climacteric: The Journal of the International Menopause Society* 2: 37–43, 1999.

Ganesan R. The aversive and hypophagic effects of estradiol. *Physiol Behav* 55: 279–285, 1994.

Gaspard UJ, Wery, Scheen, et al. Long-term effects of oral estradiol and dydrogesterone on carbohydrate metabolism in postmenopausal women. *Climacteric: The Journal of the International Menopause Society* 2(2): 93–100, June 1999.

Geary, N. Estradiol and the control of eating. *Appetite* 29: 386, 1997.

Glueck CJ, Wang P, Kobayashi S, et al. Metformin therapy throughout pregnancy reduces the development of gestational diabetes in women with polycystic ovary syndrome. *Fertility and Sterility* 77: 250–255, 2002.

Godsland I, Walton C, Stevenson J. Carbohydrate Metabolism, Cardiovascular Disease and Hormone Replacement Therapy. In *The Modern Management of the Menopause*, Proceedings of the VII International Congress on the Menopause, Stockholm, Sweden. New York: Parthenon Publishing Group, 1994, pp. 231–249.

Gordon CM. Menstrual disorders in adolescents. Excess androgens and the polycystic ovary syndrome. *Pediatr Clin North Am* 46(3): 519–543,1999.

Herzog AG. Polycystic ovarian syndrome in women with epilepsy: epileptic or iatrogenic? *Ann Neurol* 39: 559–560,1996.

Herzog AG, Seibel MM, Schomer D, et al. Temporal lobe epilepsy: an extrahypothalamic pathogenesis for polycystic ovarian syndrome? *Neurology* 34(10): 1389–1393, 1984.

Heymsfield S, Gallagher D, Poehlman E, et al. Menopausal changes in body composition and energy expenditure. *Exp Ger* 29(3/4): 377–389, 1994.

Isojarvi JIT, Laatikainen TJ, Pakarinen AJ, Juntunen KTS, Myllyla VV. Polycystic ovaries and hyperandrogenism in women taking valproate for epilepsy. *N Eng J Med* 329: 1383–1388,1993.

Kaye S, Folsom A, Soler J, Prineas R, et al. Association of body mass and fat distribution with sex hormone concentrations in postmenopausal women. *Int J Epidemiol* 20: 151–156, 1991.

Ley C, Lees B, Stevenson J. Sex and menopause-associated changes in body-fat distribution. *Am*

J Clin Nutr 55: 950–954, 1992.

Nestler J, et al. Dehydroeplandrosterone: The "missing link" between hyperinsulinemia and atherosclerosis? *FASEB J* 6: 3073–3075, 1992.

Niki E, Nakano M. Estrogens as antioxidants. *Methods Enzymol* 186: 330,1990.

Peiris A, et al. Relationship of body fat distribution to the metabolic clearance of insulin in premenopausal women. *Int J Obesity* 11: 581–589, 1985.

Pownall H, Ballantyne C, Kimball K, et al. Effect of moderate alcohol consumption on hypertriglyceridemia. *Arch Intern Med* 159: 981–987, 1999.

Rosano G. Syndrome X in women is associated with estrogen deficiency. *Eur Heart J* 16: 610–614, 1995.

Schmidt MI, Watson RL, Duncan BB, et al. Clustering of dyslipidemia, hyperuricemia, diabetes, and hypertension and its association with fasting insulin and central and overall obesity in a general population. *Metabolism* 45 (6): 699–706, 1996.

Stoll BA. Perimenopausal weight gain and progression of breast cancer precursors. *Cancer Detect Prev* 23(1): 31–36, 1999.

Tchernof A, et al. Menopause, central body fatness, and insulin resistance: Effectsl hormone-replacement therapy. *Coron Artery Dis* 9(8): 503–511, 1998.

Vandermolen DT, Ratts VS, Evans WS, et al. Metformin increases the ovulatory rate and pregnancy rate from clomiphene citrate in patients with polycystic ovary syndrome who are resistant to clomiphene citrate alone. *Fertil Steril* 75(2): 310–315, 2001.

Visser M, Bouter L, McQuillan, G. Elevated C-Reactive Protein Levels in Overweight and Obese Adults. *JAMA* 282(22): 2131,1999.

Chapter 14: The Many Faces of Infertility: Overlooked Factors

Cassidy A, Bingham S, Setchell K. Biological effects of isoflavones in young women: Importance of the chemical composition of soyabean products. *Br J Nutrition* 74: 587–601,1995.

Coyle JT, Puttfarcken P. Oxidative stress, glutamate, and neurodegenerative disorders. *Science* 262(5134): 689–695,1993.

Divi RL, Chang HC, Doerge DR. Anti-thyroid isoflavones from soybean: Isolation, characterization, and mechanisms of action. National Center for Toxicological Research, Jefferson, AR 72079, USA. *Biochem Pharmacol* 54(1): 1087–1096, Nov. 15, 1997.

Gray LE Jr, Ostby J, Marshall R, Andrews J. Reproductive and thyroid effects of low-level polychlorinated biphenyl (Aroclor 1254) exposure. *Fundamental and Applied Toxicology* 20(3): 288–294, 1993.

Knight, DC, Eden JA. A review of the clinical effects of phytoestrogens. *Obstet Gynecol* 87(5 Part 2): 897–904, 1996.

Kronenberg F, Hughes C. Exogenous and endogenous estrogens: An appreciation of biological complexity (editorial). *Menopause: The Journal of the North American Menopause Society* 6(1): 4–6, 1999.

Nagata C, Kabuto M, Kurisu Y, Shimizu H. Decreased serum estradiol concentration associated with high dietary intake of soy products in premenopausal Japanese women. *Nutrition and Cancer* 29(3): 228–233,1997.

Ondrizek RR, Chan PJ, Patton WC, King A. An alternative medicine study of herbal effects on the penetration of zona-free hamster oocytes and the integrity of sperm deoxyribonucleic acid *Fertil Steril* 71(3): 517–522,1999.

Sharara FI, Seifer DB, Flaws JA. Environmental toxicants and female reproduction. *Fertil Steril* 70(4):613–622,1998.

Thomas R, Reid RL. Thyroid disease and reproductive function: A review. *Obstet Gynecol* 70: 789–798, 1987.

Whitten PL, Lewis C, Russell E, Naftolin F. Potential adverse effects of phytoestrogens. *J Nutrition* 125 (Suppl): S 776, 1995.

Chapter 15: The Ovaries and Your Other Body Systems

Abitbol J, Abitbol B. The voice and menopause: The twilight of the divas. *Contracept Fertil Sex* 26(9): 649–655, Sept. 1998.

Abraham GE, Flechas JD, Hakala JC. Effect of daily ingestion of tablet containing 5 mg iodine and 7.5 mg iodide as the potassium salt for a period of three months on thyroid function tests and thyroid volume by ultrasonometry in ten euthyroid Caucasian women. Submitted for publication, 2002.

Aloia JF, McGowan DM, Vaswani AN, Ross P, Cohn SH. Relationship of menopause to skeletal and muscle mass. *Am J Clin Nutr* 53: 1378–1383, 1991.

Arden NK, lloyd ME, Spector TD, Hughes GR. Safety of hormone replacement therapy (HRT) in systemic lupus erythematosus (SLE). *Lupus* 3: 11–13, 1994.

Bolognia JL, Braverman IM, Rousseau ME, Sarrle PM. Skin changes in menopause. *Maturitas* 11: 295–304, 1989.

Brincat M, Kalaban S, Studd JWW, et al. A study of the decrease in skin collagen content, skin thickness, and bone mass in the postmenopausal woman. *Obstet Gynecol* 70: 840–845,1987.

Brincat M, Moniz CF, Kalaban S, et al. Decline in skin collagen content and metacarpal index after the menopause and its preventions with sex hormone replacement. *Br J Obstet Gynaecol* 94: 126–129, 1987.

Brincat M, Versi E, Moniz CF, et al. Skin collagen in postmenopausal women receiving different regimens of estrogen therapy. *Br J Obstet Gynecol* 70: 123–127,1987.

Brocklehurst JC, Fry J, Griffiths L, et al. Urinary infections and symptoms of dysuria in women aged 45–64 years: Their relevance to similar findings in the elderly. *Age Ageing* 1: 41–47,1972.

Cardozo 1. Role of estrogens in the treatment of female urinary incontinence. *J Am Geriatr Soc* 38: 326–330,1990.

Castelo-Branco C, Duran M, Gonzalea-Merlo J. Skin collagen changes related to age and hormone replacement therapy. *Maturitas* 15: 113–119,1992.

Chen Y, Dales R, Tang M, Krewski D. Obesity may increase the incidence of asthma in women but not in men: Longitudinal observations from the Canadian National Population Health Survey. *Am J Epidemiol* 155(3): 191–197, 2002.

Claude F, Allemany YR. Asthma and menstruation. *Presse Med* 38: 755–762, 1938.

Cohen A, Dubbs AW, Myers A. The treatment of atrophic arthritis with estrogenic substance. *N Engl J Med* 1222: 140–142, 1940.

Cornell Bell A, Sullivan D, Allansmith M. Gender-related difference in the morphology of the lacrimal gland. *Invest Ophthal and Vis Sci* 26: 1170–1175, 1985.

Da Silva JA, Hall GM. The effects of gender and sex hormones on outcome in rheumatoid arthritis. *Clin Rheumatol* 6: 196–219, 1992.

Davidsonn MH, Maki KC, Maryx P, et al. Effects of continuous estrogen (17 -beta estradiol) and estrogen-progestin (norethindrone) replacement regimens on cardiovascular risk markers in postmenopausal women. *Arch Int Med* 160: 3315–3325, 2000.

Elia G, Bergman A. Estrogen effects on the urethra: Beneficial effects in women with genuine stress incontinence. *Obstet Gynecol Sur* 48: 509–513, 1993.

Eliasson 0, Scherzer HH, De Graff AC. Morbidity of asthma in relation to the menstrual cycle. *J Allergy Clin Immunol* 77: 87–94, 1986.

Gharagozloo Z, Brubaker R. The correlation between serum progesterone and aqueous dynamics during the menstrual cycle. *Acta Ophthalmol* 69: 791–795, 1991.

Gibbs CJ, Courts II, Lock R, et al. Premenstrual exacerbation of asthma. *Thorax* 39: 833–836, 1984.

Goldberg VM, Moskowitz RW, Rosner IA. The role of estrogen and oophorectomy in immune oophoritis. *Semin Arthritis Rheum.* 11(Suppl.): 134–139, 1981.

Guttridge NM. Changes in ocular and visual variables during the menstrual cycle. *Ophthalmic Physiol Opt* 14(1): 38–48, 1994.

Hall GM, Daniels M, Huskisson EC, Spector TD. A randomized controlled trial of hormone replacement therapy in postmenopausal rheumatoid arthritis. *Ann Rheum Dis* 53: 112–116, 1994.

Hall GM, Spector T. The use of estrogen replacement as an adjunct therapy in rheumatoid arthritis. In *The Modern Management of the Menopause: A Perspective for the 21st Century*, eds. G. Berg and M. Hammar. Carnforth, UK: Parthenon Publishing, 1994, pp. 369–375.

Hall GM, Spector TD, Studd JWW. Carpal tunnel syndrome and hormone replacement therapy. *Br Med J* 304: 382–386, 1992.

Hanley SP. Asthma variation with menstruation. *Br J Dis Chest* 75: 306–308, 1981.

Harju T, Keistinen T, Tuuponen T, Kivela T. Hospital admissions of asthmatics by age and sex. *Allergy* 51: 693–696, 1996.

Hassager C, Jensen LT, Podenphant J, et al. Collagen synthesis in postmenopausal women during therapy with anabolic steroids or female sex hormones. *Metabolism* 39: 1167–1169, 1990.

Holmdahl R, Carlsten H, Jansson L, Larsson P. Oestrogen is a potent immunomodulator of murine experimental rheumatoid disease. *Br J Obstet Gynaecol* 99: 325–328, 1989.

Holzer G. Ovarian failure and joints. In *The Modern Management of the Menopause: A Perspective for the 21st Century*, eds. G. Berg and M. Hammar. Carnforth, UK: Parthenon Publishing, 1994, pp. 359–367.

Horwitz BJ, Fisher RS. The irritable bowel syndrome (review). *N Engl J Med* 344: 1846–1850, 2001.

Hsu JT, Kim CH, O'Conner MK, et al. Effect of menstrual cycle on esophageal emptying of liquid and solid boluses. *Mayo Clin Proc* 68: 753–756, 1993.

Hu F, Stampfer M, Manson J, et al. Trends in the incidence of coronary heart disease and changes in diet and lifestyle in women. *N Engl J Med* 343: 530–537, 2000.

Jackson S, Shepherd A, Brookes S, Abrams P. The effect of oestrogen supplementation on post-menopausal urinary stress incontinence: A double-blind placebo-controlled trial. *Br J Obstet Gynaecol* 106(7): 711–718, 1999.

Karpel JP, Wait J1. Asthma in women, part 3: Perimenstrual asthma, effects of hormone therapy. *J Crit Illness* 15(5): 265–272, 2000.

Katz PO, Castrell DO. Gastroesophageal reflux disease during pregnancy. *Gastroenterology Clin North Amer* 27(1): 153–167, 1998.

Kiely PM, Carney LG, Smith G. Menstrual cycle variations of corneal topography and thickness. *Am J Optom Physiol Opt* 60(10): 822–829, 1983.

LaCharity LA. The experiences of younger women with coronary artery disease. *J Women's Health & Gender-Based Medicine* 8: 773–785, 1999.

Latman NS. Relation of menstrual cycle phase to symptoms of rheumatoid arthritis. *Am J Med* 73: 947–950.

Leach N, Wallis N, Lothringer L, et al. Corneal hydration changes during the normal menstrual cycle—a preliminary study. *J Reprod Med* 6: 15–18, 1971.

Lindholm P, Vilkman E, Raudaskoski T, Suvanto-Luukkonen E, Kauppila A. The effect of postmenopause and postmenopausal HRT on measured voice values and vocal symptoms. Department of Otolaryngology and Phoniatrics, Oulu University Hospital, Finland. *Maturitas* 28(1): 47–53, Sept. 1997.

Marrero JM, Goggin PM, de Caestecker JS, et al. Determinants of pregnancy heartburn. *Br J Ostet Gynaecol* 99: 731–734, 1992.

Mathias JR, Clench MH, Abell TL, et al. Effect of leuprolide acetate in treatment of abdominal pain and nausea in premenopausal women with functional bowel disease: a double-blind, placebo-controlled, randomized study. *Digestive Diseases and Sciences* 43: 1347–1355, 1998.

Matthews KA, Meilahn E, Kuller LH, et al. Menopause and risk factors for coronary heart disease. *N Engl J Med* 321: 641, 1989.

McClung MR, et al. Effects of risedronate on the risk of hip fracture in elderly women. *NEJM* 344: 333–340, 2001.

Metka M, Enzelsberger H, Knogler W, et al. Ophthalmic complaints as a climacteric symptom.

Maturitas 14: 3–8, 1991.

Nilas L, Christensen C. The Pathophysiology of peri- and menopausal bone loss. *Br J Obstet Gynaecol* 96: 580–585, 1989.

Pattie MA, Murdoch BE, Theodoros D, Forbes K. Voice changes in women treated for endometriosis and related conditions: The need for comprehensive vocal assessment. *J Voice* 12(3): 366–371, Sept. 1998.

Pector TD, Campion GD. Generalized osteoarthritis: A hormonally mediated disease. *Ann Rheum Dis* 48: 523, 1989.

Punnonen R, Jokela H, Aine R, et al. Impaired ovarian function and risk factors for atherosclerosis in premenopausal women. *Maturitas* 27: 231–238, 1997.

Redmond, GP. *Androgenic Disorders*. New York: Raven Press, 1995.

Rees 1. An aetiological study of premenstrual asthma. *J Psychosomatic Res* 7: 191–193, 1963.

Rejula K, Haahtela T, Klaukka T, Rantanen J. Incidence of occupational asthma in young adults has increased in Finland. *Chest* 110: 58–61, 1996.

Riss B, Binder S, Riss P, Kemeter P. Corneal sensitivity during the menstrual cycle. *Br J Ophthalmol* 66(2): 123–126, 1982.

Riss B, Riss P. Corneal sensitivity in pregnancy. *Ophthalmologica* 183(2): 57–62, 1981.

Rosano GMC, Sarrel PM, Poole-Wilson, PA, Collins P. Beneficial effect of oestrogen (17beta estradiol) on exercise-induced myocardial ischaemia in women with coronary artery disease. *Lancet* 342: 133–136, 1993.

Rosner lA, Manni A, Malemud CJ, et al. Estradiol receptors in articular chondrocytes. *Biochem Biophys Res Commun* 106: 1379–1382, 1982.

Scholes D, et al. Injectable hormone contraception and bone density: Results from a prospective study. *Epidemiology* 13: 581–587, 2002.

Schneider HPG. The International Menopause Society Report on the 10th World Congress on the menopause. *Climacteric* 5: 219–228, 2002.

Serrander AM, Peek KE. Changes in contact lens comfort related to the menstrual cycle and menopause. *J Am Optom Assoc* 64 (3): 162–166, 1993.

Shames RS, Heilbron DC, Janson SL, et al. Clinical differences among women with and without self-reported perimenstrual asthma. *Ann Allergy Asthma Immunol* 8: 65–72, 1998.

Shuster S, Black MM, McVitie E. The influence of age and sex on skin thickness, skin collagen, and density. *Br J Dermatol* 93: 639–643, 1975.

Skobeloff EM, Spivey WH, Silverman R, et al. The effect of the menstrual cycle on asthma presentations in the emergency department. *Arch Int Med* 156: 1837–1840, 1996.

Smith, P. Estrogens and the urogenital tract. Studies on steroid hormone receptors and a clinical study on a new estradiol-releasing vaginal ring. *Acta Obstet Gynecol Scand* 1: 157–160, 1993.

Smith P, Heimer G, Lindskog M, and Ulmsten U. Oestradiol-releasing vaginal ring for treatment of postmenopausal urogenital atrophy. *Maturitas* 16: 145–149, 1993.

Spector TD, Hochberg MC. The protective effect of the oral contraceptive pill on rheumatoid arthritis. *J Clin Epidemiol* 43: 1221–1230, 1990.

Ter RB. Gender differences in gastroesophageal reflux disease. *J Gender Specific Med* 3(2): 42–44, 2000.

The Writing Group for the PEPI Trial. Effects of estrogen or estrogen/progestin regimens on heart disease risk factors in postmenopausal women: The postmenopausal estrogen/progestin intervention (PEPI) trial. *JAMA* 273: 199–208, 1995.

Van Thiel DH, Gravaler JS, Stremple GJ. Lower esophageal sphincter pressure during the normal menstrual cycle. *Am J Obstet Gynecol* 134: 64–67, 1979.

Van Thiel DH, Gavaler JS, Stremple GJ. Lower esophageal sphincter pressure in females using sequential oral contraceptives. *Gastroenterology* 71: 232–234, 1976.

Viskin S. Long QT. Syndromes and torsade de pointes. *Lancet* 354: 1625–1633, 1999.

Vliet EL. Hormone connections in urinary incontinence in women. *Top Ger Rehab* 15(4):

16–30, 2000.

Ward M, Stone S, Sandman C. Visual perception in women during the menstrual cycle. *Physiol and Behav* 20: 239–243, 1978.

Watts NB, Notelovitz M, Timmons MC, et al. Comparison of oral estrogens and estrogens plus androgen on bone mineral density, menopausal symptoms, and lipid-lipoprotein profiles in surgical menopause. *Obstet Gynecol* 85: 529–537, 1995.

Wenger NK. Cardiovascular disease in menopausal women: The benefits of HRT are not restricted to improving lipid profiles. *Medicographia* 21: 223–228, 1999.

Yamanishi T, Yasuda K, Suda S, et al. Effect of functional continuous magnetic stimulation for urinary incontinence. *J Urology* 163: 456–459, 2000.

Chapter 16: Balancing Ovarian Hormones for Optimal Health

Akamatsu T, Akiyama T, Kimura T, Saito H, Yanaihara T. Menopausal insomnia and hormone replacement therapy. Third International Symposium, Women's Health and Menopause, June 1998.

Araujo DAC, Farias MLF, Andrade ATL. Effects of transdermal and oral estrogen replacement on lipids and glucose metabolism in postmenopausal women with type 2 diabetes mellitus. *Climacteric* 5: 286–292, 2002.

Benyon HL, Garbett ND, Barnes PJ. Severe premenstrual exacerbations of asthma: Effect of intramuscular injection of progesterone. *Lancet* 2: 370–372, 1988.

Bjorn I, Backstrom T. Drug-related side effects is a common reason for poor compliance in hormone replacement therapy. *Maturitas* 32: 77–86, 1999.

Bush TL, Whiteman MK. Hormone replacement therapy and risk of breast cancer (editorial). *JAMA* 281: 2140–2142, 1999.

Cucinelli F; Soranna L. Murgia F; Muzj G, Perri C; Cinque B, Mancuso S, Lanzone A. Differential effect of transdermal estrogen plus progestagen replacement therapy on insulin metabolism in postmenopausal women related to their insulinemic secretion. Third International Symposium Women's Health and Menopause, June 1998.

Cullberg J. Mood changes and menstrual symptoms with different gestagenlestrogen combinations. *Acta Psychiatr Scand* (suppl) 236: 1, 1972.

Davidsonn MH, Maki KC, Maryx P, et al. Effects of continuous estrogen (17-beta estradiol) and estrogen-progestin (norethindrone) replacement regimens on cardiovascular risk markers in postmenopausal women. *Arch Int Med* 160: 3315–3325, 2000.

Davis SR, Burger HG. Use of androgens in postmenopausal women. *Curr Opinion Obstet Gynecol* 9: 177–180, 1997.

De Lignieres B, Dennerstein L, Backstrom T. Influence of route of administration on progesterone metabolism. *Maturitas* 21: 251–257, 1995.

Dickey, MD, Richard P. *Managing Contraceptive Pill Patients*, 9th ed, 2002. Available from: Essential Medical Information Systems, Inc., P.O. Box 1607, Durant, OK 74702–1607.

Ditkoff EC, Crary WG, Cristo M, Lobo RA. Estrogen improves psychological function in asymptomatic postmenopausal women. *Obstet Gynecol* 78: 991–995, 1991.

Duncan A, Lyall H, Roberts R, et al. The effect of 17-beta estradiol and norethisterone on insulin sensitivity in postmenopausal women. Third International Symposium Women's Health and Menopause, June 1998.

Falkeborn M, Lithell H, Persson I, et al. Lipids and antioxidative effects of 17-beta estradiol and sequential norethisterone acetate treatment in a 3–month randomized controlled trial. *Climacteric* 5: 240–248, 2002.

Fitzpatrick L, Pace C, Wiita B. Comparison of regimens containing oral micronized progesterone or medroxyprogesterone acetate on quality of life in postmenopausal women: A cross-sectional survey. *J Wos Hlth & Gender Based Med* 9(4): 381–387, 2000.

Gaspard UI.. Wery OJ, Scheen AJ, et al. Long-term effects of oral estradiol and dydrogesterone on carbohydrate metabolism in postmenopausal women. *Climacteric* 2(2): 93–100, 1999.

Gelfand MM. Estrogen-androgen hormone replacement therapy. *European Menopause Journal* 2:22–26, 1995.

Genazzani, AR (president of the International Menopause Society). HRT and breast cancer: Is there any news? A clinician's perspective (editorial). *Climacteric: The Journal of the International Menopause Society*, 3: 13–16, 2000.

Genazzani AR, Gadducci A, Gamnacciani M. Controversial issues in climacteric medicine II: Hormone replacement therapy and cancer. International Menopause Society Expert Position Paper. *Gynecol Endocrinol* 15: 453–465, 2001.

Godsland IF, Crook D, Wynn V. Clinical and metabolic considerations of long-term oral contraceptive use. The Wynn Institute for Metabolic Research. *Am J Obstetrics Gynecology* 166(6) Part 2: 1955–1966, June 1992.

Grabrick DM, Hartmann LC, Cerhan JR, et al. Risk of breast cancer with oral contraceptive use in women with a family history of breast cancer. *JAMA* 284: 1791–1798, 2000. (Editorial comment, pp. 1837–1838.)

Grady D, Herrington D, Bittner V, et al. for the HERS Research Group. Heart and estrogen/progestin replacement study follow-up (HERS II): Part 1: cardiovascular outcomes during 6.8 years of hormone therapy. *J Am Med Assoc* 288: 49–57, 2002.

Halbreich, U. Menopause and psychopharmacology: Signs, symptom and treatment. Third International Symposium Women's Health and Menopause, June 1998.

Henderson AF, Gregoire AJP, Kumar R, Studd JWW. The treatment of severe postnatal depression with oestradiol skin patches. *Lancet* 338: 816, 1991.

Holst J, Backstrom T, Hammerbach S, et al. Progestogen addition during oestrogen replacement therapy--effects on vasomotor symptoms and mood. *Maturitas* 11: 13–19, 1989.

Hulley S, Grady D, Bush T, et al. Randomized trial of estrogen plus progestin (HERS) for secondary prevention of coronary heart disease in postmenopausal women. *J Am Med Assoc* 280: 6–5 613, 1998.

Jensen J, Christensen C, Rodbro P. Estrogen-progesterone replacement therapy changes body composition in early postmenopausal women. *Maturitas* 8: 209–216, 1986.

Klaiber E, Broverman D, Vogel W, et al Relationships of serum oestradiol levels, menopausal duration and mood during hormone replacement therapy. *Psychoneuroendocrinology* 22: 549–558, 1997.

Kritz-Silverstein D, Barrett-Conner E. Long-term postmenopausal hormone use, obesity, and fat distribution in older women. *JAMA* 275(1): 46–49, Jan. 3, 1996.

Low biologic aggressiveness in breast cancer in women using hormone replacement therapy. *J Clin Oncol* 16(9): 3115–3120, 1998.

Lloyd T, et al. Oral contraceptive use by teenage women does not affect body composition. *Obstet Gynecol* 100: 235–239, 2002.

Magos AL, Brewster E, Singh R, O'Dowd T, Brincat M, Studd JWW. The effects of norethisterone in postmenopausal women on oestrogen replacement therapy: A model for the premenstrual syndrome. *Br J Obstet Gynaecol* 93: 1290–1296, 1986.

Magos AL, Brincat M, Studd JWW. Treatment of the premenstrual syndrome by subcutaneous oestradiol implants and cyclical oral norethisterone: A placebo controlled study. *Br Med J* 1: 1629–1631, 1986.

Montgomery JC, Brincal M, Tapp A, Appleby L, Versi E, Fenwick PBC, Studd JWW. Effects of oestrogen and testosterone implants on psychological disorders in the climacteric. *Lancet* 1: 297–299, 1987.

O'Meara ES, Rossing MA, Daling JR, et al. Hormone replacement therapy after a diagnosis of breast cancer in relation to recurrence and mortality. *J Nat Cancer Inst* 93: 754–762, 2001.

Polo-Kantola P, Erkkola R, Irjala K, Polo O. When does oestrogen replacement therapy improve sleep quality? Third International Symposium Women's Health and Menopause, June 1998.

Powers MS, Schenkel L, Darley PE, et at Pharmacokinetics and pharmacodynamics of transdermal dosage forms of 17-beta estradiol: Comparison with conventional oral estrogens used for hormone replacement therapy. *Am J Obstet Gynecol* 152: 1099–1106, 1985.

Prang AJ. Estrogen may well affect response to antidepressant. *JAMA* 219: 143–144, 1972.

Raudaskoski T, et al. Insulin sensitivity during postmenopausal hormone replacement with transdermal estradiol and intrauterine levonorgestrel. *Acta Obstet Gynecol Scand* 78(6): 540–545, July 1999.

Reubinoff B, Wurtman J, Adler D, et al. Effect of hormone replacement therapy on body composition fat distribution and food intake in early postmenopausal women: A prospective study. *Fertil Steril* 64(5): 963–968, 1995.

Ripley HS, Shorr E, Papanicolaou GN. The effect of treatment of depression in the menopause with estrogenic hormone. *Amer J Psychiat* 96: 905–915, 1940.

Rosano GMC, Sarrel PM, Poole- Wllson, PA, Collins P. Beneficial effect of oestrogen (17-beta estradiol) on exercise-induced myocardial ischaemia in women with coronary artery disease. *Lancet* 342: 133–136, 1993.

Sayegh RA, Kelly L, Wurtman J, Deitch A, et al. Impact of hormone replacement therapy on the body mass and fat compositions of menopausal women: A cross-sectional study. *Menopause* 6(4): 312–315, 1999.

Schneider HPG. The view of the International Menopause Society on the women's health initiative (WHI). *Climacteric* 5: 211–216, 2002.

Selby PI., Peacock M. Dose dependent response of symptoms, pituitary and bone to transdermal oestrogen in postmenopausal women. *Br Med J* 293: 1337–1339, 1986.

Sellers TA, Mink PJ, Cerhan JR, et al. The role of hormone replacement therapy in the risk for breast cancer and total mortality in women with a family history of breast cancer. *Ann Intern Med* 127: 973–980, 1997.

Seuroeren I. Weight gain and hormone replacement therapy: Are women's fears justified? *Maturitas* 34(Suppl 1): S3–S8, 2000.

Sherwin BB, Gelfand MM. Differential symptom response to parenteral estrogen and/or androgen administration in surgical menopause. *Am J Obstet Gynecol* 151: 153–158, 1985.

Speroff L. Postmenopausal estrogen-progestin therapy and breast cancer: A clinical response to epidemiological reports. *Climacteric: The Journal of the International Menopause Society* 3: 3–12, 2000.

Sulak PJ, et al. Acceptance of altering the standard 21-day/7-day oral contraceptive regimen to delay menses and reduce hormone withdrawal symptoms. *Am J Obstet Gynecol* 186: 1142–1149, 2002.

Sulak P. Using OCs to manage perimenopause. *OBGyn Management* 41–50, 2000.

Talone Ep, Lello S, Caporali M, Sotgia T, Pasqua C, Guardianelli F, Romanini C. Postmenopausal depressive symptoms: Psychopharmacological treatment and hormonal replacement therapy. Third International Symposium Women's Health and Menopause, June 1998.

Tchernof A, et al. Menopause, central body fatness, and insulin resistance: Effects of hormone-replacement therapy. *Coron Artery Dis* 9(8): 503–511, 1998.

Van Vollenhoven RF, McGuire JL. Estrogen, progesterone and testosterone: Can they be used to treat autoimmune diseases? *Cleve Clin J Med* 61: 276–284, 1994.

Vassilopoulou-Sellin R, et al. Estrogen replacement therapy after localized breast cancer: Clinical outcome of 319 women followed prospectively. *J Clin Oncol* 17: 1482–1487, 1999.

Vintamaki T, Tuimala R. Can climacteric women self-adjust therapeutic estrogen doses using symptoms as markers? *Maturitas* 199–203, 1998.

Watson NR, Studd JWW, Savvas M, et al. Treatment of severe premenstrual syndrome with oestradiol patches and cyclical oral norethisterone. *Lancet* 2: 730–732, 1989.

Whitehead M. Oestrogens: Relative potencies and hepatic effects after different routes of administration. *J Obstet Gynecology* 3(suppl): S11–16, 1982.

Wren BG, McFarland K, Edwards P, et al. Effect of sequential transdermal progesterone cream on endometrium, bleeding pattern, and plasma progesterone and salivary progesterone levels in postmenopausal women. *Climacteric* 3: 155–160, 2000.

Chapter 17: Test-and- Treat Strategies for Optimal Thyroid, Adrenal, and Glucose-Insulin Balance

Batukan C, Baysal B. Metformin improves ovulation and pregnancy rates in patients with polycystic ovary syndrome. *Arch Gynecol Obstet* 265(3): 124–127, 2001.

Boscaro M, Barzon L, Sonino N. The diagnosis of Cushing's syndrome. *Arch Int Med* 160:3045–3053, 2000.

Bunevicius R, Kazanavicius G, Zalinkevicius R, et al. Effects of thyroxine as compared with thyroxine plus triiodothyronine in patients with hypothyroidism. *N Engl J Med* 340(6): 424–429, 1999.

Chen Y, et al. Why do low-fat high-carbohydrate diets accentuate postprandial lipemia in patients with NIDDM? *Diabetes Care* 18(1): 10–16, 1995.

Coulston A, et al. Persistence of hypertriglyceridemic effect of low- fat high-carbohydrate diets in NIDDM patients. *Diabetes Care* 12(2): 94–101, 1989.

Coulston A, et al. Plasma glucose, insulin and lipid responses to high-carbohydrate lowfat diets in normal humans. *Metabolism* 32(1): 52–56, 1983.

DeFronzo RA, Ferrannini E. Insulin resistance: A multifaceted syndrome responsible for NIDDM, obesity, hypertension, dyslipidemia, and atherosclerotic cardiovascular disease. *Diabetes Care* 14(3): 173, 1991.

De Leo V, La Marca A, Ditto A, et al. Effects of metformin on gonadotropin-induced ovulation in women with polycystic ovary syndrome. *Fertil Steril* 72(2): 282–285, 1999.

Despres JP, Lamarche B, Mauriege P, et al. Hyperinsulinemia as an independent risk factor for ischemic heart disease. *N Engl J Med* 334: 952–957, 1996.

Dimanti-Kandarakis E, Louli C, Tsianateli T, Bergiele A. Therapeutic effects of metformin on insulin resistance and hyperandrogenism in polycystic ovary syndrome. *Eur J Endocrinol* 138(3): 269–274, 1998.

Dong B, Hauck W, Gambertoglio J. Bioequivalence of generic and brand-name levothyroxine products in the treatment of hypothyroidism. *JAMA* 277(15): 1205–1213, 1997.

Fogelholm M, Kukkonen-Harjula K, Nenonen A, et al. Effects of walking training on weight maintenance after a very-low-energy diet in premenopausal obese women. *Arch Intern Med* 160: 2177–2184, 2000.

Goodwin FK, Prange AJ, Post RM, et al. Potentiation of antidepressant effects by L-triiodothyronine in tricyclic non-responders. *Amer J Psychiat* 139: 34–38, 1982.

Kaplan NM. The deadly quartet: upper-body obesity, glucose intolerance, hypertriglyceridemia and hypertension. *Arch Int Med* 149: 1514–1520, 1989.

Kocak M, Caliskan E, Simsir C, Haberal A. Metformin therapy improves ovulatory rates, cervical scores, and pregnancy rates in clomiphene citrate-resistant women with polycystic ovary syndrome. *Fertil Steril* 77 (1): 101–106, 2002.

Lipworth B. Systemic adverse effects of inhaled corticosteroid therapy. *Arch Internal Med* 159:941–955, 1999.

Ludwig D, et al. Relation between consumption of sugar-sweetened drinks and childhood obesity: A prospective, observational analysis. *Lancet* 1187: 505–508, 2001.

Manson J, Hu F, Rich-Edwards J, et al. A prospective study of walking as compared with vigorous exercise in the prevention of coronary heart disease in women. *N Eng J Med* 341(9): 650–658, 1999.

Moller D, ed. *Insulin Resistance.* Chicester: John Wiley and Sons, 1993.

Morin-Papunen LC, Koivunen RM, Rukonen A, Martikainen HK. Metformin therapy improves the menstrual pattern with minimal endocrine and metabolic effects in women with polycystic ovary syndrome. *Fertil Steril* 69(4): 691–696, 1998.

Vandermolen DT, Ratts VS, Evans WS, et al. Metformin increases the ovulatory rate and pregnancy rate from clomiphene citrate in patients with polycystic ovary syndrome who are resistant to clomiphene citrate alone. *Fertil Steril* 75(2): 310–315, 2001.

Chapter 18: Starting Your "Clean-Up" Campaign: Get Rid of Ovarian Disruptors You Can Control

Abt AB, Oh JY, Huntington RA, Burkhart KK. Chinese herbal medicine induced acute renal failure. *Arch Intern Med* 155: 211–212, Jan. 1995.

Davis SR, et al. The effects of Chinese medicinal herbs on postmenopausal vasomotor symptoms of Australian women: a randomized controlled trial. *Med J Australia* 174: 68–71, 2001.

Grandjean, P. and Landrigan, P.J. Chemical exposure and risk of autism and ADHD in children. *The Lancet*, Nov. 8, 2006; Vol. 368

Koff RS. Herbal hepatotoxicity: Revisiting a dangerous alternative. *JAMA* 273: 502–503, Feb. 1995.

Milewicz A, Mikulski E, Bidzinska B. Satiety and appetite stimulating peptides in ageing women. Third International Symposium Women's Health and Menopause, June 1998.

The Practice Committee of the American Society of Reproductive Medicine. Smoking and Infertility. *Fertility and Sterility*:86(suppl 4), Nov. 2006: S172–177

The Practice Committee of the American Society of Reproductive Medicine, Status of environmental and dietary estrogens—are they significant estrogens? *Fertility and Sterility*:86(suppl 4), Nov. 2006: S218–220.

Prior J, Vigna Y, Alojada N. Conditioning exercise decreases premenstrual symptoms. *Eur J Appl Phyiol* 55:349–355, 1986.

Racette S, et al. Effects of aerobic exercise and dietary carbohydrate on energy expenditure and body composition during weight reduction in obese women. *Amer J Clin Nutr* 61: 486–494, 1995.

Yudkin J. Dietary fat and dietary sugar in relation to ischaemic heart-disease and diabetes. *Lancet* 4–5, 1964.

Yudkin J. Sucrose, coronary heart disease, diabetes, and obesity: Do hormones provide a link? *Am Heart J* 115(2): 493–498, 1988.

Chapter 19: Create Your Own Path

Cameron, D.R, & Braunstein GD. (2004). Androgen replacement therapy in women. *Fertility and Sterility*, 82, 273–289.

Executive Committee of the International Menopause Society. (2004, August 28). Guidelines for the hormone treatment of women in the menopausal transition and beyond. (Position Statement) Original Statement, February 13, 2004 Climacteric, 7, 8–11. Available online at www.imsociety.org

Stickler, R.C. (2003). Women's health initiative results: A glass more empty than full. *Fertility and Sterility*, 80, 488-490

Vliet, E.L. (2002). Menopause and perimenopause: The role of ovarian hormones in common neuroendocrine syndromes in primary care. *Primary Care Clinics in Office Practice*, 29, 43–67.

Vliet, E.L. The Savvy Woman's Guide to Testosterone. HER Place Press, Tucson and Dallas. 2005.

Vliet, E.L. The Savvy Woman's Guide to PCOS. HER Place Press, Tucson and Dallas, 2006.

Medical Textbooks

While there are many excellent medical textbooks, I recommend these because they provide well-researched, up-to-date information from the worldwide literature on women's reproductive hormones and health. They are useful for health professionals and further reading for interested consumers:

Brain: Source and Target for Sex Steroid Hormones, The. A. R. Genazzani, F. Petraglia, and R. H. Purdy (eds.). New York and London: Parthenon Publishing Group, 1996.

Clinical Guide for Contraception: 4th Edition, A. Speroff L, Darney PD. Lippincott Williams and Wilkins, New York, 2005.

DHEA: A Comprehensive Review. J.H.H. Thijssen and H. Nieuwenhuyse (eds.). New York and London: Parthenon Publishing Group, 1999.

Endocrine Disruptors: Effects on Male and Female Reproductive Systems. Rajesh K. Naz, Ph.D. (ed.). New York and London: CRC Press, 1999.

Facts of Hormone Therapy for Menopausal Women, The. Sturdee DW. Parthenon Publishing Group, New York, 2004.

Future of Hormone Therapy: What Basic Science and Clinical Studies Teach Us, 2005, The. Singh M, Simpkins JW (editors). Annals of NY Academy of Sciences, volume 1052.

Gender Differences in Metabolism: Practical and Nutritional Implications. Mark Tarnopolsky, M.D., Ph.D., FRCP(C). New York and London: CRC Press, 1999.

Hormone Therapy and the Brain: A Clinical perspective on the Role of Estrogen. Victor W. Henderson, M.D., M.S. New York and London: Parthenon Publishing Group, 2000.

Hormone Replacement Therapy and The Skin. Brincat MP (editor). Parthenon Publishing, New York, 2001.

Management of the Menopause, 3rd edition, The. Studd J (editor). Parthenon Publishing Group (CRC Press), New York, 2003

Menopause and the Heart. M. Neves-e-Castro, M. Birkhauser, T. B. Clarkson, P. Collins (eds.). New York and London: Parthenon Publishing Group, 1999.

Testosterone: Action, Deficiency, Substitution, 3rd edition. E. Nieschlag, H. M. Behre (eds.). Cambridge University Press, 2004.

Appendix III

Dr. Vliet's Programs and How to Contact Us

For Individual Medical Consultations:

1. We have a centralized appointment scheduling process for our consultations managed from the Tucson office.

Please contact the Patient Services Coordinator in Tucson at *HER Place®: Health, Enhancement and Renewal for Women, Inc.* To receive an information package, you may mail request to P.O. Box 64507, Tucson, AZ 85728, or call 520-797-9131, Fax 520-797-2948.

2. You may check our website at www.herplace.com. Read about our services on the website, and you may also request to be added to our email "alert" notification list to receive periodic health notices. Then contact the Tucson office as shown above. Legal issues and state regulations prevent us from answering medical questions via the web. All new patients are seen in person for a comprehensive evaluation at one of our offices.

For Medical Professionals and Organizations:

To arrange SPEAKING ENGAGEMENTS, SEMINARS, or WORK-SHOPS by Dr. Vliet, or a discuss PRECEPTORSHIP or Consulting Services FOR HEALTH PROFESSIONALS, please contact:

Kathryn A. Kresnik
Vice President, Business Development
HER Place®
Phone: 520-797-9131, Fax 520-797-2948.
Email: via our website www.herplace.com
Regular Mail: Use Tucson office address above